Medical Robotics

Achim Schweikard • Floris Ernst

Medical Robotics

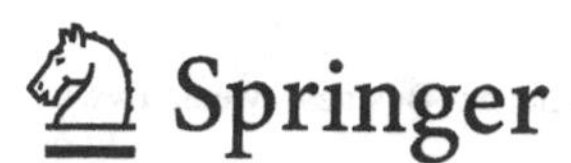

Achim Schweikard
Institute for Robotics
and Cognitive Systems
University of Lübeck
Lübeck, Germany

Floris Ernst
Institute for Robotics
and Cognitive Systems
University of Lübeck
Lübeck, Germany

ISBN 978-3-319-34674-8 ISBN 978-3-319-22891-4 (eBook)
DOI 10.1007/978-3-319-22891-4

Springer Cham Heidelberg New York Dordrecht London

Softcover re-print of the Hardcover 1st edition 2015

Printed on acid-free paper

Springer International Publishing AG Switzerland is part of Springer Science+Business Media (www.springer.com)

Preface

Medical robotics is an interdisciplinary field, with methods from computer science, mathematics, mechanical engineering, and medicine. The field emerged in the 1980s as a new branch of robotics. Robotics itself was then a branch of artificial intelligence. However, a number of technical and mathematical problems had to be solved to bring robots to routine clinical use. These problems were far outside the scope of artificial intelligence, and this supported the emergence of the new field.

When comparing medical robotics to industrial robotics, we see that the latter field is the one that sells most robots. By contrast, some of the most challenging research problems arise in medical robotics: there is a need for improving the accuracy of surgical procedures, and image guidance has become a central element of this. If we imagine that robotic exoskeletons can help paralyzed patients, it becomes clear that we will need methods for motion learning and brain-computer interfaces.

We wrote this book as a textbook for a one-semester class on medical robotics. When writing this book, we were guided by two thoughts:

- Computer scientists and engineers should learn to understand application domains, and medicine is an ideal application domain for this purpose.
- The book should be suitable as a first course in robotics.

Comparing to standard textbooks on robotics, four elements have been added here: (1) seven-joint robots; (2) navigation, calibration, and registration; (3) connection to machine learning; and (4) applications in surgical robotics, rehabilitation robotics, and neuroengineering. The text relies entirely on the most elementary mathematical tools, and we give a detailed introduction for each new method. At the end of each chapter, we provide exercises, preparing the grounds for the tools in the next chapters, while linking to the methods in the current chapter.

Chapter 1 introduces the main applications of medical robotics.

Chapter 2 presents basic methods for describing position and orientation as well as forward robot kinematics. This includes matrices, angles, and the analysis of simple linkages.

Chapter 3 introduces inverse kinematics for robots. We develop the inverse kinematics for a seven-joint lightweight robot, called the DLR-Kuka arm. This robot is designed for applications requiring direct interaction with an operator. To obtain an inverse solution, we first solve the kinematic equations for a standard six-joint robot with revolute joints, called the elbow manipulator with spherical wrist. We obtain a building-block strategy with which common types of robots can be analyzed.

Geometric methods for inverse kinematics are an alternative to algebraic methods. We illustrate geometric methods for the kinematic analysis of common medical devices.

In Chap. 4, we consider Jacobi-matrices. There are two types of Jacobians: the analytic Jacobian and the geometric Jacobian. The analytic Jacobian offers alternative methods for the inverse analysis of robots. The geometric Jacobian is a basic tool for velocity kinematics and for analyzing the relationship between joint torques and static forces/torques acting at the tool. We apply the geometric Jacobian to problems involving C-arm X-ray imaging and robot design.

Chapter 5 establishes a connection to the classical tools from medical imaging, i.e., MR, CT, ultrasound, and X-ray imaging. With this tool set, we address several problems, such as navigation, registration, image calibration, and robotic hand-eye calibration.

Chapter 6 describes methods for treatment planning. Computer programs have been used for treatment planning in radiation oncology since the 1950s. Until the 1990s, conventional systems for radiation oncology irradiated tumors from a small set of beam directions (typically three to five directions). To move the beam source, five-joint mechanisms with revolute and prismatic joints were used. This changed with the introduction of robotic radiosurgery. Up to 1000 distinct directions can now be used in a single treatment. This greatly increased the complexity of treatment planning.

Chapter 7 is the first chapter (in a series of three chapters) with basic methods from machine learning. We address the problem of tracking anatomical motion (heartbeat, respiration) with a robot. To this end, we learn the motion of a difficult-to-image anatomical target via the motion of a surrogate.

In Chap. 8, we predict respiratory motion to compensate for the time lag of the robot, while tracking a target. Again, machine learning is one of the main elements. In addition, we need a connection to basic methods from signal processing.

In Chap. 9, we consider motion replication. Robots for motion replication are the most commonly used surgical robots. The surgeon moves a passive robot, and thereby issues motion commands to a small replicator robot. We apply tools from machine learning to classify different types of motions, i.e., intended motion, tremor, and noise. In the replication process, we must separate these types of motions (all of which are part of the motion signal). In the same context, we apply the geometric Jacobian to the analysis of static forces and torques.

The three applications in Chaps. 7–9 all converge to a set of methods, which we term "motion learning." Humans learn motion, and it is obvious that we need dedicated tools for motion learning not only in medical robotics.

Chapter 10 discusses integrated systems in medical robotics. The methods developed in Chaps. 1–9 are the building blocks for such systems. It should be noted that the methods in Chaps. 1–9 have already found their way to the clinic, and have become routine tools, especially in oncology, but also in orthopedics and neurology, most of them via the connection to medical imaging and motion learning.

Chapter 11 gives an overview of methods for neuroprosthetics, brain-machine interfaces, and rehabilitation robotics.

In the appendix, we derive the geometric Jacobian matrix for the six-joint elbow manipulator and for the DLR-Kuka seven-joint robot. We also include solutions to selected exercises.

Additional material is available at https://medrob-book.rob.uni-luebeck.de.

Acknowledgements

We thank Max Wattenberg for converting many of the drawings to TikZ-format, Robert Dürichen for implementing several of the methods for motion prediction and for discussions on the subject, Ulrich Hofmann and Christian Wilde for their help with writing the text on brain-machine interfaces, Ivo Kuhlemann for his help with implementing and testing inverse kinematics algorithms, and Cornelia Rieckhoff for proof-reading.
We offer special thanks to Rainer Burgkart for discussions and suggestions on orthopedic navigation, John R. Adler for many discussions on navigation in neurosurgery and radiosurgery, and our doctoral students Norbert Binder, Christoph Bodensteiner, Christian Brack, Ralf Bruder, Markus Finke, Heiko Gottschling, Max Heinig, Robert Hanne, Matthias Hilbig, Philip Jauer, Volker Martens, Lars Matthäus, Christoph Metzner, Lukas Ramrath, Lars Richter, Stefan Riesner, Michael Roth, Alexander Schlaefer, Stefan Schlichting, Fabian Schwarzer, Birgit Stender, Patrick Stüber, Benjamin Wagner, and Tobias Wissel for their help with experiments and graphics and for reading drafts of the book.
Finally, we thank Mohan Bodduluri, Gregg Glosser, and James Wang for their help with implementing robotic respiration tracking and treatment planning for a clinical standard system.

Lübeck, Germany

Achim Schweikard
Floris Ernst

Contents

Chapter 1
Introduction

Robots are now used in many clinical sub-domains, for example: neurosurgery, orthopedic surgery, dental surgery, eye surgery, ear-nose and throat surgery, abdominal surgery/laparoscopy, and radiosurgery. This gives rise to a large number of new methods. However, medical robotics is not limited to surgery. In recent years, four main types of medical robots have emerged:

1. Robots for Navigation. The surgical instrument is moved by a robot arm. This allows precise positioning, based on pre-operative imaging. The motion of anatomic structures (e.g. caused by respiration and pulsation) can be tracked.
2. Robots for Motion Replication. The robot replicates the surgeon's hand motion, via a passive robotic interface. Thus we can downscale the motion, reduce tremor and improve minimally invasive methods.
3. Robots for Imaging. An imaging device is mounted to a robotic arm, to acquire 2D or 3D images.
4. Rehabilitation and Prosthetics. Mechatronic devices can support the recovery process of stroke patients. Robotic exoskeletons controlled by brain-computer interfaces can replace or support damaged anatomical structures.

We will discuss basic methods for each of the four cases. In the following section, we will begin by looking at several examples for surgical navigation.

A. Schweikard, F. Ernst, *Medical Robotics*,
DOI 10.1007/978-3-319-22891-4_1

1.1 Robots for Navigation

A first example of a medical robot is shown in Fig. 1.1. A robot guides a surgical saw. Before the intervention, the surgeon defines a cutting plane for a bone cut. During the operation, the robot places the saw in the predefined plane, and the surgeon can move the saw within this plane. This restricts the motion of the saw, and allows for placing the cuts with high precision.
In the figure, we see two types of robot joints: revolute joints and prismatic joints. For a revolute joint, a rigid link rotates about an axis. A prismatic link slides along a translational axis. The last joint in Fig. 1.1 is a prismatic joint. Here, the prismatic joint is passive, i.e. it is not actuated by a motor. Thus, the surgeon moves the saw by hand, while the motion plane is given by the robot.

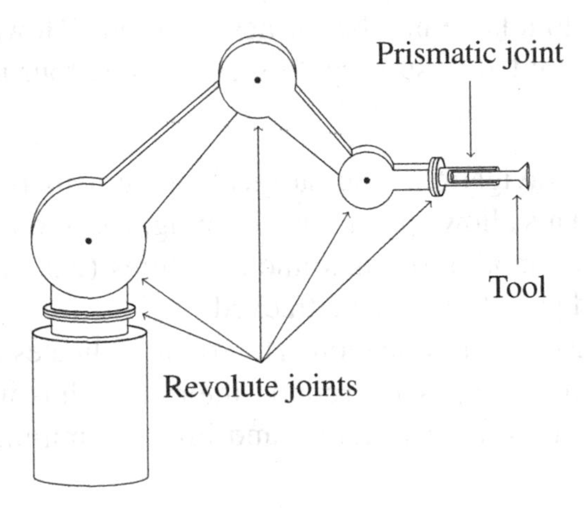

Fig. 1.1: Surgical saw mounted to a robotic arm. The arm itself consists of revolute joints. The saw is mounted to a passive component (prismatic joint). The surgeon moves the saw manually (sliding motion only). By construction, the manual motion of the saw is restricted to a single axis [6]

Remark 1.1

Fig. 1.2 illustrates a schematic notation for jointed mechanisms, for the robot in Fig. 1.1. Revolute joints are denoted by cylinders, where the cylinder axis specifies the axis of rotation. Prismatic joints are denoted by boxes. The lid of the box indicates the direction of motion.

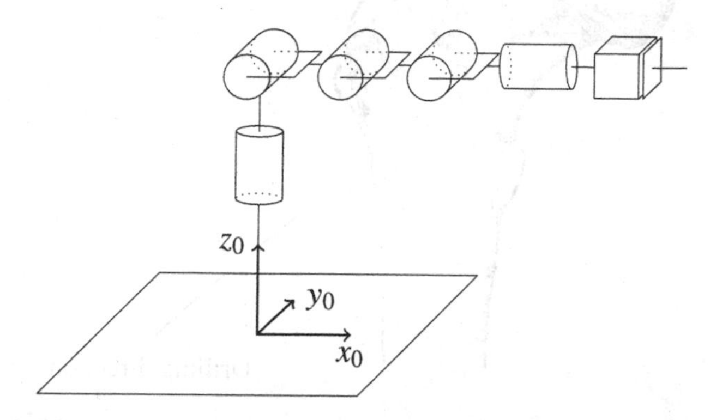

Fig. 1.2: Schematic notation for the robot in Fig. 1.1

In the figure, notice that the first two joint axes (revolute joints) intersect in space. Furthermore, the axes of joints two, three and four are parallel. We also see the axes x_0, y_0 and z_0 of a *base coordinate system*.

(End of Remark 1.1)

1.1.1 Navigation for Orthopedic Surgery

We will now show several examples for navigation problems arising in orthopedic surgery.
Figure 1.3 shows a femur bone. The region shown with the dashed pattern is the target area (e.g. a tumor). The instrument for removing the tumor is a surgical drill. The skin cut is made on the right side (an arrow indicates the drilling direction). The target is on the left side. The tumor is well visible in the CT image, but often not visible in an X-ray image. To remove the tumor, we must guide the drill. Notice also that the drill must not penetrate the joint surface. Here, the preoperative 3D images must be matched to the intra-operative situation.
Figure 1.4 shows the head of a femur bone. A small gap between the head and the rest of the bone is visible (see arrow). Epiphyseolysis is

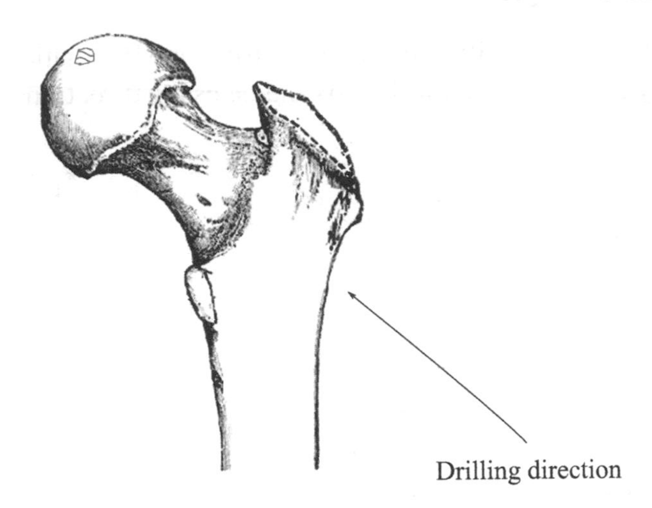

Fig. 1.3: Navigating a surgical drill. Femur figure from [3, Fig. 245]

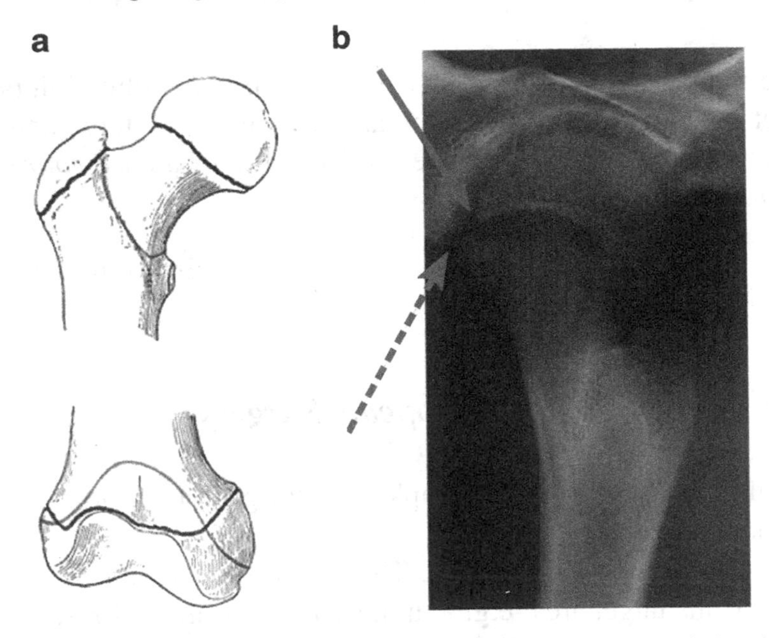

Fig. 1.4: Epiphyseolysis. *Left images*: epiphysial lines of the femur. *Source*: [3, Fig. 253]. *Right image*: X-ray image of epiphyseolysis. The femur bone is displaced against the head, the tips of the two arrows should coincide. (**a**) Epiphysial lines of the femur, shown in black. *Source*: [3, Fig. 253]. (**b**) X-ray of the femur, showing the epiphysial line at the femur head (*solid arrow*)

a condition, in which a fracture along this gap results in a downward slippage of the femur head (Fig. 1.4) [7].

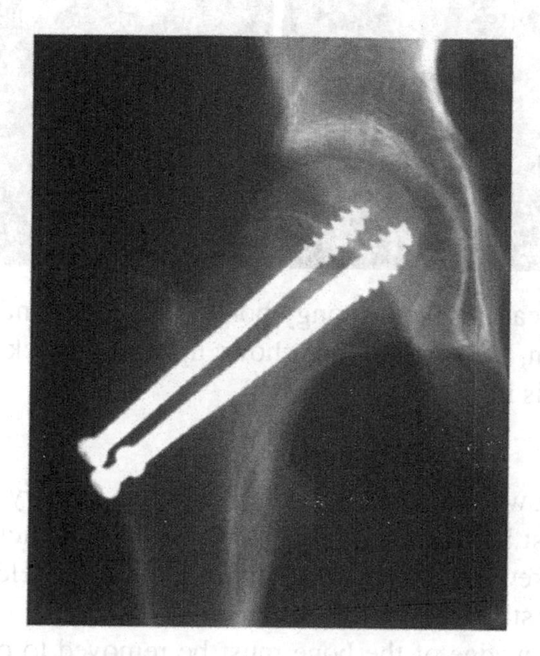

Fig. 1.5: Treatment of epiphyseolysis

To stabilize the femur head, screws are used (Fig. 1.5). However, placing the screws is difficult. The reason is that only the surface of the bone consists of hard material, the *cortical bone*. The interior of the bone, called *cancellous bone*, or spongy bone, is much softer. The screw tip must reach (but not penetrate) the cortical bone surface.
Figure 1.6 shows a cross-section (slice) of a CT-data set, side-by-side with the corresponding MRI slice. The cortical bone is visible as a ring (white/light grey in the CT image, and black in the MRI data). The spongy bone is inside this ring. When placing a screw (as in Fig. 1.5), the tip of the screw should reach, but not penetrate the thin cortical bone layer.

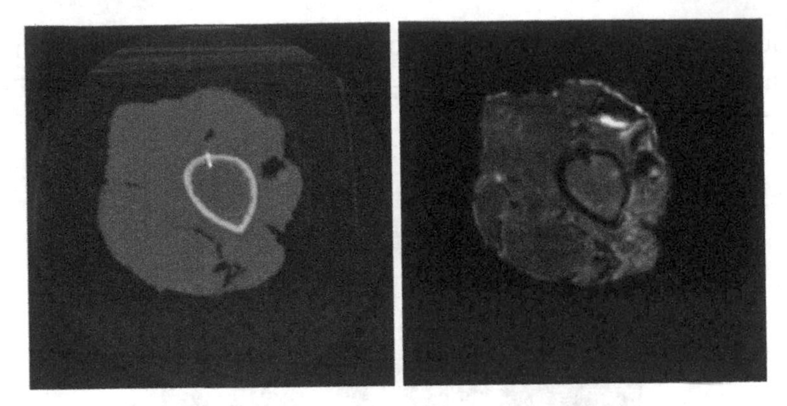

Fig. 1.6: Cortical bone and spongy bone in CT (*left*) and MRI (*right*). In the CT scan, the cortical bone shows up white (black in MRI). The spongy bone is inside

Figure 1.7 shows a similar application in spine surgery. Two or more vertebrae must be stabilized. Screws through the pedicle hold a fixation plate. Likewise, in dental surgery, implants are held by screws in delicate bony structures of the chin.
In Fig. 1.8, a wedge of the bone must be removed to obtain a better positioning of the bone axis. The navigation system guides the surgeon to locate the cutting planes during the operation.

1.1.2 Radiologic Navigation

During an intervention, the visibility of anatomic target structures is often limited. Thus, for example, a CT image is taken before an operation. During the actual operation, only X-ray imaging is available. The CT image shows more detail than an intraoperative X-ray image, but does not show the current position of the surgical instrument. For precise navigation, we would need a CT image showing *both* the instrument and the target at the same time. Thus, we need a virtual marker visualizing the instrument position in the CT image.
One first method for surgical navigation is called *radiologic navigation*. Radiologic navigation is based on X-ray imaging. During the operation, X-ray images are taken with a *C-arm* (Fig. 1.9). A C-arm is a

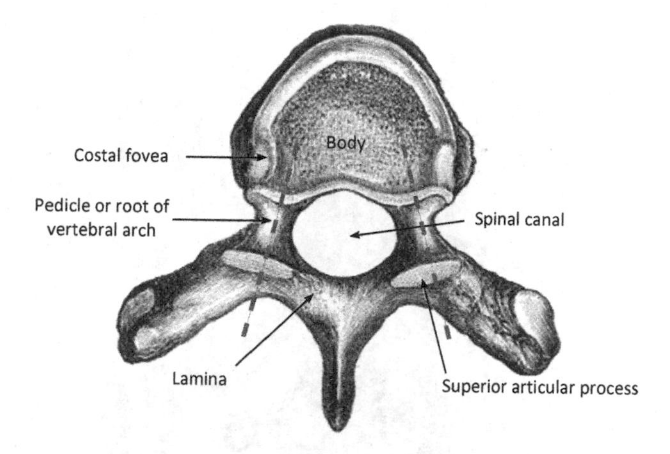

Fig. 1.7: Placement of pedicle screws. The insertion path for the screws (*dashed lines*) must not touch the spinal canal. Source of drawing [3, Fig. 82]

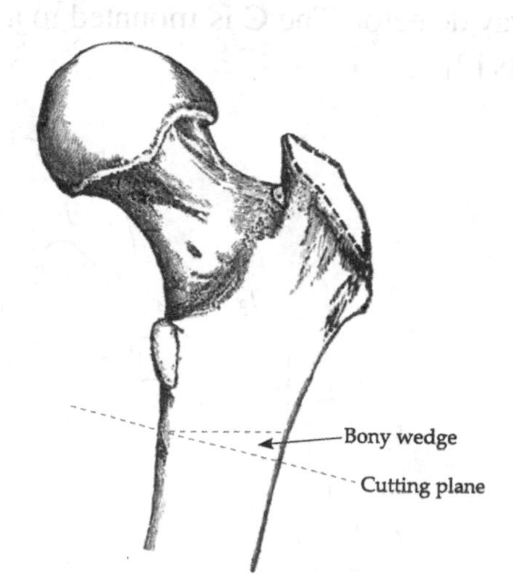

Fig. 1.8: Corrective osteotomy for the femur bone. Source of the drawing: [3, Fig. 245]

mobile X-ray imaging device with five joints. There are two prismatic joints, and three revolute joints. A C-arm allows for taking X-ray images from varying angles during an operation.
Figure 1.10 shows the joints of a C-arm, in the notation introduced in Remark 1.1.

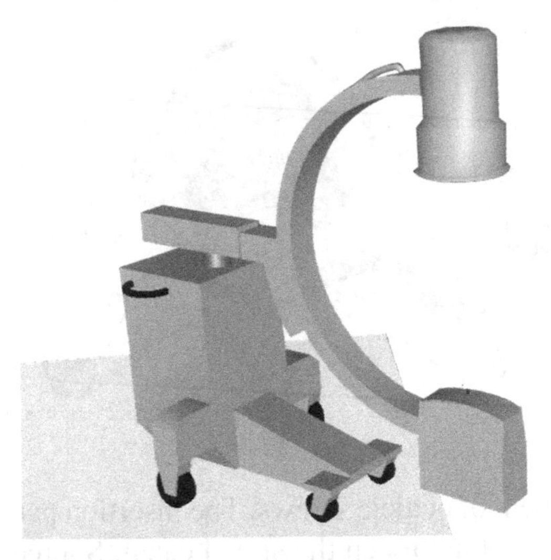

Fig. 1.9: C-arm X-ray imaging. A C-shaped structure carries an X-ray source and an X-ray detector. The C is mounted to a jointed mechanism with five joints [2]

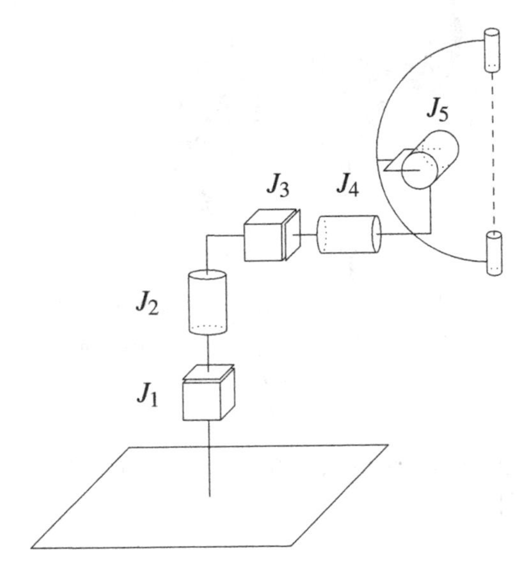

Fig. 1.10: Joints of a C-arm. J_2, J_4 and J_5 are revolute joints. J_1 and J_3 are prismatic

A second tool needed for radiological navigation is *infrared tracking* (IR tracking). An infrared tracking system consists of a camera, and one or more infrared markers, either reflective (i.e. illuminated by the camera) or active IR-LEDs (Fig. 1.11). The system tracks positions and orientations of the markers in space. Markers can be attached to objects and tools in the operating room. The camera of the tracking system is attached to the wall of the operating room, and provides the *base coordinate system*. Notice that infrared tracking not only outputs the *position* of the pointer tip of the marker, but also the *orientation* of the marker in space. This means we not only know the tip coordinates (e.g. as x-, y-, z-coordinates) with respect to the camera coordinate system, but we also obtain information about the angle and the pointing direction of the marker in space. To output such angular information, standard tracking systems use *matrices* or *quaternions*. Typical systems report the marker position to within 0.1 mm.

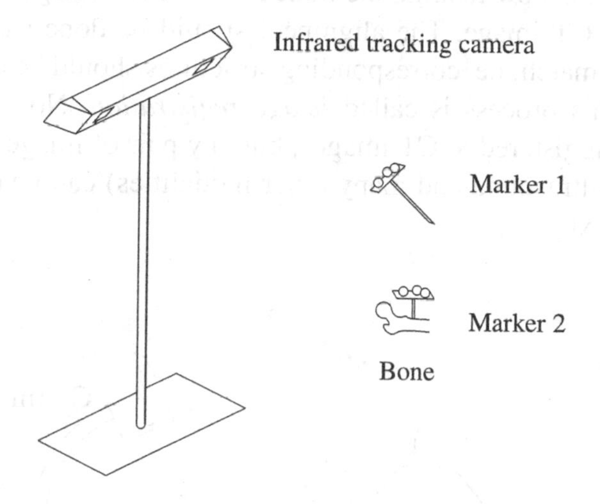

Fig. 1.11: Infrared tracking system with two markers. One of the markers is attached to a bone

Figure 1.12 shows the principle of radiological navigation. A first marker of the infrared tracking system is attached to the C-arm. The second marker is attached to the saw. After making a skin incision (opening the skin), a third marker is rigidly attached to the bone. Then an X-ray image of the bone is taken with the C-arm. Given the position

of the C-arm in space, we can compute the exact spatial coordinates of points on the bone visible in the C-arm image. These coordinates are computed with respect to the (infrared) camera coordinate system. We can now steer the robot to a predefined point on the bone surface, or guide the robot to find a pre-planned angle with respect to the bone. If the bone moves during the procedure, we can calculate and correct the displacement by subtraction.
When attaching a marker to the robot or the saw, we do not know the spatial reference between the robot's coordinate system, and the internal coordinate system of the infrared tracking camera. The process of finding the spatial mapping between the two coordinate systems is called *hand-eye calibration.* A similar problem occurs when calibrating C-arm images with respect to the infrared marker.
As noted above, tumors are often not visible in X-ray images, but well visible in 3D CT images taken before the operation. The navigation problem is now to align the bone in the X-ray image to the same bone in the CT image. The alignment should be done such that the two images match, i.e. corresponding structures should be at the same position. This process is called *image registration.* Not only X-ray images are registered to CT images, but any pair of image modalities (CT, MRI, ultrasound and many other modalities) can be considered in this context.

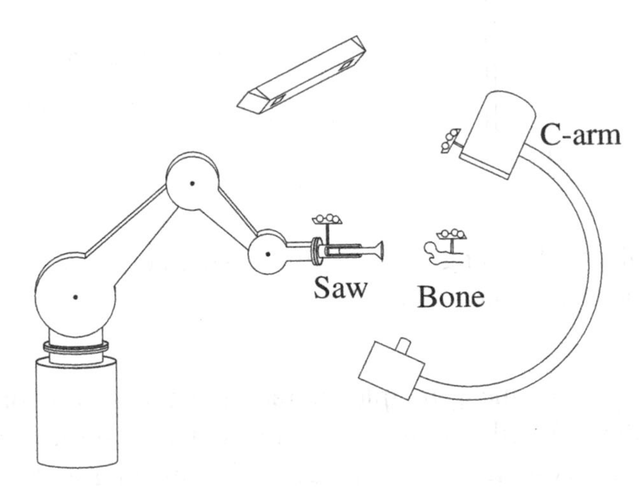

Fig. 1.12: Radiologic navigation. Markers for the infrared tracking system are attached to the saw, the C-arm and the bone

1.1.3 Stereotaxic Navigation

A second method for navigation is *stereotaxic navigation*. It is typically used in neurosurgery and allows for reaching targets in the brain with high precision.

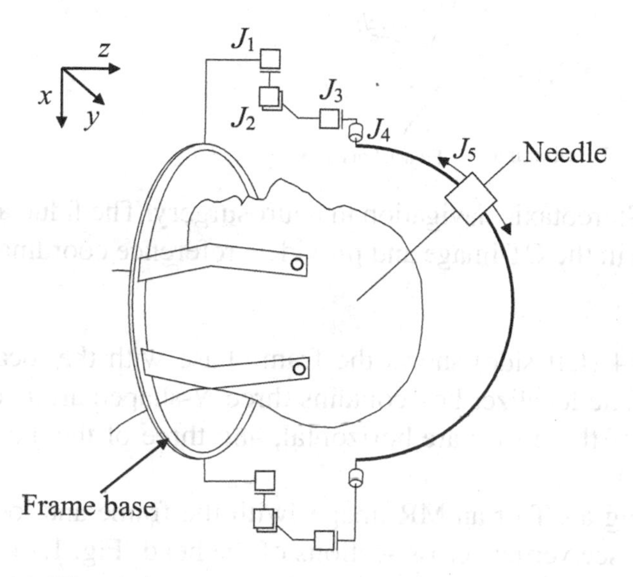

Fig. 1.13: Five-joint mechanism for stereotaxic neurosurgery

To this end, a small robotic mechanism with five joints is rigidly attached to the head of the patient (Fig. 1.13). The instrument is a needle, and can be moved by changing the settings of the joint angles. Recall the schematic notation for robot joints. In the figure, the joints are called $J_1, J_2, ..., J_5$. Here, J_1, J_2 and J_3 are prismatic, and J_4, J_5 are revolute joints.

During the procedure, the patient's head is fixed in space with a stereotaxic frame (Fig. 1.14). The frame has three parts (A, B and C). Part A is the frame base. This part directly attaches to the head. Part B is a box with localizers for CT/MR imaging, and attaches to the base. The localizers are also called *fiducials*. Part C is the passive jointed mechanism in Fig. 1.13, and part C can also be rigidly attached to the frame base. To this end, we remove the localizer frame B.

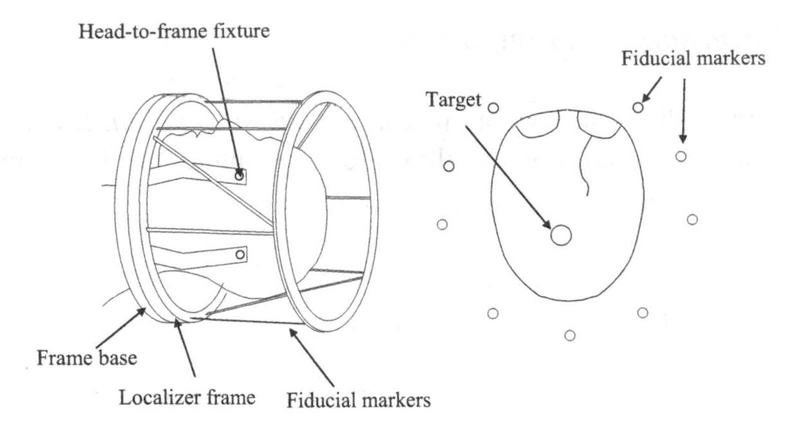

Fig. 1.14: Stereotaxic navigation in neurosurgery. The fiducial markers are visible in the CT image and provide a reference coordinate system

Figure 1.14 (left side) shows the frame base with the localizer box attached. The localizer box contains three *N*-shaped arrangements of rods. Six of these rods are horizontal, and three of them are oblique (see figure).
After taking a CT or an MR image (with the frame and localizers in place), we see vertical cross sections of the head (Fig. 1.14, right).
Vertical cross sections (with the patient on the treatment table, as in Fig. 1.14) are also called axial cross sections. The three viewing directions for imaging are shown in Fig. 1.15.
In the cross-sections, we will see points (indicated as small circles in Fig. 1.14, right), stemming from the fiducial rods. From the distance between two adjacent points (one from an oblique rod and one from a horizontal rod) we derive the z-coordinate of the image cross-section. With similar methods, we can obtain x- and y-coordinates of the target in the image.
In the next step of the procedure, we remove the localizer box with the fiducial rods, and attach the jointed mechanism to the frame base. As noted above, the jointed mechanism carries the instrument (e.g. a biopsy needle or an electrode).
Having determined the coordinates of the target in the images, we can compute the angle settings for the jointed mechanism and insert a

needle along a predefined path. Again, calibration methods are needed to map the CT/MR coordinate system to the frame coordinate system.

Example 1.1

The joints J_4 and J_5 in Fig. 1.13 are revolute joints. The joint angles of J_4 and J_5 determine the orientation of the needle. The needle tip moves when we change the values of the angles. Let θ_4 and θ_5 be the values of the joint angles for J_4 and J_5. The current values for θ_4 and θ_5 can be read from a scale imprinted onto the metal frame. We can compute the position of the needle tip for given θ_4, θ_5. The position is described with respect to the coordinate system shown in the figure. We can also derive a closed form expression, stating the coordinates of the needle tip as a function of θ_4, θ_5. Similarly, we can include the prismatic joints into the computation. This derivation of a closed formula is one example of a *forward kinematic analysis* of a mechanism. Conversely, computing angle values from a given tip position and needle orientation is called an *inverse kinematic analysis* (see also Exercise 1.1 at the end of this chapter).

(End of Example 1.1)

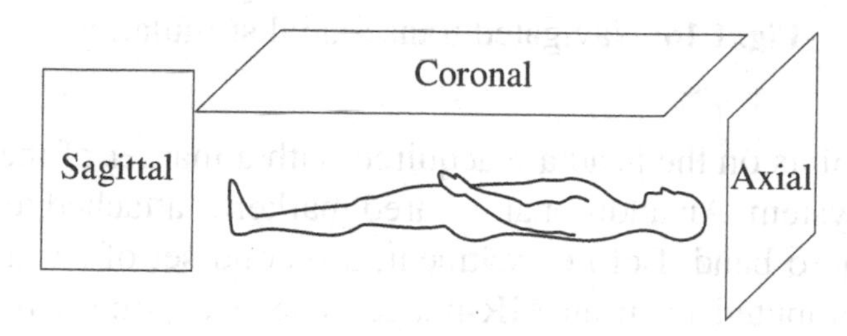

Fig. 1.15: Imaging directions: axial, sagittal, coronal

1.1.4 Non-invasive Navigation for the Head

Stereotaxic navigation with a head-frame is invasive and painful for the patient. The frame must be attached under local anesthesia. The next example shows a less invasive (but also less accurate) alternative for applications in neurology (Fig. 1.16). In transcranial magnetic stimulation (TMS), a magnetic coil stimulates small regions in the brain. For diagnostic applications, the coil is held by the surgeon. This becomes difficult if the coil must remain in the same place (with respect to the head) for extended periods of time in certain cases more than 30 min. In robotic TMS, we navigate the coil with a robot.

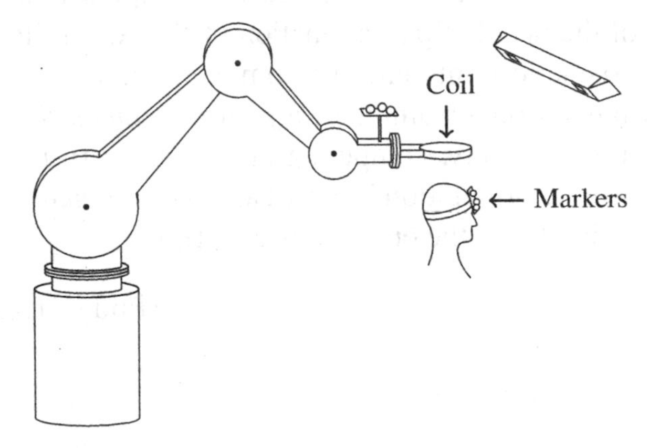

Fig. 1.16: Navigated transcranial stimulation

Surface points on the head are acquired with a marker of the infrared tracking system. An additional infrared marker is attached to the head with a velcro band. Before treatment, a second set of surface points can be computed from an MR-image. The two point sets are then matched in a registration step. In this way, we can locate a target inside the brain, given in MR-coordinates. During the procedure, the robot can compensate for small motions of the head.
Beyond the fields mentioned above (orthopedic surgery, neurosurgery and neurology), navigation methods are used in many other fields (e.g. ENT surgery, radiosurgery, abdominal surgery and heart surgery). The applications described above are simpler than many others, because the target does not deform.

1.1.5 Navigation for Moving Targets

In radiosurgery, robots are used to move the radiation source. This source weighs 200 kg and cannot be moved by the surgeon. Lung tumors move as the patient breathes. The robot compensates for this motion, i.e. the robot tracks the tumor motion, see Fig. 1.17.
Real-time tracking of internal organs is difficult, especially in this application. Methods for *motion correlation* can overcome this problem: suppose that the skin of the patient moves with respiration, and the target tumor also moves with respiration. The skin motion may be small (i.e. in a range of 1–2 mm), but we can track it with fast cameras or infrared tracking. Now assume the observable skin motion of the patient correlates to the tumor motion. Then we can use skin motion as a surrogate signal, to track the internal target.

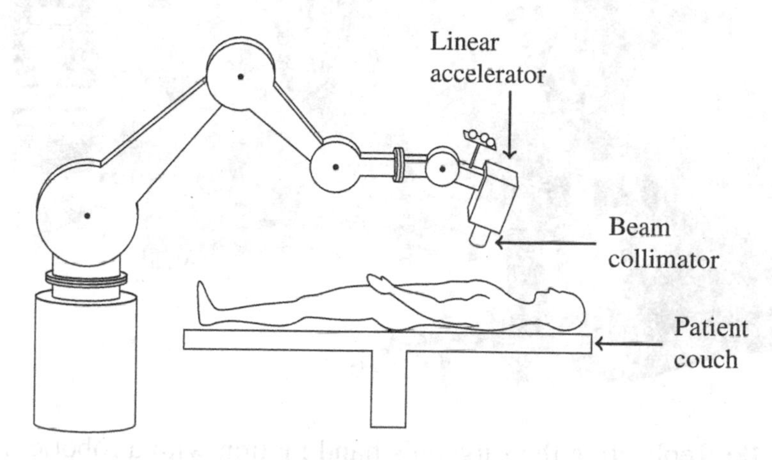

Fig. 1.17: Radiosurgery: a robotic arm or a jointed mechanism moves a medical linear accelerator. The linear accelerator generates a beam of photon radiation

In the same application (robotic radiosurgery), the motion of the robot must be planned. The plan must take into account the geometry and location relationships in the area surrounding the tumor. Hence, planning must be done on an individual basis for each treatment.

1.2 Movement Replication

As noted above, robots are not only used for navigation. Using appropriate sensors, it is not difficult to record all hand motions of a surgeon during an intervention. One can then replicate hand motion by a robotic arm. With this, a number of problems in microsurgery can be addressed. An example is shown in the next figure. The motion of the surgeon can be down-scaled. Assume the motion range of the surgeon's hand is 1 cm, and our robot replicates the same motion, but down-scales it to a range of 1 mm. Thus, delicate interventions can be performed with very high accuracy, see Fig. 1.18.

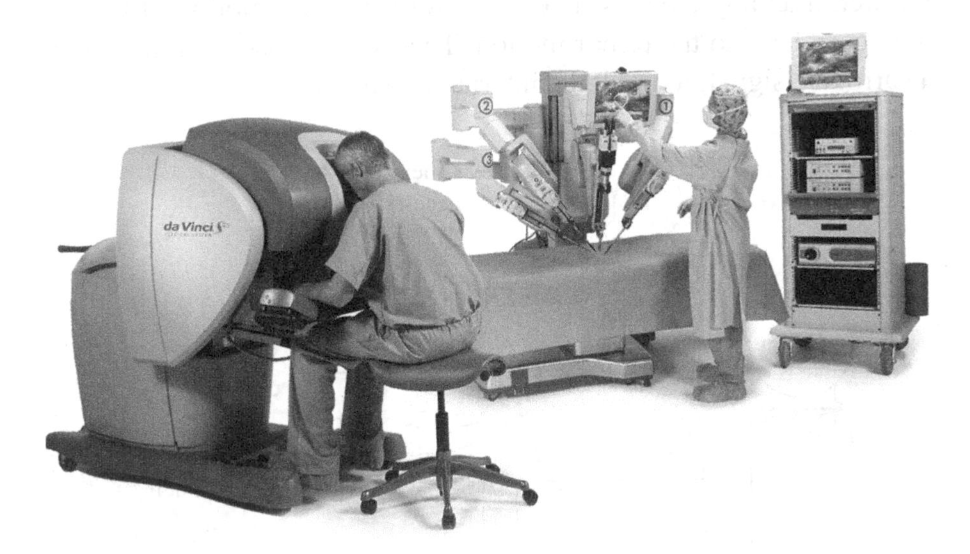

Fig. 1.18: Replicating the surgeon's hand motion with a robotic interface mounted to the patient couch (da Vinci Surgical System, ©2015 Intuitive Surgical, Inc.)

A second example is the placement of heart catheters [1]. The surgeon pushes the catheter through the blood vessel tree under image guidance. A robotic interface transmits motion commands to the tip of the catheter. The catheter tip is articulated, and can thus be steered.

1.3 Robots for Imaging

A further application of medical robots is image acquisition. The process of computing a CT image from a set of X-ray images is one instance of *image reconstruction* (see Fig. 1.19). As an example, we can move the C-shaped structure of the C-arm. Then the source-detector assembly will move along a circular arc in space. By taking a series of X-ray images during this circular motion (Fig. 1.20), we obtain the raw data for a three-dimensional CT image. A reconstruction algorithm then computes the 3D image.

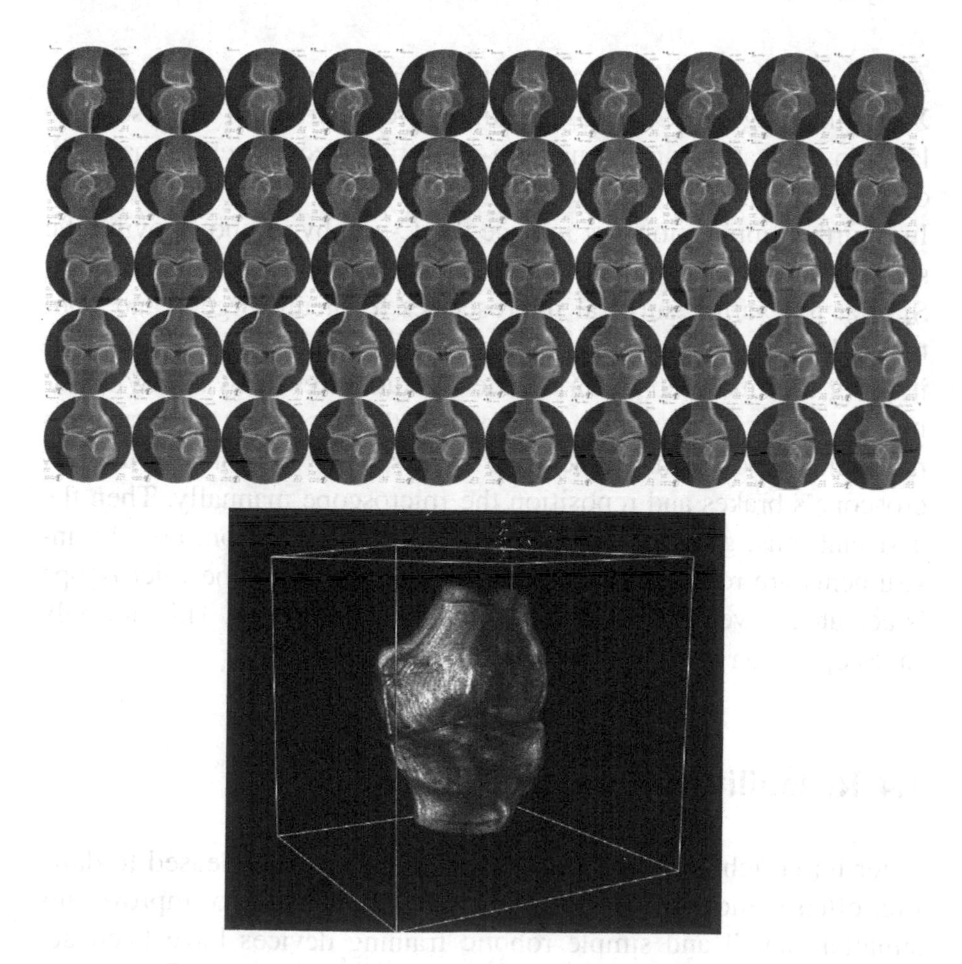

Fig. 1.19: Reconstruction. *Top*: 2D projection images taken from a series of angles. *Bottom*: Reconstructed 3D image

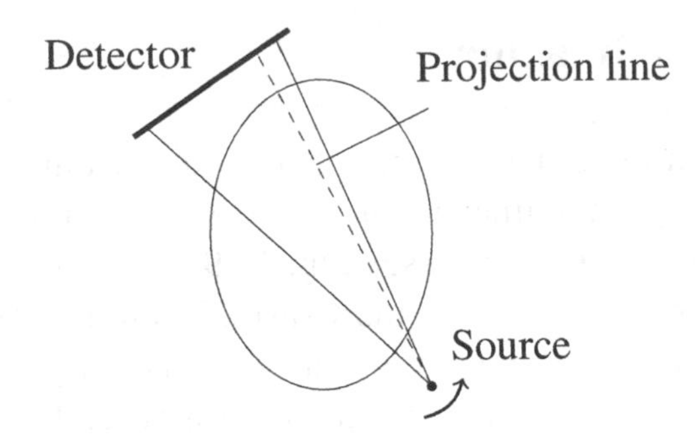

Fig. 1.20: Rotating source-detector assembly for CT imaging or 3D imaging with a C-arm

Above we discussed radiologic navigation. We saw that it combines X-ray imaging and CT imaging. Image reconstruction is closely related to navigation, since our intra-operative reconstruction may rely on partial or modified image data.
In a further application, we replace the C-arm by a robot moving the source and the detector (Fig. 1.21).
Similar to C-arms, surgical microscopes for neurosurgery and ophthalmology are mounted to jointed mechanisms (Fig. 1.22). Repositioning the microscope during the operation, even by a few millimeters, forces the surgeon to interrupt the operation. The surgeon must first hand the instruments to an assistant, then unlock the microscope's brakes and reposition the microscope manually. Then the assistant must give the instruments back to the surgeon, and the instruments are reinserted into the operation cavity. If the microscope is actuated, several of these steps become unnecessary. This not only saves operation time, but reduces infection risk.

1.4 Rehabilitation and Prosthetics

After initial rehabilitation, most stroke patients are released to daily life, often without regaining their original mobility. To improve this situation, small and simple robotic training devices have been developed. Stroke patients can use these robots at home. The robots perform simple and repetitive movements to help the patient regain mobility.

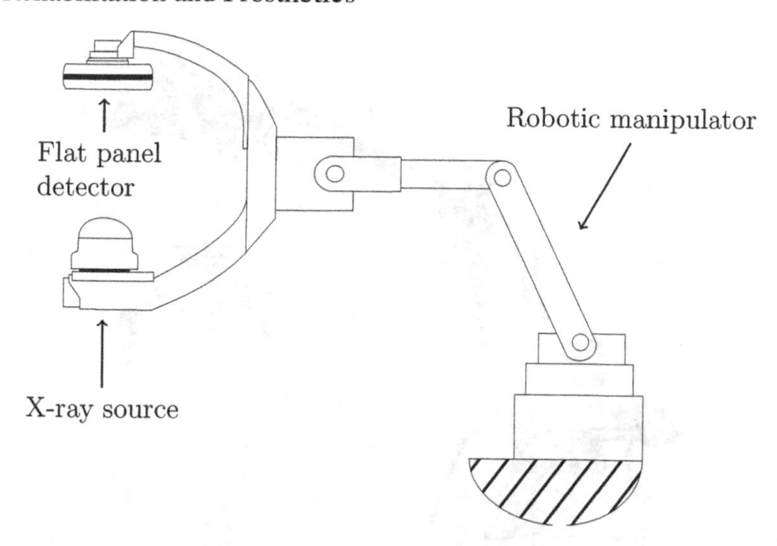

Fig. 1.21: Robotic C-arm imaging system for angiography [4]

In neuro-prosthetics, intelligent actuator systems directly assist patients in performing motion tasks, e.g. after paralysis (see Fig. 1.23). The systems can be reconfigured for various tasks, such as finger turning operations, bottle opening and grasping. In each case, the patient applies forces and torques, which can be measured to adjust the system parameters.

An exoskeleton is an external skeleton supporting the body. A first application is to reduce tremor during microsurgery. A major research goal is to provide actuated exoskeletons for paralyzed patients.

Targeted muscle reinnervation (TMR) is a surgical procedure for establishing a control channel between the patient and an exoskeleton. In TMR, several independent nerve-muscle units are created in the chest. These units can then be used for signal recording with external electromyography (EMG). EMG is non-invasive, and electrodes on the skin surface record signals from muscle contractions. With TMR, patients can control a robotic arm prosthesis. With the artificial arms, patients who lost both arms in accidents are able to perform a variety of tasks such as eating, putting on glasses and using a pair of scissors [5]. Methods from machine learning can be applied to improve the motion patterns on the side of the robot arm.

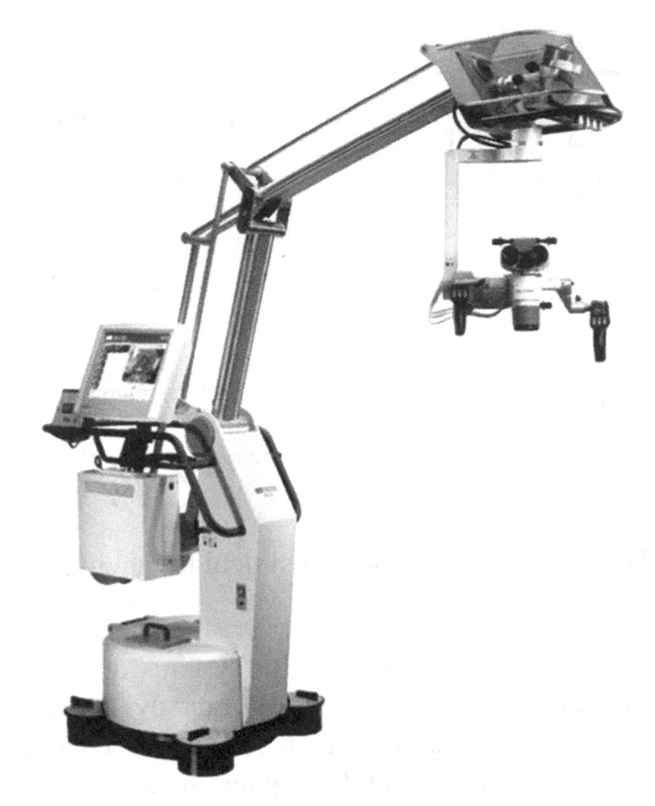

Fig. 1.22: Surgical microscope (MÖLLER 20-1000, Möller-Wedel GmbH)

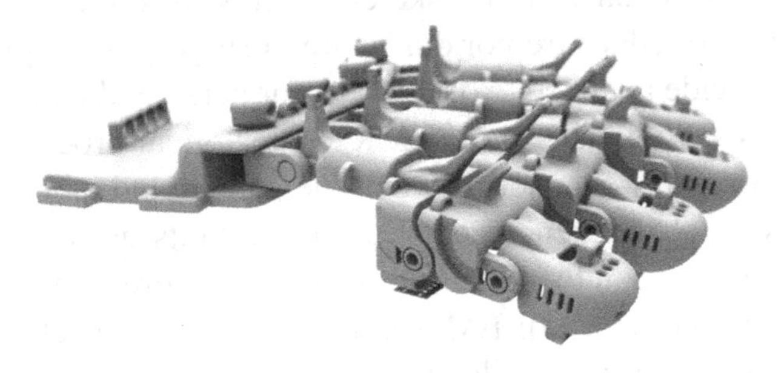

Fig. 1.23: Robotic hand for stroke rehabilitation [8]

Exercises

Exercise 1.1

The joint angles (θ_4 and θ_5) for the neurosurgical frame in Fig. 1.13 are shown in Figs. 1.24 and 1.25.

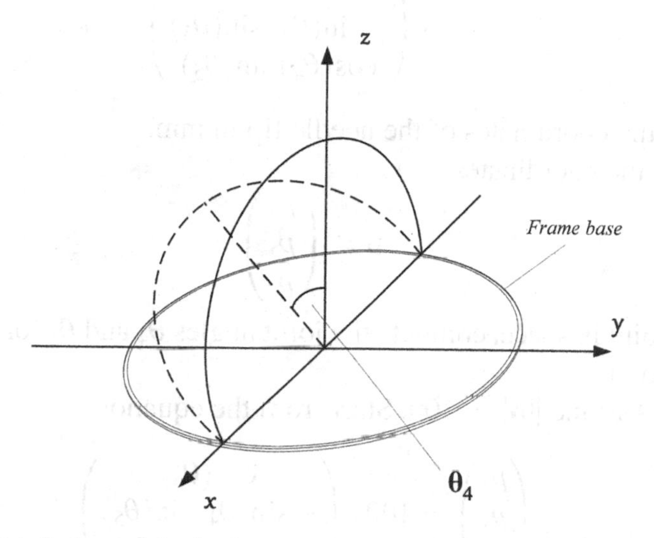

Fig. 1.24: Joint angle θ_4 for the neurosurgical frame in Fig. 1.13

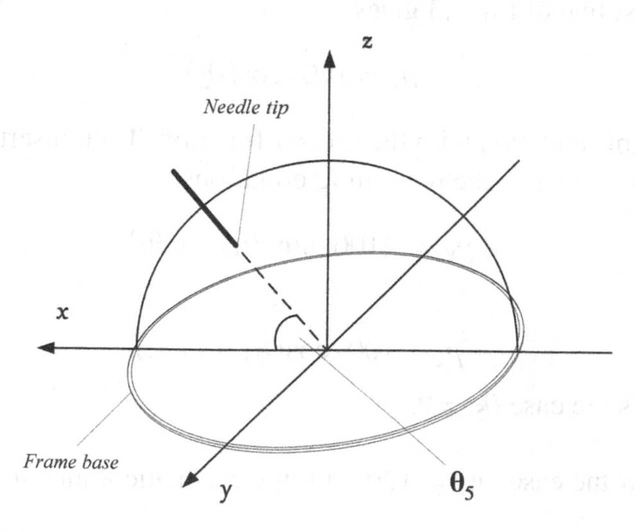

Fig. 1.25: Joint angle θ_5 for the frame in Fig. 1.13

Place a coordinate system at the centroid of the frame base, with axes (*x*-,*y*-,*z*-) as shown in Fig. 1.25.
Assume the distance of the needle tip (Fig. 1.25) from the coordinate origin is 100 mm.

a) For angle values taken from the set $\theta_4 \in \{-90,0,90\}$ and $\theta_5 \in \{0,90,180\}$verify that the expression

$$100 \cdot \begin{pmatrix} \cos(\theta_5) \\ -\sin(\theta_4)\sin(\theta_5) \\ \cos(\theta_4)\sin(\theta_5) \end{pmatrix} \tag{1.1}$$

gives the coordinates of the needle tip in mm.

b) Given the coordinates

$$\mathbf{p} = \begin{pmatrix} p_x \\ p_y \\ p_z \end{pmatrix} \tag{1.2}$$

of a point in space, compute the joint angles θ_4 and θ_5 for reaching this point.
Hint: Assume $||\mathbf{p}|| = 100$. Start from the equation

$$\begin{pmatrix} p_x \\ p_y \\ p_z \end{pmatrix} = 100 \cdot \begin{pmatrix} \cos(\theta_5) \\ -\sin(\theta_4)\sin(\theta_5) \\ \cos(\theta_4)\sin(\theta_5) \end{pmatrix} \tag{1.3}$$

The first line of Eq. 1.3 gives

$$p_x = 100 \cdot \cos(\theta_5) \tag{1.4}$$

Solve this equation with the arccos-function. Then insert the solution into either of the remaining equations

$$p_y = -100 \cdot \sin(\theta_4)\sin(\theta_5) \tag{1.5}$$

and

$$p_z = 100 \cdot \cos(\theta_4)\sin(\theta_5) \tag{1.6}$$

Discuss the case $\theta_5 = 0$.

c) Discuss the case $||\mathbf{p}|| \neq 100$ with the prismatic joints in Fig. 1.13.

d) Implement your solution for part b) in a short program. Input: point **p** with $||\mathbf{p}|| = 100$.
Output: point **p'**
p' is computed as follows: Extract angles θ_4 and θ_5 from the input point according to the solution in part b). Then reinsert the angles θ_4 and θ_5 into Eq. 1.3, giving **p'**.

e) Extend your program to the general case with prismatic joints.

Exercise 1.2

a) Set up a flow chart for the navigation process illustrated in Fig. 1.12.
b) Describe the difference between radiologic navigation and stereotaxic navigation.
c) The terms navigation, calibration, reconstruction and registration and their applications were described above. The process of delineating organs in a medical image is called segmentation. Describe a situation in which registration could be used to facilitate segmentation. Conversely, describe a scenario in which segmentation could help registration. Describe similar interactions between calibration and registration.

Exercise 1.3

As an example for image reconstruction, we consider the process of computing a three-dimensional CT image from a series of X-ray images. You can think of a C-arm (Fig. 1.9) taking images from different angles as it rotates the source-detector assembly.
In Fig. 1.20, a projection line is shown dashed. The anatomy along this projection line attenuates the X-rays. Each voxel along the projection line contributes to the attenuation. The sum of these contributions (of each voxel) will then be measured at the detector. Hence, the sum of the resulting attenuation is known. The goal is to estimate the unknown gray level at each voxel, given all the sum values from different angles.

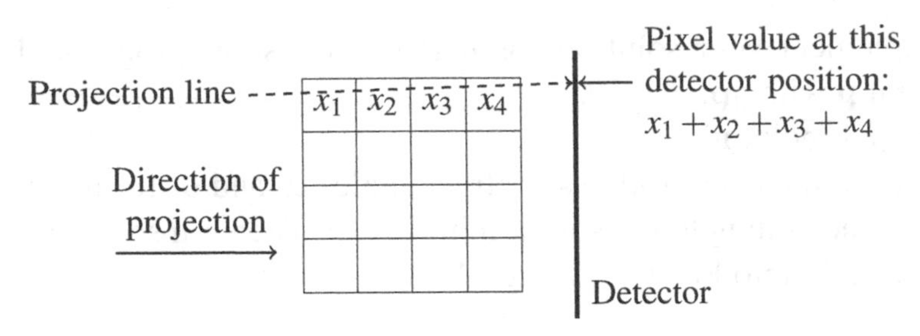

Fig. 1.26: Input data for reconstruction. Variables x_i correspond to voxels (one variable for each voxel). A variable represents the attenuation at this voxel

Figure 1.26 illustrates the input data for reconstruction. For each angle, we have a projection image. The goal is to compute a gray level for each voxel, i.e. values for the variables x_i. Input data are the pixel values measured at the detector. In the figure, the pixel value for the topmost pixel is the sum of the values $x_1,\ldots,x_4$ in the first row. In the case of several projection images, we obtain a linear system of equations of the following form

$$\begin{aligned} a_{11}x_1+a_{12}x_2+\cdots+a_{1n}x_n &= b_1 \\ &\vdots \\ a_{m1}x_1+a_{m2}x_2+\cdots+a_{mn}x_n &= b_m \end{aligned} \tag{1.7}$$

Here, the values b_i are the pixel values measured at the detector, the coefficients a_{ij} are constant, and each a_{ij} is either 0 or 1. (We could use other values for a_{ij}, for example a factor expressing the length of the path of the ray through the corresponding voxel.) The resulting linear equation system can be solved in many ways. The ART (algebraic reconstruction technique) algorithm is particularly useful for this application. To simplify the notation, we assume there are only two equations and two variables.

$$\begin{aligned} a_{11}x_1+a_{12}x_2 &= b_1 \\ a_{21}x_1+a_{22}x_2 &= b_2 \end{aligned} \tag{1.8}$$

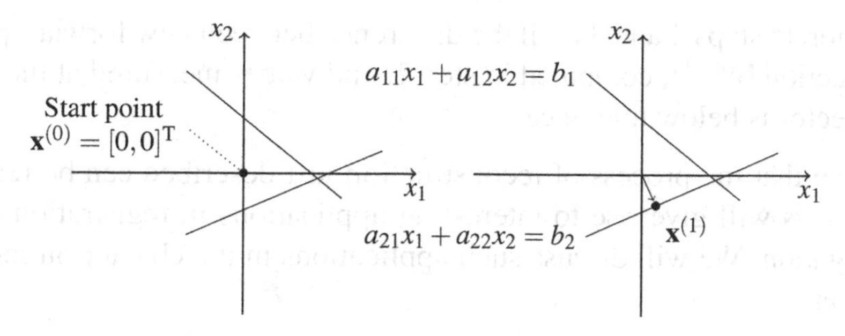

Fig. 1.27: ART algorithm. *Left*: visualization of the two lines in Eq. 1.8. *Right*: Projecting the start point (0,0) onto one of the lines

Each of the two equations corresponds to one line in the visualisation. Start with an arbitrary estimate for the solution, for example the point $(0,0)^{\mathrm{T}}$ (Fig. 1.27).
Now project this start point onto the first line (Fig. 1.27). Call this new point $\mathbf{x}^{(1)}$. Proceed by projecting $\mathbf{x}^{(1)}$ onto the second line. Iteratively repeat, until the intersection point between the two lines is reached. This is the solution of the equation system. We need to give a closed formula for computing the projections. Set $\mathbf{a}_i = (a_{i1}, a_{i2})$. Then

$$\mathbf{x}^{(n+1)} = \mathbf{x}^{(n)} - \frac{\mathbf{a}_i\mathbf{x}^{(n)} - b_i}{\mathbf{a}_i^2}\mathbf{a}_i \tag{1.9}$$

We write the scalar product of $\mathbf{a}_i$ and $\mathbf{x}^{(n)}$ as $\mathbf{a}_i\mathbf{x}^{(n)}$ instead of $\mathbf{a}_i^{\mathrm{T}}\mathbf{x}^{(n)}$ (see also the notation page in Appendix E). Likewise, $\mathbf{a}_i^2$ denotes the scalar product $\mathbf{a}_i^{\mathrm{T}}\mathbf{a}_i$. This iteration formula computes the $(n+1)$-th estimate $\mathbf{x}^{(n+1)}$ from the n-th $\mathbf{x}^{(n)}$, i.e. it projects the point $\mathbf{x}^{(n)}$ onto the i-th line of the system, which is given by $\mathbf{a}_i$ and b_i. The line index i can be chosen at random. The coefficients a_{ij} form a matrix which will be called $\mathbf{A}$.
Instead of Eq. 1.8, we can thus write $\mathbf{Ax} = \mathbf{b}$. The ART algorithm is now given by:

1. Start by setting $\mathbf{x}^{(0)} = (0,0)^{\mathrm{T}}$.
2. Choose a random index i and compute $\mathbf{x}^{(n+1)}$ from $\mathbf{x}^{(n)}$ via Eq. 1.9
3. Compute the forward projection from the $(n+1)$-th estimate, i.e. $\mathbf{b}^{(n+1)} = \mathbf{A}\mathbf{x}^{(n+1)}$

4. Iterate steps 2 and 3 until the difference between new forward projection $\mathbf{b}^{(n+1)}$, computed in step 2, and values measured at the detector is below tolerance

Notice that the process of reconstruction just described can be reverted. This will give rise to interesting applications in registration and navigation. We will discuss such applications in the chapter on registration.

a) Explain the difference between the two types of projections (projection in Fig. 1.26) and projection in Fig. 1.27 in the ART algorithm.
b) Explain why reconstruction is needed to compute 2D slice images (i.e. regular CT image stacks) from 2D X-ray images.
c) Explain why we cannot cancel some of the $\mathbf{a}_i$'s in Eq. 1.9.
d) Prove Eq. 1.9.
e) Implement the ART algorithm for planar images. For simplicity, first use synthetic images such as the binary image of a rectangle shown in Fig. 1.28 (left) as input.
f) Compare different implementations of linear equation solvers, such as the one provided in MATLAB (`linsolve()`) (or any other linear equation system solver) to the implementation of the ART algorithm for larger images.

```
0000000000000   000*000000000
0000000000000   000*000000000
0011111111100   001*111111100
0010000000100   0010*00000100
0010000000100   0010*00000100
0010000000100   0010*00000100
0011111111100   00111*1111100
0000000000000   00000*0000000
0000000000000   00000*0000000
```

Fig. 1.28: *Left*: Synthetic binary image of a rectangle, *right*: projection line through the image, voxels along the projection line marked with *asterisk*

References

[1] J. Bismuth, E. Kashef, N. Cheshire, and A. B. Lumsden. Feasibility and safety of remote endovascular catheter navigation in a porcine model. *Journal of Endovascular Therapy*, **18**(2): 243–249, 2011. DOI 10.1583/10-3324R.1.

[2] R. Graumann, O. Schütz, and N. Strobel. C-arm X-ray system with adjustable detector positioning, 2004.

[3] H. Gray and W. H. Lewis. *Anatomy of the Human Body*. Lea & Febiger, Philadelphia, PA, 20th edition, 1918.

[4] S. Groß and D. Heinl. C-arm mounted on a robotic arm, 2009.

[5] T. A. Kuiken, G. A. Dumanian, R. D. Lipschutz, L. A. Miller, and K. A. Stubblefield. The use of targeted muscle reinnervation for improved myoelectric prosthesis control in a bilateral shoulder disarticulation amputee. *Prosthetics and Orthotics International*, **28**(3):245–253, 2004.

[6] M. Roth, C. Brack, A. Schweikard, H. Götte, J. Moctezuma, and F. Gossé. A new less invasive approach to knee surgery using a vision-guided manipulator. In *International Symposium on Robotics and Manufacturing (ISRAM'96), World Automation Congress (WAC'96)*. ASME Press, 1996, pages 731–738.

[7] R. B. Salter and W. R. Harris. Injuries involving the epiphyseal plate. *The Journal of Bone and Joint Surgery*, **45**(3):587–622, 1963.

[8] P. Weiss, M. Heldmann, T. F. Münte, A. Schweikard, and E. Maehle. A rehabilitation system for training based on visual feedback distortion. In J. L. Pons, D. Torricelli, and M. Pajaro, editors, *Converging Clinical and Engineering Research: Proceedings of the International Conference on Neurorehabilitation (ICNR) 2012*. Springer. Published in *Biosystems & Biorobotics*, **1**:299–303, 2013. DOI 10.1007/978-3-642-34546-3_47.

References

Chapter 2
Describing Spatial Position and Orientation

Coordinate systems describe the position of objects in space. For example, we can define a fixed coordinate system in the room (e.g. one corner of the room) and then refer to this coordinate system when stating coordinates of a point. If we agree that all coordinates are given in millimeters, we obtain a common frame of reference.
Consider Figs. 1.2 and 1.3 in the introduction chapter. We need to state the coordinates of the target point on the bone, and we also need to know the current position of the drill tip. Furthermore, we will need to specify the angle at which to hold the drill. In this chapter, we will discuss the basic mathematical methods for this purpose.

2.1 Matrices

Assume we have defined a base coordinate system. Call this system B. We are now given a second coordinate system S (Fig. 2.1).
In the figure, the displacement of S relative to B is denoted by the vector $\mathbf{p}$. The system S has the same orientation as the base system B, meaning that the x-, y- and z-vectors of S point into the same directions as the respective base vectors.
A 4×4 matrix $\mathbf{M}$ describes the position and orientation of S with respect to the base coordinate system.

A. Schweikard, F. Ernst, *Medical Robotics*,
DOI 10.1007/978-3-319-22891-4_2

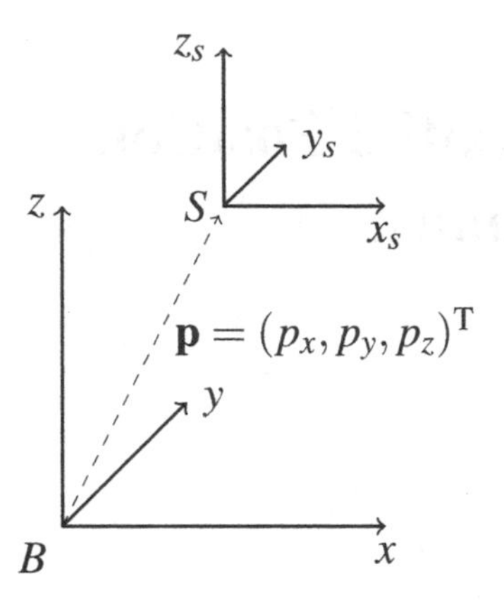

Fig. 2.1: Vector **p** describes the position of the coordinate system S with respect to the base coordinate system B

For the case in Fig. 2.1, the matrix **M** is

$$\mathbf{M} = \begin{pmatrix} 1 & 0 & 0 & p_x \\ 0 & 1 & 0 & p_y \\ 0 & 0 & 1 & p_z \\ 0 & 0 & 0 & 1 \end{pmatrix}. \tag{2.1}$$

But what if we change the orientation of the second system S? This is shown in Fig. 2.2.
We must change **M** accordingly:

$$\mathbf{M}' = \begin{pmatrix} 0 & 0 & -1 & p_x \\ 0 & 1 & 0 & p_y \\ 1 & 0 & 0 & p_z \\ 0 & 0 & 0 & 1 \end{pmatrix} \tag{2.2}$$

We look at the upper left 3×3 part of this matrix. This part of the matrix has a very simple interpretation, visible already in the above examples. Specifically, the three columns of this 3×3-matrix each represent a 3D-vector. The first such vector gives the direction of x_S (in terms of the base), the second gives the direction of y_S, and the third shows the direction of z_S. You should verify this simple observation in the examples of Figs. 2.1 and 2.2. Thus, we have rotated about the y_S-axis, which is reflected in the fact that the y_S-axis does not change.

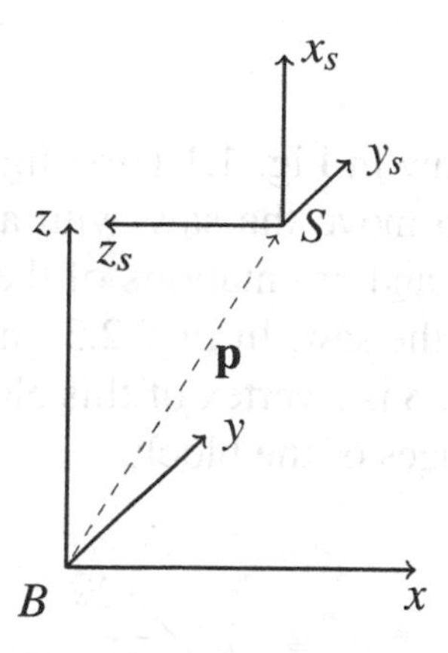

Fig. 2.2: Coordinate system S after a change of orientation. We have rotated S about the axis y_S by $-90°$. The vector x_S now points into the z-direction of the base, and z_S points into the negative x-direction of the base

The last line of the matrix has an interesting geometric interpretation as well, but here we ignore this, simply assuming we have added the last line to make the matrix square.
In general, a 4×4 matrix representing the position of a system S with respect to the base B has the following form:

$$\mathbf{M}' = \begin{pmatrix} n_x & o_x & a_x & p_x \\ n_y & o_y & a_y & p_y \\ n_z & o_z & a_z & p_z \\ 0 & 0 & 0 & 1 \end{pmatrix} \tag{2.3}$$

To distinguish the matrices of this form from other 4×4 matrices, they are also called homogeneous 4×4 matrices.
We will sometimes use a shorter term for coordinate systems. Since a coordinate system provides a frame of reference, we will simply call it a frame.
Following the above observations, the three matrix entries n_x, n_y, n_z specify the orientation of x_S. Likewise, the entries $o_x, o_y, o_z, a_x, a_y, a_z$ specify y_S and z_S, respectively. Finally p_x, p_y, p_z again specify the position of the origin of S. Notice again that only the 12 values $n_x, \ldots, p_z$ carry the matrix information. The values in the last row of the matrix are constant.

Example 2.1

Consider the surgical saw in Fig. 1.1 (first figure of the introduction chapter). Our goal is to move the saw with a robot. Thus, we must command the positions and orientations of the saw. First we attach a coordinate system S to the saw. In Fig. 2.3, the saw is simply shown as a block. The origin of S is a vertex of this block. The axes x_S, y_S and z_S of S coincide with edges of the block.

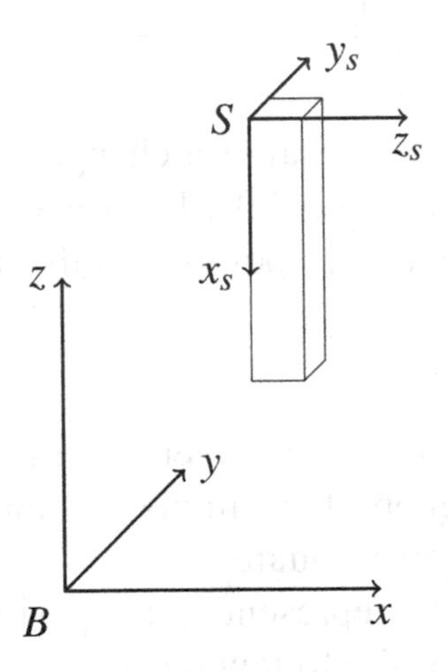

Fig. 2.3: Coordinate system S for a surgical saw

According to our notation, we find that the following matrix ${}^B\mathbf{M}_S$ describes the position of the saw:

$$
{}^B\mathbf{M}_S = \begin{pmatrix} 0 & 0 & 1 & p_x \\ 0 & 1 & 0 & p_y \\ -1 & 0 & 0 & p_z \\ 0 & 0 & 0 & 1 \end{pmatrix} \tag{2.4}
$$

The notation ${}^B\mathbf{M}_S$ indicates that the matrix gives the position and orientation of S with respect to B.

Notice that here we have again rotated about the y-axis, but now in the opposite direction. We see that we need a convention indicating the direction of rotation. We will do this next, after introducing conventions for rotations about fixed axes.

2.2 Angles

An alternative way to describe the orientation of the object coordinate system S is to use angles. Thus in Fig. 2.3, we state that the saw's coordinate system is rotated by an angle of 90° about the y-axis of the base. To describe an arbitrary orientation in space, we use the three angle values α, β, γ. They refer to rotations about the three axes x, y and z of the base coordinate system. To represent a position of the saw, we thus have the coordinates $(p_x, p_y, p_z)^{\mathrm{T}}$ of S, and the three angles α, β, γ.

We must now define a convention for the direction of rotation. Thus we must agree on the positive sense of rotation. Here we set forth the following convention. A positive rotation about the x-axis will move the y-axis towards the z-axis. Likewise, positive revolute motion about the z-axis will move the x-axis towards the y-axis. The full conventions are:

pos. sense	$x \to y$	$y \to z$	$z \to x$
neg. sense	$y \to x$	$z \to y$	$x \to z$

With this convention, our system in Fig. 2.3 is described by

$$(p_x, p_y, p_z, 0, 90, 0)^{\mathrm{T}} \tag{2.5}$$

In general, the six-vector

$$^{B}YPR_{S} = (p_x, p_y, p_z, \alpha, \beta, \gamma)^{\mathrm{T}} \tag{2.6}$$

is called the Yaw-Pitch-Roll vector, or YPR-vector. However, there are several other conventions (see the exercises at the end of this chapter). We will soon see that the matrix representation is often preferable over the YPR-representation.

The medical literature has its own naming conventions for rotations. They are:

Medicine	Engineering
Flexion (+)/extension (−)	Yaw
Varus (+)/valgus (−)	Pitch
Rotation (+)/derotation (−)	Roll

2.2.1 Relative Position and Orientation

Suppose we replace the saw by a drill (see Fig. 2.4). The drill has its own coordinate system S. At the tip of the drill, we place a new coordinate system S'. We have the position of S with respect to the base B. Now we would like to compute the position of S' with respect to the base system B. Thus, suppose we have defined two matrices ${}^{B}\mathbf{M}_{S}$ and ${}^{S}\mathbf{M}_{S'}$.

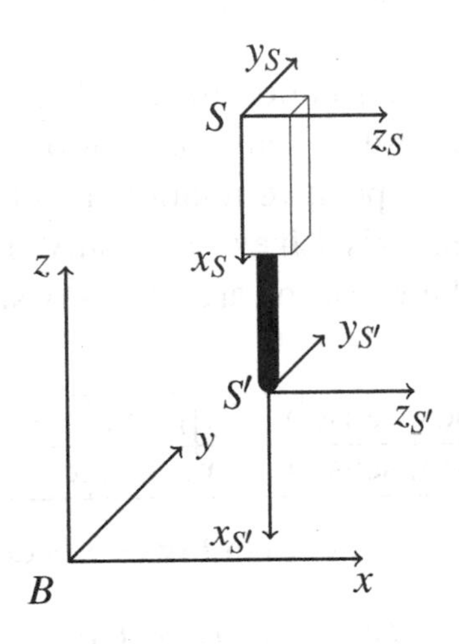

Fig. 2.4: Drill tip coordinate system

Here we have again used the convention that the matrix ${}^{B}\mathbf{M}_{S}$ describes a transition from coordinate system B to coordinate system S. The first of the two matrices (${}^{B}\mathbf{M}_{S}$) has been computed above. The second matrix is also easy to compute. From the figure, we see that it is simply given by:

$$ {}^{S}\mathbf{M}_{S'} = \begin{pmatrix} 1 & 0 & 0 & p'_x \\ 0 & 1 & 0 & p'_y \\ 0 & 0 & 1 & p'_z \\ 0 & 0 & 0 & 1 \end{pmatrix} \tag{2.7} $$

Here $\mathbf{p'} = (p'_x, p'_y, p'_z)^{\mathrm{T}}$ denotes the origin of S', given in coordinates of S.

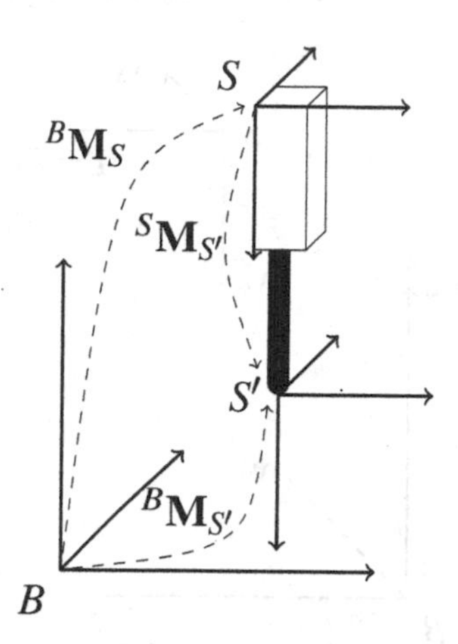

Fig. 2.5: Matrix transformations. The matrix describing position and orientation of the drill tip with respect to the base is the product of two matrices $^B\mathbf{M}_S$ and $^S\mathbf{M}_{S'}$

Now the matrix we are looking for (drill tip with respect to base) is simply given by the product of the two matrices already computed, i.e.

$$^B\mathbf{M}_{S'} = {^B\mathbf{M}_S}\ {^S\mathbf{M}_{S'}}. \tag{2.8}$$

This is illustrated in Fig. 2.5. It is easy to verify this equation with the above interpretation of matrix columns.
Above we looked at relative transformations between coordinate systems. The following example discusses a different situation: a vector is given in a coordinate system S, and our goal is to express its coordinates in another coordinate system.

Example 2.2

Assume the vector $\mathbf{q}$ in Fig. 2.6 is given with respect to the drill coordinate system S. $\mathbf{q}$ points along the z-direction of S, and

$$^S\mathbf{q} = \begin{pmatrix} 0 \\ 0 \\ 1 \end{pmatrix}. \tag{2.9}$$

To express the fact that $\mathbf{q}$ is given in terms of S, we have used the above notation with superscripts and subscripts.

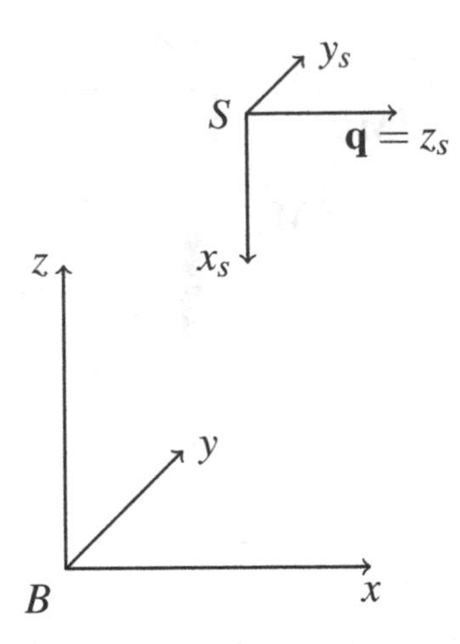

Fig. 2.6: Transforming the coordinates of a point given with respect to S

Now from the figure we also see that $\mathbf{q}$ points along the positive x-axis of the base coordinate system. Thus, in base coordinates $\mathbf{q}$ is given as

$$^{B}\mathbf{q} = \begin{pmatrix} 1 \\ 0 \\ 0 \end{pmatrix}. \tag{2.10}$$

The matrix $^{B}\mathbf{M}_{S}$ transforming from the base system B to S was derived in Eq. 2.4. In principle, we can use this matrix to compute $^{B}\mathbf{q}$ from the given $^{S}\mathbf{q}$.
However, we cannot directly multiply $^{S}\mathbf{q}$ with $^{B}\mathbf{M}_{S}$. The reason is that $^{S}\mathbf{q}$ is a three-vector and $^{B}\mathbf{M}_{S}$ is a 4×4-matrix. To overcome this difficulty, we extend $^{S}\mathbf{q}$. Hence, we add a fourth coordinate, with the value zero, i.e. we replace the three-vector $^{S}\mathbf{q} = (q_x, q_y, q_z)^{\mathrm{T}}$ by

$$^{S}\mathbf{q} = \begin{pmatrix} q_x \\ q_y \\ q_z \\ 0 \end{pmatrix}. \tag{2.11}$$

Multiplying, we obtain

$$^{B}\mathbf{q} = ^{B}\mathbf{M}_{S}\ ^{S}\mathbf{q}. \tag{2.12}$$

(End of Example 2.2)

2.3 Linkages

A linkage consists of several links and joints. The linkage moves if we change the joint angles. Assume we mount a gripper to the tip of the linkage. Our goal is to find a 4×4 matrix expressing the position and orientation of the gripper, given the joint angles. Thus the matrix we are looking for is a function of the joint angles. We will first look at a one-joint linkage.

Example 2.3

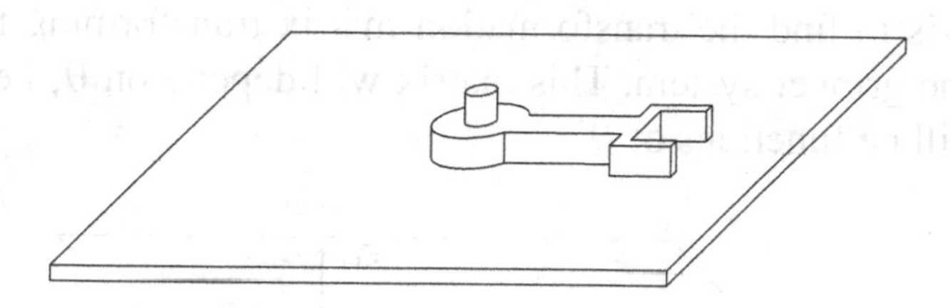

Fig. 2.7: Planar robot with a single revolute joint

Consider the robot shown in Fig. 2.7. It only has a single joint, and a single link. But it does have a gripper, mounted to the end of the single link.

This robot is not very interesting (it cannot even close its gripper) but it illustrates how we apply coordinate systems. A null position of a robot is a fixed reference position. Assume the null position of our one-joint robot is the position shown. In this null position, the joint angle is zero. If we change the joint angle, our robot will start to move. We place a base coordinate system in our standard orientation with the origin on the robot plane (Fig. 2.8). The rotation axis of this joint is the axis z_B of our standard base system, i.e. z_B is orthogonal to the robot plane. We measure the angle of rotation by the angle θ. At the position shown, we have $\theta = 0$, i.e. the null position of our robot.

Thus our z_B axis is the rotation axis of the joint. Also place a gripper coordinate system with its origin into the center of the gripper (Fig. 2.9). Call the gripper system G. In the null position, G has the same orientation as B. We assume G is rigidly attached to the grip-

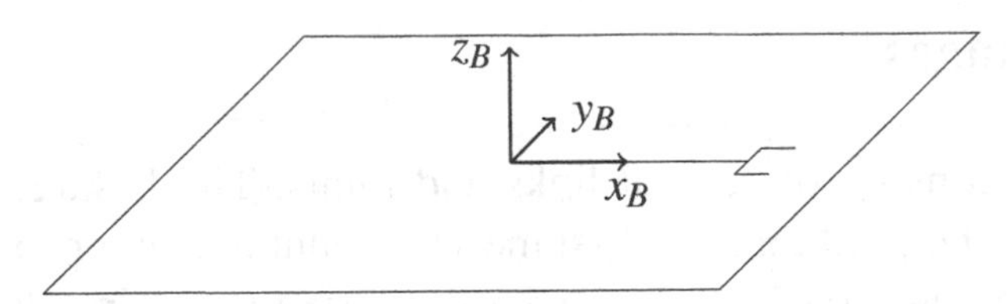

Fig. 2.8: Base coordinate system for the robot in Fig. 2.7. The robot has a single revolute joint. The axis of rotation of this joint is the z-axis of the base system

per and moves with the robot. B does not move, since it is our base system.
Our goal is to find the transformation matrix transforming from the base to the gripper system. This matrix will depend on θ, i.e. matrix entries will be functions of θ.

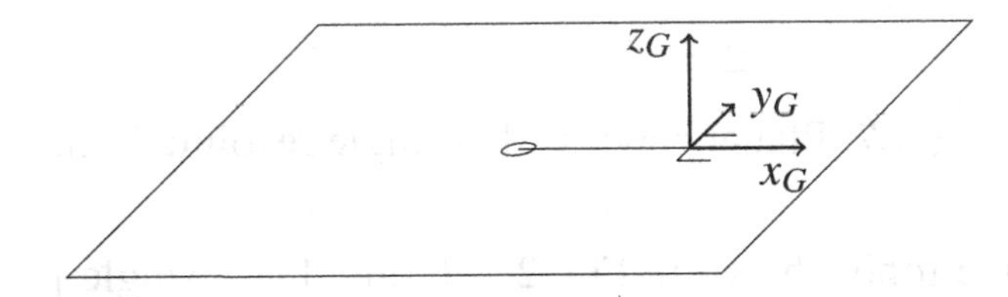

Fig. 2.9: Gripper coordinate system for the robot in Fig. 2.7

To find the transformation we use a two-step process. The process resembles the computation of the drill tip matrix (see above). However, we will need an additional step. We introduce an intermediate coordinate system S_1, which moves with the robot as it rotates (Fig. 2.10). Note again that the base system will always stay fixed. The origin of

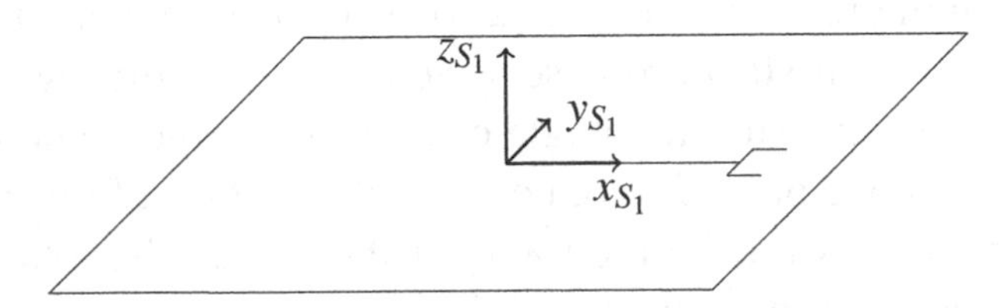

Fig. 2.10: Intermediate coordinate system S_1 for the robot in Fig. 2.7. Notice that the origin of S_1 coincides with the origin of B. S_1 rotates with the robot, while B remains fixed

this intermediate system S_1 remains at the origin of the base system, but otherwise S_1 rotates with the robot.
The gripper system is fixed at a point in the center between the two gripper jaws. This point is called the tool center point, and depends on the tool we use, e.g. a saw, a drill, or a gripper.
Throughout this book, we will often use the term *effector* instead of gripper. We can replace the gripper by a saw or a drill, or some other tool. An effector can thus be any tool mounted to the end of a kinematic chain.
The placement of the system S_1, as the robot moves, is shown in Fig. 2.11.

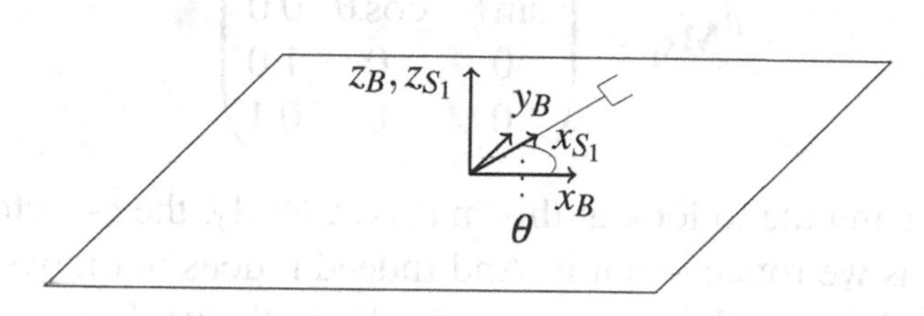

Fig. 2.11: The intermediate coordinate system S_1 rotates with the robot, (angle θ). The two z-axes (of B and S_1) coincide. The y-axis of S_1 is not shown

We now look at the scene from above: the placement of S_1 within the base system is shown in Fig. 2.12:

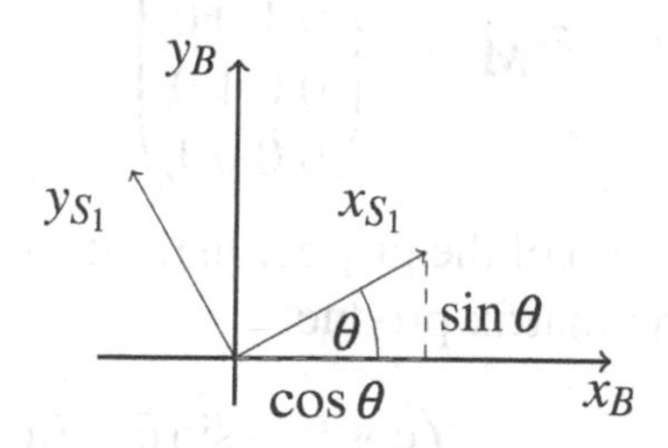

Fig. 2.12: Placement of intermediate coordinate system S_1 with respect to the base coordinate system, depending on the angle θ of rotation of the robot in Fig. 2.7

We consider the vector x_{S_1} in the figure. In terms of the base, this vector has the x-coordinate $\cos\theta$, and the y-coordinate $\sin\theta$. Likewise, we see that the y-vector of S_1 is given by

$$\begin{pmatrix} -\sin\theta \\ \cos\theta \end{pmatrix} \tag{2.13}$$

Putting this into a 4×4-matrix as described above, we obtain the position of the intermediate system S_1 with respect to the base, depending on the joint angle θ:

$$^{B}\mathbf{M}_{S_1} = \begin{pmatrix} \cos\theta & -\sin\theta & 0 & 0 \\ \sin\theta & \cos\theta & 0 & 0 \\ 0 & 0 & 1 & 0 \\ 0 & 0 & 0 & 1 \end{pmatrix} \tag{2.14}$$

We pause a minute to look at this matrix. Clearly, the z-vector should not move as we rotate about it. And indeed it does not move, namely the third column of the matrix simply shows the unchanged z-vector. The first and second columns of the matrix show the motions of the x- and y-vectors, depending on the angle θ.
This completes the first step of our computation. For the second step, we find the transformation from S_1 to the gripper. Since this transformation is only a translation by the link length (called L), the matrix is given by:

$$^{S_1}\mathbf{M}_{G} = \begin{pmatrix} 1 & 0 & 0 & L \\ 0 & 1 & 0 & 0 \\ 0 & 0 & 1 & 0 \\ 0 & 0 & 0 & 1 \end{pmatrix} \tag{2.15}$$

Thus the desired position of the gripper in terms of the base coordinate system is given by the matrix product

$$^{B}\mathbf{M}_{S_1} \cdot {}^{S_1}\mathbf{M}_{G} = \begin{pmatrix} \cos\theta & -\sin\theta & 0 & L\cos\theta \\ \sin\theta & \cos\theta & 0 & L\sin\theta \\ 0 & 0 & 1 & 0 \\ 0 & 0 & 0 & 1 \end{pmatrix} \tag{2.16}$$

Note that this matrix contains the angle θ. It expresses the location of the gripper coordinate system, depending on the joint angle of the robot. We have completed the *forward kinematic analysis* in a simple example. In general, the goal of forward analysis is to find the location of the effector, given values for each joint angle.

(End of Example 2.3)

To summarize things, we have used three coordinate systems in our analysis: the base B, the gripper G, and the intermediate system S_1. Introducing the intermediate system was indeed the main step, and it will be extremely useful when analyzing more complex robots.
The next example shows that we can repeat the same construction to obtain transformations for n-joint robots.
But before we get to the next example, we again look at Eq. 2.14. In this equation we have derived a matrix describing a simple rotation about the z-axis. It is now straightforward to derive the two other elementary rotation matrices, namely matrices describing rotations about x and y. Take a minute to verify the following matrices, and note the placements of the minus-signs in the matrices.

$$R(x,\theta) = \begin{pmatrix} 1 & 0 & 0 & 0 \\ 0 & \cos\theta & -\sin\theta & 0 \\ 0 & \sin\theta & \cos\theta & 0 \\ 0 & 0 & 0 & 1 \end{pmatrix} \qquad R(y,\theta) = \begin{pmatrix} \cos\theta & 0 & \sin\theta & 0 \\ 0 & 1 & 0 & 0 \\ -\sin\theta & 0 & \cos\theta & 0 \\ 0 & 0 & 0 & 1 \end{pmatrix}$$

$$R(z,\theta) = \begin{pmatrix} \cos\theta & -\sin\theta & 0 & 0 \\ \sin\theta & \cos\theta & 0 & 0 \\ 0 & 0 & 1 & 0 \\ 0 & 0 & 0 & 1 \end{pmatrix} \tag{2.17}$$

Even more straightforward is the derivation of the elementary translation matrices:

$$T(p_x,0,0) = \begin{pmatrix} 1 & 0 & 0 & p_x \\ 0 & 1 & 0 & 0 \\ 0 & 0 & 1 & 0 \\ 0 & 0 & 0 & 1 \end{pmatrix} \qquad T(0,p_y,0) = \begin{pmatrix} 1 & 0 & 0 & 0 \\ 0 & 1 & 0 & p_y \\ 0 & 0 & 1 & 0 \\ 0 & 0 & 0 & 1 \end{pmatrix}$$

$$T(0,0,p_z) = \begin{pmatrix} 1 & 0 & 0 & 0 \\ 0 & 1 & 0 & 0 \\ 0 & 0 & 1 & p_z \\ 0 & 0 & 0 & 1 \end{pmatrix} \tag{2.18}$$

2.4 Three-Joint Robot

Suppose now we have a robot with three joints. Such a robot is shown in Fig. 2.13. We call this robot the *elbow manipulator*. Our goal is to express the position and orientation of the gripper with respect to the base coordinate system. We place a coordinate system into each link of the robot. We obtain a chain of coordinate systems, leading from the base system to the gripper system in several steps. Notice that this robot has only three joints, and typical robots have six joints. However, all computations for the three-joint robot can later be used for more complex robots.

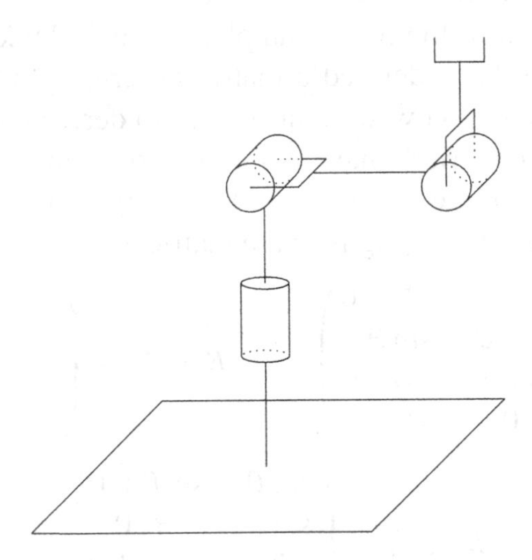

Fig. 2.13: Three-joint robot (elbow manipulator). All three joints are revolute joints

The three joint angles are called $\theta_1, \theta_2, \theta_3$. The position shown in the figure is the null position of the robot, meaning $\theta_1 = \theta_2 = \theta_3 = 0$.
As above, we define intermediate coordinate systems $S_0 = (x_0, y_0, z_0)$ and $S_i = (x_i, y_i, z_i)$, $i = 1, \ldots, 3$ (see Fig. 2.14).
Think of the first system $B = S_0 = (x_0, y_0, z_0)$ as the base system. It is attached to the table, and does not move, although it rests with its origin at the upper tip of the first link. This may seem odd, but we do this to simplify the overall matrix product, i.e. we thus do not need an extra transformation leading from the table to the tip of the first link.

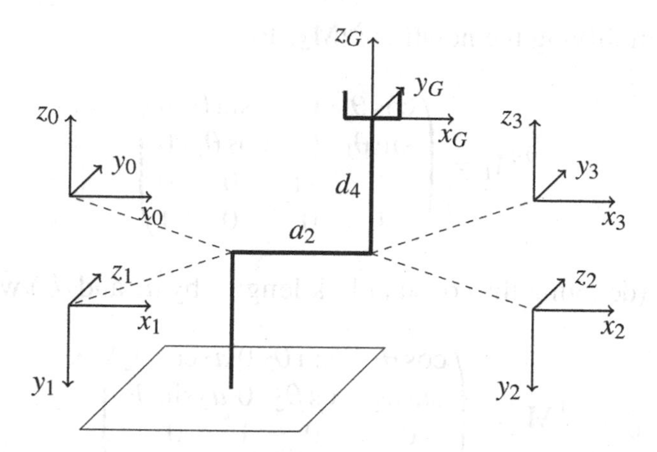

Fig. 2.14: Joint coordinate systems for transforming between base system $S_0 = (x_0, y_0, z_0)$ via $S_i = (x_i, y_i, z_i)$ to the gripper coordinate system $S_G = (x_G, y_G, z_G)$

Our goal is to derive a matrix which transforms from the base coordinate system $B = S_0$ to the gripper system S_G. Having defined the intermediate matrices S_i, we can partition this goal into a series of small steps. The first step is the transformation from S_0 to S_1. We will do this next.
The rotation axis of the first joint is the axis z_0. To get from S_0 to S_1, we must take into account any rotations about this first axis. As in the case of our single joint robot in the above example, the matrix $R(z,\theta)$ in Eq. 2.17 describes this rotation. But now we are not done, since we have not reached S_1 yet. To do so, we must rotate about the x_0-axis by the fixed angle of $-90°$ (see Fig. 2.14). Overall, the following matrix product gives the transformation from S_0 to S_1.

$$
{}^{S_0}\mathbf{M}_{S_1} = R(z,\theta_1)R(x,-90) = \begin{pmatrix} \cos\theta_1 & -\sin\theta_1 & 0 & 0 \\ \sin\theta_1 & \cos\theta_1 & 0 & 0 \\ 0 & 0 & 1 & 0 \\ 0 & 0 & 0 & 1 \end{pmatrix} \begin{pmatrix} 1 & 0 & 0 & 0 \\ 0 & 0 & 1 & 0 \\ 0 & -1 & 0 & 0 \\ 0 & 0 & 0 & 1 \end{pmatrix} \tag{2.19}
$$

Hence (simplifying the notation ${}^{S_0}\mathbf{M}_{S_1}$ to ${}^{0}\mathbf{M}_1$):

$$ {}^{0}\mathbf{M}_1 = \begin{pmatrix} \cos\theta_1 & 0 & -\sin\theta_1 & 0 \\ \sin\theta_1 & 0 & \cos\theta_1 & 0 \\ 0 & -1 & 0 & 0 \\ 0 & 0 & 0 & 1 \end{pmatrix} \tag{2.20} $$

Similarly (denoting the constant link lengths by a_2 and d_4) we obtain:

$$ {}^{1}\mathbf{M}_2 = \begin{pmatrix} \cos\theta_2 & -\sin\theta_2 & 0 & a_2\cos\theta_2 \\ \sin\theta_2 & \cos\theta_2 & 0 & a_2\sin\theta_2 \\ 0 & 0 & 1 & 0 \\ 0 & 0 & 0 & 1 \end{pmatrix} \tag{2.21} $$

$$ {}^{2}\mathbf{M}_3 = \begin{pmatrix} \cos\theta_3 & 0 & \sin\theta_3 & 0 \\ \sin\theta_3 & 0 & -\cos\theta_3 & 0 \\ 0 & 1 & 0 & 0 \\ 0 & 0 & 0 & 1 \end{pmatrix} \tag{2.22} $$

$$ {}^{3}\mathbf{M}_G = \begin{pmatrix} 1 & 0 & 0 & 0 \\ 0 & 1 & 0 & 0 \\ 0 & 0 & 1 & d_4 \\ 0 & 0 & 0 & 1 \end{pmatrix} \tag{2.23} $$

Multiplying, we have (abbreviating s_1 for $\sin\theta_1$ etc.) :

$$ {}^{0}\mathbf{M}_3 = {}^{0}\mathbf{M}_1 \cdot {}^{1}\mathbf{M}_2 \cdot {}^{2}\mathbf{M}_3 \tag{2.24} $$

$$ \begin{pmatrix} c_1(c_2c_3 - s_2s_3) & -s_1 & c_1(c_2s_3 + s_2c_3) & a_2c_1c_2 \\ s_1(c_2c_3 - s_2s_3) & c_1 & s_1(c_2s_3 + s_2c_3) & a_2s_1c_2 \\ -s_2c_3 - c_2s_3 & 0 & -s_2s_3 + c_2c_3 & -a_2s_2 \\ 0 & 0 & 0 & 1 \end{pmatrix} \tag{2.25} $$

The last equation can be simplified with the trigonometric addition formulas. Therefore (setting s_{12} for $\sin(\theta_1 + \theta_2)$, etc.):

$$ {}^{0}\mathbf{M}_3 = \begin{pmatrix} c_1c_{23} & -s_1 & c_1s_{23} & a_2c_1c_2 \\ s_1c_{23} & c_1 & s_1s_{23} & a_2s_1c_2 \\ -s_{23} & 0 & c_{23} & -a_2s_2 \\ 0 & 0 & 0 & 1 \end{pmatrix} \tag{2.26} $$

For the final result, we must multiply with the constant transformation ${}^{3}\mathbf{M}_{G}$, given above, which transforms from S_3 to the gripper coordinate system:

$$ {}^{0}\mathbf{M}_{G} = \begin{pmatrix} c_1c_{23} & -s_1 & c_1s_{23} & a_2c_1c_2 + d_4c_1s_{23} \\ s_1c_{23} & c_1 & s_1s_{23} & a_2s_1c_2 + d_4s_1s_{23} \\ -s_{23} & 0 & c_{23} & -a_2s_2 + d_4c_{23} \\ 0 & 0 & 0 & 1 \end{pmatrix} \tag{2.27} $$

You may wish to check Eq. 2.27 for various settings of the angles $\theta_1, \theta_2, \theta_3$ (see also the exercises at the end of this chapter).

2.5 Standardizing Kinematic Analysis

In the previous section, we saw that kinematic equations for simple robots can become quite long. Here we only looked at a three-joint robot. Thus it is useful to simplify and standardize the notation, to make it as compact as possible. This is what was done in a paper by Denavit and Hartenberg from 1955 [4]. We have already seen an example for such a simplification: We placed the base coordinate system at the tip of the first link in our analysis of the three-joint robot (Fig. 2.14), to reduce the number of elementary matrices in the matrix product.
If we take a step back and look at the placement of the other coordinate systems in the example, we see that all z-axes (in Fig. 2.14) coincide with the rotation axes of the joints. But there is more that can be done to standardize the placement of coordinate systems. Notice that the transformation between two arbitrary coordinate systems in space can require as many as six elementary transformations (rotations and translations). The main idea in [4] is that four elementary transformations will suffice, if we place the coordinate systems in an appropriate way. We will explain this idea in a little more detail below, but let us first look at the rules for placing the coordinate systems. Place the systems such that

1. $B = S_0$ is the fixed base system.
2. The axis z_i is the rotation axis of the joint with index $(i+1)$.
3. The axis x_i is orthogonal to the axis z_{i-1}, and also orthogonal to z_i. By convention, the pointing direction of x_i is from z_{i-1} towards z_i.

4. Place y_i in such a way that S_i is a right-handed coordinate system (see also Exercise 2.2d).

These four rules are called DH-rules. You may wish to take a minute to verify that we were consistent with these rules in our example for the three-joint robot. For example, from rule 2, we see that z_0 is the axis of the first joint, as in our example.
Placing axes is not all. We also need to place the origin of each system. Let O_i denote the origin of S_i. In general, the two axes z_{i-1} and z_i are neither parallel, nor do they coincide or intersect. The DH-rules hold for any general robot, so that we assume z_{i-1} and z_i are on skew lines. We connect the two lines by their joint normal, and put the origin O_i on the intersection point of z_i and this normal (Fig. 2.15).
Our goal is now to derive a compact transformation matrix for transforming from S_{i-1} to S_i. We will see that the above rules will lead to a comparatively small matrix.
We noted above that the main observation in the original paper by Denavit and Hartenberg [4] is that four elementary transformations will always suffice for transforming from S_{i-1} to S_i. Notice that we must follow the rules when placing S_{i-1} and S_i. The four specific transformations to be given now will not suffice, if you did not follow the rules. (To understand why, you should check that the rules amount to 'removing' two degrees of freedom[1].)

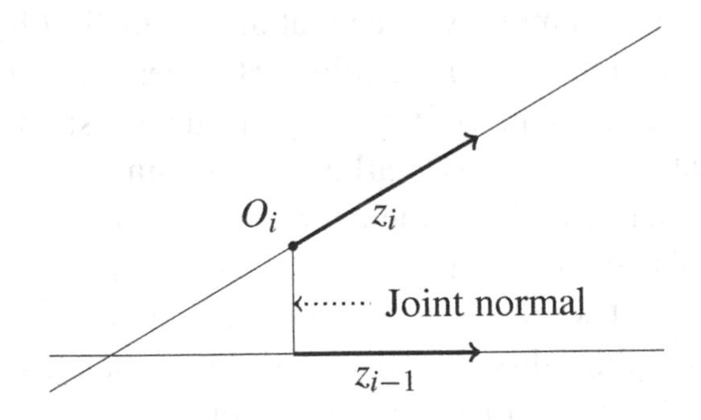

Fig. 2.15: Placement of the origin O_i of system S_i

[1] The *degree of freedom* of a mechanical system is the number of independent parameters that define its position and orientation in space.

Denavit and Hartenberg show that the following elementary translations/rotations always suffice:

1. Translate along z_{i-1} by an amount d_i
2. Rotate about z_{i-1} by θ_i
3. Translate along x_i by a_i
4. Rotate about x_i by α_i

In our example, the values d_i, a_i, α_i are constant, while θ_i is the (variable) joint angle. We will hence call θ_i the joint variable. We have given names to the elementary transformations, and we have written them as matrices in Eqs. 2.17 and 2.18. Thus the transformations can be written as follows:

$$\begin{gathered} T(0,0,d_i) \\ R(z,\theta_i) \\ T(a_i,0,0) \\ R(x,\alpha_i) \end{gathered} \tag{2.28}$$

Now we are not far from our goal. The matrix

$$^{i-1}\mathbf{M}_i = T(0,0,d_i)R(z,\theta_i)T(a_i,0,0)R(x,\alpha_i) \tag{2.29}$$

transforms from S_{i-1} to S_i.
With Eqs. 2.17 and 2.18, we can write

$$^{i-1}\mathbf{M}_i = \begin{pmatrix} 1&0&0&0 \\ 0&1&0&0 \\ 0&0&1&d_i \\ 0&0&0&1 \end{pmatrix} \begin{pmatrix} c\theta_i & -s\theta_i & 0 & 0 \\ s\theta_i & c\theta_i & 0 & 0 \\ 0&0&1&0 \\ 0&0&0&1 \end{pmatrix} \begin{pmatrix} 1&0&0&a_i \\ 0&1&0&0 \\ 0&0&1&0 \\ 0&0&0&1 \end{pmatrix} \begin{pmatrix} 1&0&0&0 \\ 0&c\alpha_i&-s\alpha_i&0 \\ 0&s\alpha_i&c\alpha_i&0 \\ 0&0&0&1 \end{pmatrix} \tag{2.30}$$

Finally, we obtain

$$^{i-1}\mathbf{M}_i = \begin{pmatrix} c\theta_i & -c\alpha_i s\theta_i & s\alpha_i s\theta_i & a_i c\theta_i \\ s\theta_i & c\alpha_i c\theta_i & -s\alpha_i c\theta_i & a_i s\theta_i \\ 0 & s\alpha_i & c\alpha_i & d_i \\ 0&0&0&1 \end{pmatrix}. \tag{2.31}$$

We see that the matrix describing a robot with six joints is a product of six matrices as in Eq. 2.31. Although we have taken care to reduce the number of elementary transformations, the matrix product is not simple. However, having set up the rules for the placement of coordinate systems, we can arrive at a yet more compact description of a robot. We simply set up a table containing the parameters $\alpha_i, a_i, d_i, \theta_i$. Each line in the table corresponds to one joint, and we obtain a table of the form in Table 2.1.

Table 2.1: DH-table

i	α_i	a_i	d_i	θ_i
1	α_1	a_1	d_1	θ_1
2	α_2	a_2	d_2	θ_2
$\vdots$	$\vdots$	$\vdots$	$\vdots$	$\vdots$

The tables for defining kinematic constructions, as in Table 2.1, can be applied to our three-joint robot. We obtain Table 2.2.

Table 2.2: DH-table for the three-joint robot

i	α_i	a_i	d_i	θ_i
1	−90	0	0	θ_1
2	0	a_2	0	θ_2
3	90	0	0	θ_3
G	0	0	d_4	0

It should be noted that a number of special cases can arise when applying the DH-rules. For example, the axes z_{i-1} and z_i can intersect or be parallel, or even coincide. In all such cases, the rules can be relaxed, and we obtain two or more equivalent ways for fixing the axis x_i or the origin O_i.

2.6 Computing Joint Angles

We saw that we can describe the position of the gripper, given angles $\theta_1, \theta_2 \ldots$. We now wish to do the opposite. Namely, given a desired position for the gripper, how do we choose the angles? In general, this is what we need to program a robot. The next example discusses a simple case.

Example 2.4

We return to the one-joint robot in example 2.2. Here the problem just stated is very simple. Fix a point on the table. Now, which angle must we prescribe to reach that point? The situation is illustrated in Fig. 2.16.
There is an easy answer to our question. We are given the target point $\mathbf{p} = (p_x, p_y)^T$, and we wish to grasp this point with our gripper. Elementary mathematics will help us to find θ, given $\mathbf{p}$. We have $\cos\theta = p_x$ and $\sin\theta = p_y$. (Here we have assumed that our robot link has unit length, i.e. $L = 1$ in Fig. 2.16 and $\|p\| = 1$) We can solve this for θ by dividing the two equations:

$$\frac{\sin\theta}{\cos\theta} = \frac{p_y}{p_x} \tag{2.32}$$

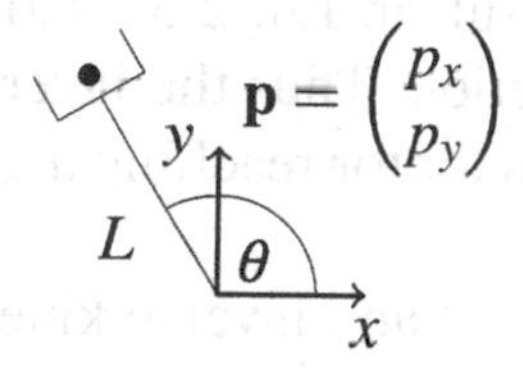

Fig. 2.16: Calculating the joint angle θ for reaching a given point $\mathbf{p}$ (*black dot*)

From this, we could conclude $\tan\theta = \frac{p_y}{p_x}$, and $\theta = \arctan\frac{p_y}{p_x}$.
But this simple solution has a drawback. By definition, the function arctan returns values in the range $(-\pi/2, \pi/2)$. Thus, it can never return a value larger than $\pi/2$. By consequence, our robot can never reach the point $\mathbf{p}$ shown in the figure, since its null position points along the x-axis. In fact, the entire half-plane to the left of the y-axis is lost for our robot.
There is a standard way to repair this. We extend the function arctan. The function atan2 is defined on the basis on the arctan-function. This function atan2 takes two arguments x and y, hence the name. It is

defined by distinguishing several cases for the values of the arguments x and y.

$$\operatorname{atan2}(y,x) = \begin{cases} 0 & \text{for } x = 0, y = 0 \\ \pi/2 & \text{for } x = 0, y > 0 \\ 3 \cdot \pi/2 & \text{for } x = 0, y < 0 \\ \arctan(y/x) & \text{for } x > 0, y \geq 0 \\ 2\pi + \arctan(y/x) & \text{for } x > 0, y < 0 \\ \pi + \arctan(y/x) & \text{for } x < 0, y \geq 0 \\ \pi + \arctan(y/x) & \text{for } x < 0, y < 0 \end{cases} \tag{2.33}$$

With this definition, we obtain

$$\theta = \operatorname{atan2}(p_y, p_x). \tag{2.34}$$

You should verify that our one-joint robot can reach all positions on a full circle with this definition.
A matrix equation as in Eq. 2.27 is called the forward kinematic solution of the robot. The result in Eq. 2.34 shows a simple example of an inverse kinematic solution. Thus the inverse solution states the required joint angles necessary for reaching a given position and orientation.
We will discuss the forward and inverse kinematics for medical linkages in more detail in Chap. 3.

2.7 Quaternions

In a typical navigation scenario, we combine a robot arm with a tracking device. Most tracking systems are equipped with a pointer tool. Then the tracking system works like this: we hold the pointer in a fixed position in space. The tracking system outputs the coordinates of this point. (It also outputs the spatial direction of the pointer.) When we move the pointer, the system follows with a high sampling rate, which can be as high as 4 kHz. Internally, most tracking systems do not work with matrices or YPR-angles. Instead, they work with *quaternions*.

Thus, they will output a quaternion to the host computer, not a matrix, while the robot usually works with matrices or YPR angles. With quaternions we can represent orientations just as with 3×3-matrices or YPR-angles.
A quaternion is a 4-vector of the form

$$\mathbf{a} = (a_1, a_2, a_3, a_4)^{\mathrm{T}} \tag{2.35}$$

We can add quaternions just like regular 4-vectors i.e.

$$\mathbf{a} + \mathbf{b} = (a_1 + b_1, a_2 + b_2, a_3 + b_3, a_4 + b_4)^{\mathrm{T}} \tag{2.36}$$

We would like to define a multiplication for quaternions. One may argue that we already have a multiplication, i.e. the standard scalar product for two vectors. However, this is not what we need. We need a multiplication for two quaternions such that the result is also a quaternion, i.e. a 4-vector. The cross-product for 3-vectors could be a candidate, but it is only defined for 3-vectors. Here we define for two quaternions **a**, **b**:

$$\mathbf{ab} = \begin{pmatrix} a_1b_1 - a_2b_2 - a_3b_3 - a_4b_4 \\ a_1b_2 + a_2b_1 + a_3b_4 - a_4b_3 \\ a_1b_3 - a_2b_4 + a_3b_1 + a_4b_2 \\ a_1b_4 + a_2b_3 - a_3b_2 + a_4b_1 \end{pmatrix} \tag{2.37}$$

This is certainly not easy to memorize. To simplify memorizing the formula in Eq. 2.37, quaternions can be written in a slightly different, but equivalent way.
Instead of $\mathbf{a} = (a_1, a_2, a_3, a_4)^{\mathrm{T}}$, we write

$$\mathbf{a} = a_1 + a_2 i + a_3 j + a_4 k \tag{2.38}$$

Note that i, j and k are *symbols*, not numbers, and we have a table stating symbolic product rules for i, j and k. The symbolic rules are

$$\begin{array}{lll} ii = -1 & jj = -1 & kk = -1 \\ ij = k & jk = i & ki = j \\ ji = -k & kj = -i & ik = -j \end{array} \tag{2.39}$$

Now we can multiply i, j and k just as they were numbers, and one can easily verify that the product **ab** for quaternions defined in this way is equivalent to this new definition.

The new rules are somewhat easier to memorize than the original definition in Eq. 2.37, and they are reminiscent of the rules for the positive/negative sense of rotation. For all purposes other than remembering the specific multiplication above, we will remain with our first definition in Eq. 2.37. Hence, from now on, a quaternion is simply a 4-vector.

Notice that in general $\mathbf{ab} \neq \mathbf{ba}$.

Just as for any 4-vector, we have a norm, namely

$$\|\mathbf{a}\| = \sqrt{a_1^2 + a_2^2 + a_3^2 + a_4^2} \tag{2.40}$$

Unit quaternions are quaternions having norm 1. We represent rotations in the following way. Given a 3-vector $\mathbf{p} = (p_x, p_y, p_z)^{\mathrm{T}}$. Set $\mathbf{p} = (0, p_x, p_y, p_z)^{\mathrm{T}}$, and we have turned our 3-vector $\mathbf{p}$ into a quaternion. For convenience, we will also call it $\mathbf{p}$. We noted above that quaternions are similar to matrices, and one similarity is that a quaternion also has an inverse.

Namely, set

$$\mathbf{a}^{-1} = \frac{(a_1, -a_2, -a_3, -a_4)^{\mathrm{T}}}{\|a\|}, \tag{2.41}$$

for $\mathbf{a} = (a_1, a_2, a_3, a_4)^{\mathrm{T}}$. (You should check that $\mathbf{aa}^{-1}$ really gives the quaternion $\mathbf{e} = (1, 0, 0, 0)^{\mathrm{T}}$.)

Now we can define the three-product $\mathbf{apa}^{-1}$, and its result is a quaternion $\mathbf{q}$. Here, $\mathbf{q}$ will always have the form $\mathbf{q} = (0, q_2, q_3, q_4)^{\mathrm{T}}$, i.e. its first element will always be zero. Hence we can regard $\mathbf{q}$ as a 3-vector. We interpret $\mathbf{q}$ as the vector obtained by rotating $\mathbf{p}$ under the rotation defined by $\mathbf{a}$.

Hence, to summarize

$$\mathbf{q} = \mathbf{apa}^{-1} \tag{2.42}$$

defines quaternion rotation, where $\mathbf{a}$ is the (unit) quaternion by which we rotate, and $\mathbf{p}$ is the object of rotation. Thus the quaternion $\mathbf{a}$ takes the role of a 3×3-rotation matrix. Notice that a quaternion is much more compact than a 3×3-matrix, which is why quaternions are also often used in graphics.
To understand exactly which rotation is represented by a given unit quaternion, we observe that for $\mathbf{a} = (a_1, a_2, a_3, a_4)^T$, the component a_1 defines the angle, and the 3-vector $(a_2, a_3, a_4)^T$ defines the axis of the rotation. Details are explained in the following example.
For more information about quaternions, refer to [1].

Example 2.5

Suppose we wish to rotate about the z-axis of the base system by the angle $\theta = \pi$. To select the axis of rotation, we set $\mathbf{p} = (0, 0, 1)^T$. Then the quaternion

$$\mathbf{a} = \left(\cos \pi/2, \sin \pi/2 \frac{\mathbf{p}}{\|\mathbf{p}\|} \right)^T \tag{2.43}$$

describes this rotation. In our case $\mathbf{p}$ is already normalized, so that $\mathbf{a} = (0, 0, 0, 1)^T$ describes the desired rotation. Equation 2.43 describes the general case, i.e. how to get from an angle and an axis to the corresponding quaternion.

(End of Example 2.5)

We will further discuss quaternions in the exercises for this chapter. Specifically, we will need a method for converting the different representations (angles, matrices, quaternions). This will be done in Exercise 2.7.

Exercises

Exercise 2.1 *Matrix Transformation*

In Eq. 2.11, we added a fourth component with the constant value zero to the vector **q**. Discuss the effect of adding a fourth component with value 1 instead. With this result, provide an interpretation for the last row of a homogeneous 4×4-matrix.

Exercise 2.2 *Coordinate Systems*

Imaging directions for medical imaging are specified in reference to the human body. Figure 1.15 shows the conventions.

a) Define a base coordinate system B as in Fig. 2.1. Derive YPR angle values for the three imaging directions in Fig. 1.15. In each case, the z-axis should be orthogonal to the image plane.
b) Derive the same orientations as in part a), but now according to the conventions for matrices.
c) Assume the five joints of a C-arm are given as in Fig. 1.10. Derive joint angle values for $J_1, ..., J_5$ corresponding to the orientations in Fig. 1.15, (ignoring the issues of mechanical reachability). The angle values should refer to the null position of the C-arm shown in Fig. 1.10.
d) Typical coordinate systems in engineering are so-called right-handed coordinate systems. However, medical imaging often relies on left-handed coordinate systems. The base coordinate system in Fig. 2.1 is a right-handed system. This means: x-axis of the system = thumb of your right hand, y-axis = index finger right hand, z-axis = middle finger right hand. Derive a mathematical test for deciding whether three given orthogonal unit vectors form a right-handed system or a left-handed system.

Exercise 2.3 *Orthogonal matrices and the inverse of a homogeneous* 4×4 *matrix*

The 3×3 matrix

$$\mathbf{R} = \begin{pmatrix} n_x & o_x & a_x \\ n_y & o_y & a_y \\ n_z & o_z & a_z \end{pmatrix} \tag{2.44}$$

is called orthogonal if the product $\mathbf{RR}^{\mathrm{T}}$ is the 3×3 unit matrix. Here $\mathbf{R}^{\mathrm{T}}$ denotes the transpose of $\mathbf{R}$. The upper left 3×3 matrix in a homogeneous matrix must always be orthogonal, since the first three columns in the homogeneous matrix represent vectors in an orthogonal coordinate system.

a) Show that for an orthogonal matrix $\mathbf{R}$ as in Eq. 2.44, we have $\mathbf{RxRx} = \mathbf{xx}$ for any 3-vector $\mathbf{x}$. Interpret this observation.
b) From the definition of an orthogonal matrix, we see that the inverse of an orthogonal matrix is its transpose, i.e. $\mathbf{R}^{\mathrm{T}} = \mathbf{R}^{-1}$. Based on this, derive the inverse of a homogeneous 4×4 matrix.
c) Show that $\mathbf{RxRy} = \mathbf{xy}$ for any 3-vectors $\mathbf{x}$, $\mathbf{y}$, if $\mathbf{R}$ is orthogonal.

Exercise 2.4 *Linkages*

a) Verify the result in Eq. 2.16 for $\theta = 0$ and $\theta = \pi/2$.
b) Verify the result in Eq. 2.27 for the settings $\theta_1 = 0, \theta_2 = 0, \theta_3 = 0$, and $\theta_1 = \pi/2, \theta_2 = 0, \theta_3 = -\pi/2$, and $\theta_1 = 0, \theta_2 = -\pi/2, \theta_3 = \pi/2$.

Exercise 2.5 *Angle/matrix conversion*

a) Given the three angles α, β, γ (defined as YPR-angles), find the 3×3 rotation matrix

$$\begin{pmatrix} n_x & o_x & a_x \\ n_y & o_y & a_y \\ n_z & o_z & a_z \end{pmatrix} \tag{2.45}$$

corresponding to these angles.
b) Given the rotation matrix in Eq. 2.45, extract the YPR-angles from that matrix.
Hint: The YPR angles all refer to rotations in the base coordinate system! In this case, we multiply the corresponding matrices from right to left, i.e. we start from the matrix equation

$$\mathbf{R}(z,\gamma)\mathbf{R}(y,\beta)\mathbf{R}(x,\alpha) = \begin{pmatrix} n_x \; o_x \; a_x \\ n_y \; o_y \; a_y \\ n_z \; o_z \; a_z \end{pmatrix} \tag{2.46}$$

Here, the x-rotation is the *first* rotation, followed by the y-rotation, then the z-rotation.
Now insert the elementary rotation matrices from Eq. 2.17, and evaluate the matrix product on the left side of Eq. 2.46. You will then have nine equations containing the three angles α, β, and γ. To solve for the angles in the resulting set of equations, you may find the procedure in the derivation of the function atan2 helpful.

c) Implement the conversions from part a) and part b) of this exercise, and test your implementation for appropriate angle ranges. Comment on the case $\beta = \pm\pi/2$.

Exercise 2.6 ***Euler angles***

Euler angles are an alternative to YPR-angles. We again define three angles α, β and γ. But here we choose the axes of rotation in the following way: Now α is a rotation about the z-axis of the base system, β is a rotation about the *new* y-axis, and γ is a rotation about the *new* z-axis. You may wonder why one would rotate about the same axis (z) twice. But notice that now our rotations do *not* refer to the axes of the base system, but in each case we rotate about the *new* axes. In this case (as opposed to the YPR angles in the previous exercise), we multiply the matrices from left to right.

a) Given base and saw coordinate systems as in Fig. 2.3, derive the Euler angles for the saw coordinate system.
Compare to the YPR angles for the same systems.
b) Derive and implement a conversion between 3×3 rotation matrices and Euler angles. The derivation closely follows Exercise 2.4, with one difference: you will have to start from

$$\mathbf{R}(z,\alpha)\mathbf{R}(y,\beta)\mathbf{R}(z,\gamma) = \begin{pmatrix} n_x \; o_x \; a_x \\ n_y \; o_y \; a_y \\ n_z \; o_z \; a_z \end{pmatrix} \tag{2.47}$$

Notice here that the matrices appear in *reverse* order from what you would expect! This corresponds to the fact that now we rotate about the *new* axes each time.
Notice also that some text books define Euler angles with the angle conventions z,x,z instead of z,y,z. In fact there are 12 different ways to define the Euler angles, all equivalent.

Exercise 2.7 ***Quaternions***

a) Verify the rotation results in Example 2.4 for the input vectors $(1,0,0)^{\mathrm{T}}$ and $(0,0,1)^{\mathrm{T}}$.
b) Derive a conversion from a quaternion to a 3×3 rotation matrix. Hint: If $\mathbf{u} = (u_x, u_y, u_z)^{\mathrm{T}}$ is a given axis, and θ is a given angle, we set $c = \cos\theta$ and $s = \sin\theta$.
Then the 3×3 matrix

$$\mathbf{R} = \begin{pmatrix} c + u_x^2(1-c) & u_x u_y(1-c) - u_z s & u_x u_z(1-c) + u_y s \\ u_y u_x(1-c) + u_z s & c + u_y^2(1-c) & u_y u_z(1-c) - u_x s \\ u_z u_x(1-c) - u_y s & u_z u_y(1-c) + u_x s & c + u_z^2(1-c) \end{pmatrix} \tag{2.48}$$

describes a rotation about $\mathbf{u}$ by θ. Given a quaternion $\mathbf{q}$, extract the axis $\mathbf{u}$ and the angle θ, and insert into the definition for $\mathbf{R}$.
c) Derive a conversion from a 3×3 rotation matrix to a quaternion. Hint: Start from the equation

$$\begin{pmatrix} n_x & o_x & a_x \\ n_y & o_y & a_y \\ n_z & o_z & a_z \end{pmatrix} = \mathbf{R} \tag{2.49}$$

where $\mathbf{R}$ is the angle-axis matrix defined in Eq. 2.48.
Solve this matrix equation for the angle θ in $c = \cos\theta$ and $s = \sin\theta$, and then for the axis $(u_x, u_y, u_z)^{\mathrm{T}}$.

Exercise 2.8 ***Six-joint robot***

a) The robot in Fig. 2.17 is very similar to the three-joint robot in Fig. 2.13, and also has three revolute joints. The only difference

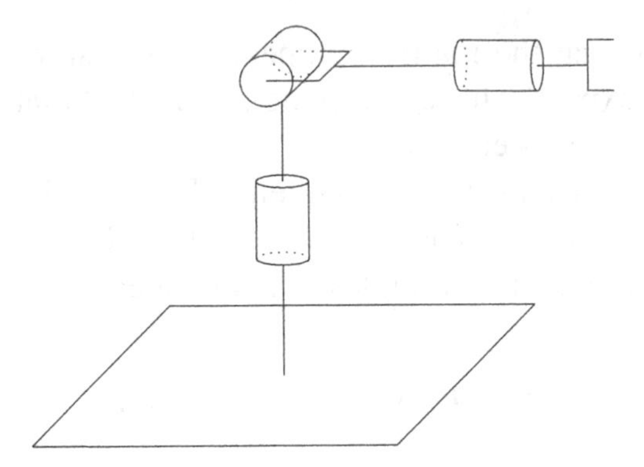

Fig. 2.17: Variant of the three-joint robot in Fig. 2.13

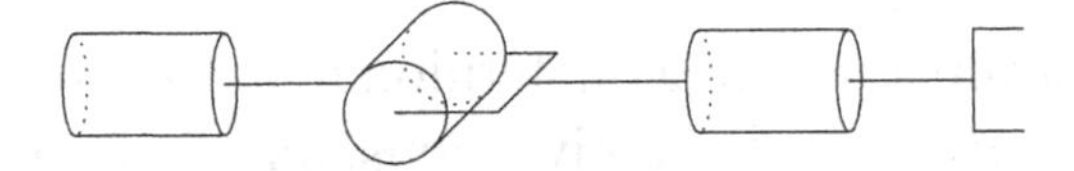

Fig. 2.18: Hand assembly with three revolute joints

is that the last joint has a different axis of rotation. Set up the coordinate systems and the DH-matrix for this robot.

b) Replace the gripper of the elbow manipulator in Fig. 2.13 by a tool flange, i.e. a disk for mounting tools. Assume now a small copy of the robot in Fig. 2.17 was mounted to this tool flange. This results in a six-joint robot. This six-joint robot has the mechanical structure of standard commercial robots (KUKA, Mitsubishi, Kawasaki, GM Fanuc, Adept and Stäubli robots). The transformation matrix expressing the position of the full six joint robot can now be obtained in a very simple way. We simply multiply the two transformation matrices. Set up this matrix for the six-joint robot and verify your result for a small set of angles.

c) The robot in Fig. 2.18 is the wrist of the six-joint robot in b). The three joint axes of the wrist intersect in a single point **q**. The tool center point (TCP) is the center of the gripper. As we move the joints of the wrist, we see that the TCP remains on a sphere. For this reason, we call this wrist a spherical wrist. Following the YPR-convention for angles, joints 1 and 3 of the wrist will be called roll-joints (*R*-joints) and joint 2 is called a pitch joint

(P-joint). Thus the wrist has an $R-P-R$ structure. Discuss the alternatives for three-joint wrists with intersecting axes, following this $R-P$ alphabet.

Exercise 2.9 ***Kinematics of the Neurosurgical Frame***

Derive the forward equation (Eq. 1.3) for the neurosurgical frame in Fig. 1.13.

Summary

A homogeneous 4×4 matrix describes the position and orientation of a coordinate system S with respect to the base system B.
According to the YPR-convention, the position and orientation of S with respect to B is represented by a 6-tuple (Eq. 2.6).
To analyze linkages and jointed mechanisms, we distinguish between forward and inverse kinematics. Forward kinematic analysis is the process of finding the matrix, depending on the joint angle values, which describes the position of the gripper. Inverse kinematics finds the joint angles for a given position and orientation. Inverse kinematics typically requires a forward analysis. Stated in simpler terms (with the notation in Fig. 2.16), forward kinematics finds the position and orientation of the effector, given the joint angles, while inverse kinematics finds the joint angles given the target position and orientation.
For the kinematic analysis of a single-joint robot, we introduced three coordinate systems, namely the base system, gripper system and an intermediate system. The coordinate systems thus form a chain. We assign a matrix to each pair of consecutive systems in this chain. Then the product matrix gives the transformation from the base to the gripper. The analysis is very similar for robots with several joints.
The atan2-function is an extension of the arctan function. It takes two arguments and implements the inverse kinematics for a robot with a single revolute joint. More complex robots can be analyzed with this function as well, again on the basis of a forward analysis. Furthermore, the atan2-function is a general tool for solving kinematic equations.

Quaternions are 4-vectors. To add two quaternions, we simply add their components. The multiplication of two quaternions resembles the cross-product for 3-vectors. Quaternion multiplication is not commutative. The rotation defined by a quaternion is derived from Eq. 2.42 and Eq. 2.43. If $\mathbf{a} = [a_1, a_2, a_3, a_4]^{\mathrm{T}}$ is a quaternion, then the first element a_1 describes the angle of rotation, while $[a_2, a_3, a_4]^{\mathrm{T}}$ describe the axis. To convert from a (unit) quaternion to a 3×3-rotation matrix, we must set up a rotation matrix given an angle and an axis (Exercise 2.7b). The reverse direction of the conversion consists of extracting an angle and an axis from a rotation matrix (Exercise 2.7c).

Notes

The DH-convention in the form discussed above is also called the *standard* DH-convention (see also [2, 4–6]). The text book by John Craig [3] uses a modified version, referred to as the *modified* DH-notation. Given an unknown DH-table, you should make sure to find out which of the two conventions it refers to.

References

[1] S. L. Altmann. *Rotations, Quaternions, and Double Groups.* Dover Publications, dover publications 2005 edition, 1986.
[2] P. Corke. *Robotics, Vision and Control: Fundamental Algorithms in MATLAB*, volume 73 of *Springer Tracts in Advanced Robotics*. Springer Science, New York, Berlin, Heidelberg, 2011.
[3] J. J. Craig. *Introduction to Robotics: Mechanics and Control.* Prentice Hall, 3rd edition, 2005.
[4] J. Denavit and R. S. Hartenberg. A kinematic notation for lower-pair mechanisms based on matrices. *Transactions of the ASME: Journal of Applied Mechanics*, **22**(2):215–221, 1955.

[5] B. Siciliano, L. Sciavicco, L. Villani, and G. Oriolo. *Robotics: Modelling, Planning and Control.* Advanced Textbooks in Control and Signal Processing. Springer, New York, Berlin, Heidelberg, 2009.
[6] M. W. Spong, S. Hutchinson, and M. Vidyasagar. *Robot Modeling and Control.* John Wiley & Sons, Inc., New York, 1st edition, 2005.

Chapter 3
Robot Kinematics

We saw that forward kinematics gives us the position (and orientation) of the gripper, when we have the joint angles. Inverse kinematics does the opposite, namely, we get the joint angles for reaching a given position. In this chapter, we will discuss inverse kinematics. The kernel of this chapter is the closed-form inverse analysis of a seven-joint robot, called the DLR-Kuka robot. To prepare this analysis, we will first analyze a six-joint robot. At the end of the chapter, we will derive the inverse kinematics for a C-arm.
We start with a simple example, namely the three-joint robot from Chap. 2. This example shows how we can get from the forward analysis to the inverse analysis, and illustrates some basic methods.

3.1 Three-Joint Robot

We start from the forward matrix ${}^0\mathbf{M}_G$ of the three-joint robot in Eq. 2.27. We set up the matrix product ${}^0\mathbf{M}_G$ from the matrices derived in Eqs. 2.20–2.23.

$$ {}^0\mathbf{M}_G = {}^0\mathbf{M}_1 \cdot {}^1\mathbf{M}_2 \cdot {}^2\mathbf{M}_3 \cdot {}^3\mathbf{M}_G = \begin{pmatrix} n_x & o_x & a_x & p_x \\ n_y & o_y & a_y & p_y \\ n_z & o_z & a_z & p_z \\ 0 & 0 & 0 & 1 \end{pmatrix} = \mathbf{T} \qquad (3.1) $$

A. Schweikard, F. Ernst, *Medical Robotics*,
DOI 10.1007/978-3-319-22891-4_3

Here, the matrix on the right hand side is the target matrix, and we denote it by **T** for short. Evaluating the matrix expression ${}^0\mathbf{M}_1 \cdot {}^1\mathbf{M}_2 \cdot {}^2\mathbf{M}_3 \cdot {}^3\mathbf{M}_G$, we must solve the equation

$$\begin{pmatrix} c_1c_{23} & -s_1 & c_1s_{23} & a_2c_1c_2 + d_4c_1s_{23} \\ s_1c_{23} & c_1 & s_1s_{23} & a_2s_1c_2 + d_4s_1s_{23} \\ -s_{23} & 0 & c_{23} & -a_2s_2 + d_4c_{23} \\ 0 & 0 & 0 & 1 \end{pmatrix} = \begin{pmatrix} n_x & o_x & a_x & p_x \\ n_y & o_y & a_y & p_y \\ n_z & o_z & a_z & p_z \\ 0 & 0 & 0 & 1 \end{pmatrix} \tag{3.2}$$

Recall also that we set $c_i = \cos\theta_i$, $s_i = \sin\theta_i$, $c_{ij} = \cos(\theta_i + \theta_j)$ and $s_{ij} = \sin(\theta_i + \theta_j)$, so that the above matrix equation becomes an equation in the variables θ_i. Our goal is to solve for these variables, given constants for the values $n_x, ..., p_z$ on the right side.
To solve this equation, first note that we can directly solve for θ_1. From the second entry of the first matrix line, we obtain

$$-s_1 = o_x \tag{3.3}$$

From the second entry of the second matrix line, we obtain

$$c_1 = o_y \tag{3.4}$$

Again, we use our function *atan*2, which we have already applied in several examples and exercises in Chap. 2.
Set

$$\theta_1 = \text{atan2}(-o_x, o_y) \tag{3.5}$$

Once we have solved for θ_1, the value for θ_1 becomes a constant. There is an easy way to move θ_1 from the left side of the equation to the right side. We multiply both sides of the matrix equation with the matrix ${}^0\mathbf{M}_1^{-1}$ (see Eq. 2.20). This ensures that all variables are on the left side, and the matrix on the left side is simplified considerably. To further simplify the expressions, we remove the constant matrix ${}^3\mathbf{M}_G^{-1}$ from the left side of the equation.
We thus transform the equation from which we started (see Eq. 3.1)

$${}^0\mathbf{M}_1 \cdot {}^1\mathbf{M}_2 \cdot {}^2\mathbf{M}_3 \cdot {}^3\mathbf{M}_G = \mathbf{T} \tag{3.6}$$

into

$$^1\mathbf{M}_2 \cdot {}^2\mathbf{M}_3 = {}^0\mathbf{M}_1^{-1}\mathbf{T} \cdot {}^3\mathbf{M}_G^{-1}. \tag{3.7}$$

We have

$$^3\mathbf{M}_G^{-1} = \begin{pmatrix} 1 & 0 & 0 & 0 \\ 0 & 1 & 0 & 0 \\ 0 & 0 & 1 & -d_4 \\ 0 & 0 & 0 & 1 \end{pmatrix} \tag{3.8}$$

and

$$\mathbf{T} \cdot {}^3\mathbf{M}_G^{-1} = \begin{pmatrix} n_x & o_x & a_x & -a_x d_4 + p_x \\ n_y & o_y & a_y & -a_y d_4 + p_y \\ n_z & o_z & a_z & -a_z d_4 + p_z \\ 0 & 0 & 0 & 1 \end{pmatrix} \tag{3.9}$$

and set

$$\begin{pmatrix} n_x & o_x & a_x & -a_x d_4 + p_x \\ n_y & o_y & a_y & -a_y d_4 + p_y \\ n_z & o_z & a_z & -a_z d_4 + p_z \\ 0 & 0 & 0 & 1 \end{pmatrix} = \begin{pmatrix} n_x & o_x & a_x & p'_x \\ n_y & o_y & a_y & p'_y \\ n_z & o_z & a_z & p'_z \\ 0 & 0 & 0 & 1 \end{pmatrix} = \mathbf{T}'. \tag{3.10}$$

Now

$$^0\mathbf{M}_1^{-1} \cdot \mathbf{T} \cdot {}^3\mathbf{M}_G^{-1} = {}^0\mathbf{M}_1^{-1} \cdot \mathbf{T}' =$$

$$\begin{pmatrix} n_x c_1 + n_y s_1 & o_x c_1 + o_y s_1 & a_x c_1 + a_y s_1 & p'_x c_1 + p'_y s_1 \\ -n_z & -o_z & -a_z & -p'_z \\ -n_x s_1 + n_y c_1 & -o_x s_1 + o_y c_1 & -a_x s_1 + a_y c_1 & -p'_x s_1 + p'_y c_1 \\ 0 & 0 & 0 & 1 \end{pmatrix} \tag{3.11}$$

We evaluate the matrix $^1\mathbf{M}_2 \cdot {}^2\mathbf{M}_3$ on the left side to

$$^1\mathbf{M}_2 \cdot {}^2\mathbf{M}_3 = \begin{pmatrix} c_{23} & 0 & s_{23} & a_2 c_2 \\ s_{23} & 0 & -c_{23} & a_2 s_2 \\ 0 & 1 & 0 & 0 \\ 0 & 0 & 0 & 1 \end{pmatrix} \tag{3.12}$$

We thus have all the ingredients of Eq. 3.7, i.e. we have evaluated both sides of this equation.
From the last column of this equation, we obtain

$$\begin{aligned} a_2 s_2 &= -p'_z \\ a_2 c_2 &= p'_x c_1 + p'_y s_1 \end{aligned} \tag{3.13}$$

Thus

$$\theta_2 = \text{atan2}\left(\frac{-p'_z}{a_2}, \frac{p'_x c_1 + p'_y s_1}{a_2}\right), \tag{3.14}$$

where

$$\begin{aligned} p'_x &= -a_x d_4 + p_x, \\ p'_y &= -a_y d_4 + p_y, \\ p'_z &= -a_z d_4 + p_z. \end{aligned} \tag{3.15}$$

Finally, from the matrix equation 3.2, we have

$$\begin{aligned} \cos(\theta_2 + \theta_3) &= a_z \\ \sin(\theta_2 + \theta_3) &= -n_z \end{aligned} \tag{3.16}$$

so that

$$\theta_3 = \text{atan2}(-n_z, a_z) - \theta_2 \tag{3.17}$$

This completes our inverse analysis of the three-joint robot.
Before we look into the analysis of more complex robots, we briefly summarize the overall procedure in the analysis of our three-joint robot for future reference: we first set up the forward matrix equation. In this equation, we found a pair of equations of the form $s_i = u$, and $c_i = v$, with constants u, v. We solved for the i-th joint angle on the basis of the atan2-function. Then we moved the matrix ${}^{i-1}\mathbf{M}_i$ to the right-hand side of the equation, since it no longer contained any unsolved variables. To find an initial pair of equations (of the form $s_i = u$, and $c_i = v$), we could be somewhat more systematic. We could

generate several matrix equations by moving matrices to the right side, while looking for appropriate pairs of equations. We will call this simple technique equation-searching.
In the next section, we will analyze a six-joint robot. We will see that this robot can be regarded as an assembly of two three-joint robots in our analysis, i.e. we can decouple the analysis for joints 1–3 and joints 4–6.

3.2 Six-Joint Robot

Figure 3.1 shows a six-joint robot. This six-joint robot can be obtained by assembling two three-joint robots. If we take a closer look at the kinematic structure, we see that the base (first three joints) is identical to the three-joint elbow manipulator discussed above. We mount a spherical wrist (with three joints) to the base. Figure 3.2 shows the resulting kinematic structure, an elbow manipulator with spherical wrist (see also Exercise 2.8).

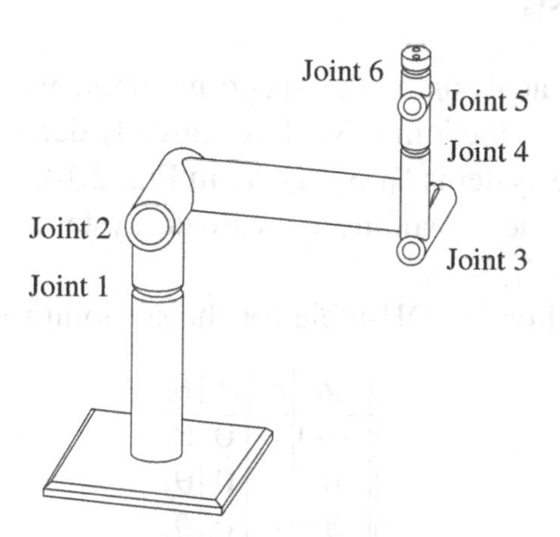

Fig. 3.1: Six-joint robot

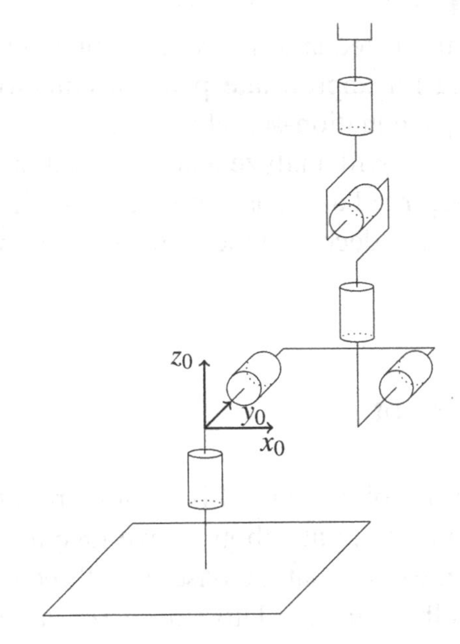

Fig. 3.2: Joint axes for the six-joint robot

Forward Analysis

For the forward analysis of the six-joint robot, we must assign coordinate systems to the joints. We have already derived the placement of the coordinate systems S_0, S_1, S_2, S_3 in Fig. 2.14.
Figure 3.3 adds the remaining coordinate systems for the hand assembly (systems S_4, S_5, S_6).
We obtain the following DH-table for the six-joint robot.

i	α_i	a_i	d_i	θ_i
1	-90	0	0	θ_1
2	0	a_2	0	θ_2
3	90	0	0	θ_3
4	-90	0	d_4	θ_4
5	90	0	0	θ_5
6	0	0	d_6	θ_6

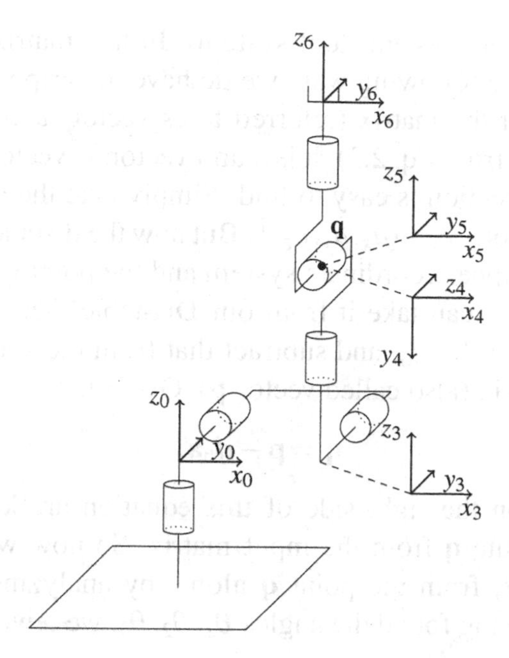

Fig. 3.3: Coordinate systems for the hand assembly of the six-joint robot

Since the hand assembly is also a (small) three joint robot, its analysis should be simple. But can we decouple the kinematic analysis of the two robots thus glued together? It is remarkable that this is indeed possible.
The main idea for the inverse analysis is the following.
We have the target coordinate system S_6 at the end of the hand assembly (Fig. 3.3). We look at the z-vector of S_6. Now revert the direction of this vector, to point into the opposite direction. We follow this opposite direction until we reach the intersection point between the axes of joints five and six. Call this intersection point $\mathbf{q}$, the wrist center. $\mathbf{q}$ is also the origin of the coordinate systems S_4 and S_5 (see Fig. 3.3). Taking a second look at the kinematics of our robot, we see that the axes for the last three joints intersect in one point. Thus $\mathbf{q}$ will not move, when we move any of the axes four, five or six. This means that the position of $\mathbf{q}$ only depends on the joints one, two and three. It is important to note that the inverse analysis takes a homogeneous 4×4-matrix as an input, which gives the position and orientation of

the last coordinate system (tool system). In this matrix, we can find the point **q** in the following way: we do have the gripper's z-vector in column three of the matrix (referred to as vector $(a_x, a_y, a_z)^{\mathrm{T}}$) in the matrix notation from Eq. 2.3). It is a unit vector. A vector pointing into the opposite direction is easy to find. Simply take the negative of the gripper's z-vector, i.e. $-(a_x, a_y, a_z)^{\mathrm{T}}$. But now the distance between the origin of the gripper coordinate system and the point **q** is a kinematic constant, and we can take it from our DH-table! Thus, multiply the gripper's z-vector by d_6, and subtract that from the vector in column four of the matrix (also called vector **p**). Overall,

$$\mathbf{q} = \mathbf{p} - d_6\mathbf{a}. \tag{3.18}$$

All elements on the right side of this equation are known, and we can thus compute **q** from the input matrix. So now we can find the angles $\theta_1, \theta_2, \theta_3$ from the point **q** alone, by analyzing a three-joint robot. After having found the angles $\theta_1, \theta_2, \theta_3$, we rewrite the forward matrix equation

$${}^{0}\mathbf{M}_1 \cdots {}^{5}\mathbf{M}_6 = \begin{pmatrix} n_x & o_x & a_x & p_x \\ n_y & o_y & a_y & p_y \\ n_z & o_z & a_z & p_z \\ 0 & 0 & 0 & 1 \end{pmatrix} \tag{3.19}$$

to

$${}^{3}\mathbf{M}_4 \cdot {}^{4}\mathbf{M}_5 \cdot {}^{5}\mathbf{M}_6 = {}^{2}\mathbf{M}_3^{-1} \cdot {}^{1}\mathbf{M}_2^{-1} \cdot {}^{0}\mathbf{M}_1^{-1} \begin{pmatrix} n_x & o_x & a_x & p_x \\ n_y & o_y & a_y & p_y \\ n_z & o_z & a_z & p_z \\ 0 & 0 & 0 & 1 \end{pmatrix} \tag{3.20}$$

This again is the kinematic equation for a three-joint robot (since everything on the right hand side is now constant), and we have already solved variants of such equations before.
This is the basic idea for solving the six-joint robot. However, some subtleties are easy to overlook here: When we analyzed the three-joint robot above, we had a full gripper matrix to start from. Now we only have a single point, namely **q**. This will cause trouble, and we shall see that we must work through the three-joint solution again, to adjust to the new situation. The new solution will be much more detailed, and will address the case of multiple solutions.

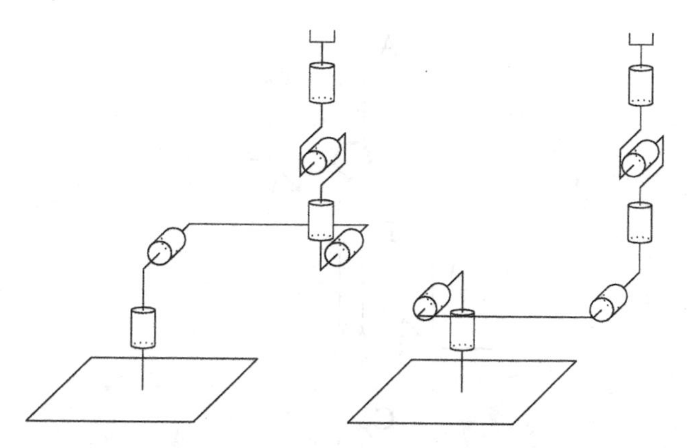

Fig. 3.4: Left-shoulder and right-shoulder configurations of the robot. The position of the tool flange with respect to the base plate is the same in both cases

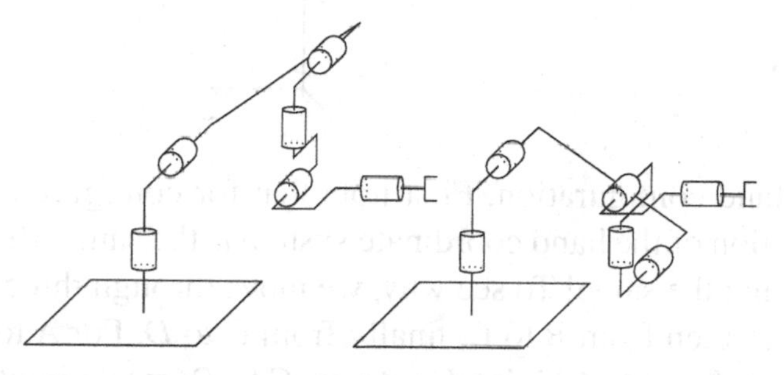

Fig. 3.5: Elbow-up and elbow-down configuration of the robot. In both cases, the robot is in left-shoulder configuration

Specifically, look at the so-called left-shoulder and right-shoulder configurations shown in Fig. 3.4.
Figure 3.5 shows two distinct configurations of the robot, where again the resulting tool position is the same. We will call the configurations in Fig. 3.5 the Elbow-up and the Elbow-down configurations.
We can now combine the elbow-configurations and the shoulder-configurations, and obtain four distinct ways for reaching a given fixed tool placement. They are: (left, up), (left, down), (right, up), (right, down). Similar to the configuration of the shoulder, we can configure

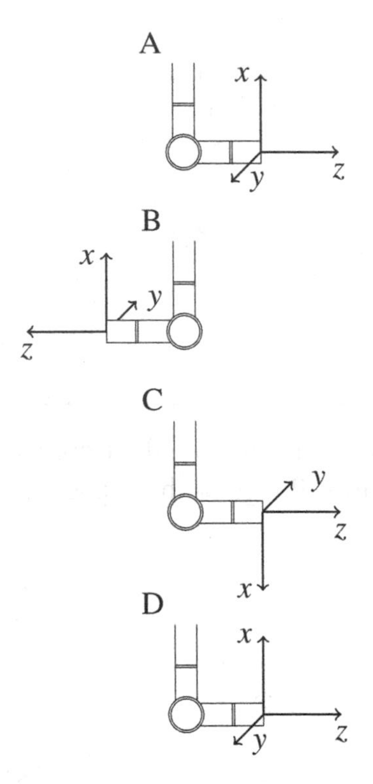

Fig. 3.6: Hand configuration. First note that for configurations A and D, the position of the hand coordinate system is the same. But the joint angles are not the same! To see why, we move through three steps, i.e. from A to B, then from B to C, finally from C to D. For A to B: rotate joint J_4 by 180°. B to C: joint J_5 rotates. C to D: rotate joint J_6, again by 180°. Hence joints four five and six have all taken new values

the hand of the robot. Thus, we can flip the hand, if we rotate joints four, five and six appropriately (Fig. 3.6).
Overall, we have three configuration parameters for the robot:

- Shoulder: (right, left) = (1,−1)
- Elbow: (up, down) = (1,−1)
- Hand: (noflip, flip) = (1,−1)

The configuration parameters are input parameters for our solution, i.e. the user must specify the desired configuration in advance. Since we have three parameters, we obtain $2^3 = 8$ distinct configurations.
As noted above, the solution for the six-joint robot proceeds in two steps. First we solve for the angles $\theta_1, \theta_2, \theta_3$. Our sole input at this stage will be the point $\mathbf{q}$ and the desired configuration. Notice that this kinematic problem is slightly different from our above solution for the three-joint robot (see Example 3.1), where our input was a target 4×4-matrix. Having found $\theta_1, \theta_2, \theta_3$, we will then solve for the remaining parameters via Eq. 3.20.
From Eq. 3.2 we see that $\mathbf{q}$ has the coordinates

$$\mathbf{q} = \begin{pmatrix} q_x \\ q_y \\ q_z \end{pmatrix} = \begin{pmatrix} a_2 c_1 c_2 + d_4 c_1 s_{23} \\ a_2 s_1 c_2 + d_4 s_1 s_{23} \\ -a_2 s_2 + d_4 c_{23} \end{pmatrix}. \tag{3.21}$$

But we have a second equation for $\mathbf{q}$, given our target position as a homogeneous 4×4 matrix $\mathbf{T}$. Given $\mathbf{T}$, we can take the two vectors $\mathbf{p}$ and $\mathbf{a}$ from this matrix, and apply Eq. 3.18, i.e. $\mathbf{q} = \mathbf{p} - d_6\mathbf{a}$. Recall that d_6 is a kinematic constant from the DH-table. Overall we have:

$$\mathbf{p} - d_6\mathbf{a} = \begin{pmatrix} a_2 c_1 c_2 + d_4 c_1 s_{23} \\ a_2 s_1 c_2 + d_4 s_1 s_{23} \\ -a_2 s_2 + d_4 c_{23} \end{pmatrix} \tag{3.22}$$

Our next goal will thus be to extract $\theta_1, \theta_2, \theta_3$ from Eq. 3.22.

Solving for θ_1

Our solution for θ_1 is very simple, and we can apply the same technique as for the one-joint robot in Chap. 2. We look at the robot from above (Fig. 3.7).
Figure 3.8 further illustrates the situation. Projecting the entire configuration onto the plane of the robot's base plate (x-y-plane), we see that the angle θ_1 can be taken from the position of the point $\mathbf{q}$ directly.

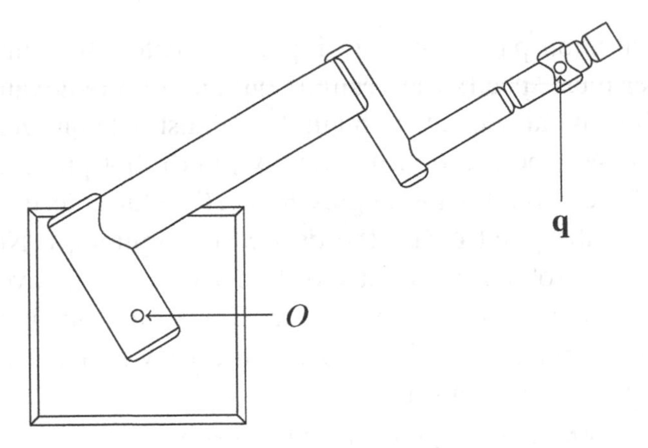

Fig. 3.7: Solving for angle θ_1. The origin of the base system (O) and $\mathbf{q}$ are marked

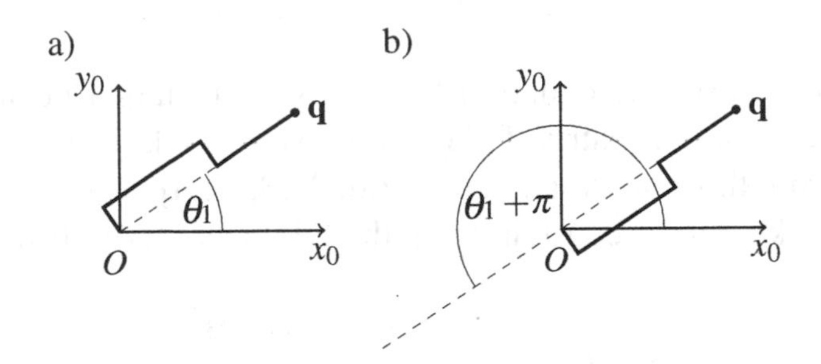

Fig. 3.8: Solutions for the angle θ_1. The robot has several ways for reaching the given point $\mathbf{q}$. Figure (**a**) shows the so-called left-shoulder configuration. To reach the right shoulder configuration (**b**) we move the first joint to the angle $\theta_1 + \pi$, and then flip the second joint

After projecting $\mathbf{q}$ onto the x-y-plane, we see that θ_1 can be computed as

$$\theta_1 = \text{atan2}(q_y, q_x) \tag{3.23}$$

Equation 3.23 refers to one possible solution for θ_1. We can obtain a second solution by changing the configuration of the shoulder (see Fig. 3.8). The process of moving from a left-shoulder configuration to a right-shoulder configuration resembles the process of flipping the hand, illustrated in Fig. 3.6. The second solution for θ_1 is given by

$$\theta_1 = \text{atan2}(q_y, q_x) + \pi. \tag{3.24}$$

From the definition of the atan2-function, we see that

$$\text{atan2}(q_y, q_x) + \pi = \text{atan2}(-q_y, -q_x). \tag{3.25}$$

We will next solve for θ_3 rather than for θ_2, since this will simplify the solution path.

Solving for θ_3

We take a step back and look at the robot. In Fig. 3.9 we see that the distance between $\mathbf{q}$ and the origin of the base system should only depend on the angle θ_3, but not on the joint angles θ_1 and θ_2.

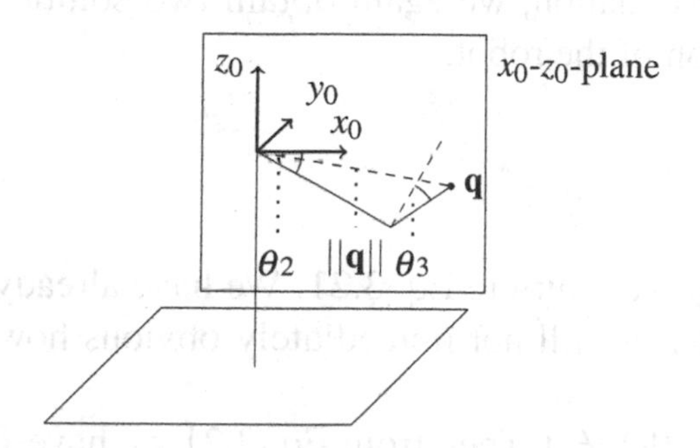

Fig. 3.9: Solving for angle θ_3. The distance $\|\mathbf{q}\|$ between the origin of the base system and the point $\mathbf{q}$ only depends on θ_3

We take the square of the norm on both sides of Eq. 3.21, and obtain:

$$\begin{aligned}\|\mathbf{q}\|^2 = q_x^2 + q_y^2 + q_z^2 = \\ (a_2c_1c_2 + d_4c_1s_{23})^2 + \\ (a_2s_1c_2 + d_4s_1s_{23})^2 + \\ (-a_2s_2 + d_4c_{23})^2\end{aligned} \tag{3.26}$$

With $\sin^2\alpha + \cos^2\alpha = 1$, the right hand side simplifies to

$$a_2^2 + d_4^2 + 2a_2d_4(c_2s_{23} - s_2c_{23}). \tag{3.27}$$

But this expression reduces to

$$a_2^2 + d_4^2 + 2a_2d_4s_3., \tag{3.28}$$

and we see that θ_2 has vanished from the expression. Thus, indeed (as expected from the figure) our distance expression only depends on θ_3.
Now

$$\begin{aligned} s_3 &= \frac{\|\mathbf{q}\|^2 - a_2^2 - d_4^2}{2a_2d_4}, \\ c_3 &= \pm\sqrt{1-s_3^2}, \\ \theta_3 &= \operatorname{atan2}(s_3, c_3). \end{aligned} \tag{3.29}$$

From the latter equation, we again obtain two solutions, controlling the configuration of the robot.

Solving for θ_2

To solve for θ_2, we return to Eq. 3.21. We have already solved for θ_1 and for θ_3, but it is still not immediately obvious how to isolate the angle θ_2.
We assume $\cos(\theta_1) \neq 0$. Then from Eq. 3.21 we have

$$\begin{aligned} x &= a_2\cos(\theta_2) + d_4\sin(\theta_2+\theta_3), \\ z &= -a_2\sin(\theta_2) + d_4\cos(\theta_2+\theta_3) \end{aligned} \tag{3.30}$$

where $x = q_x/\cos(\theta_1)$ and $z = q_z$.
In case $\cos(\theta_1) = 0$, we can base the argument which will follow on

$$\begin{aligned} y &= a_2\cos(\theta_2) + d_4\sin(\theta_2+\theta_3), \\ z &= -a_2\sin(\theta_2) + d_4\cos(\theta_2+\theta_3) \end{aligned} \tag{3.31}$$

with $y = q_y/\sin(\theta_1)$.

Furthermore, we set

$$\begin{aligned} u &= a_2 + d_4 s_3, \\ v &= d_4 c_3. \end{aligned} \tag{3.32}$$

Then we have

$$\begin{aligned} x &= u\cos(\theta_2) + v\sin(\theta_2), \\ z &= -u\sin(\theta_2) + v\cos(\theta_2). \end{aligned} \tag{3.33}$$

You may wish to check Eq. 3.33 by inserting the definitions for u, v above into Eq. 3.33. The result should lead back to Eq. 3.30 via the trigonometric addition formulas.
Now we set

$$r = \sqrt{u^2 + v^2}. \tag{3.34}$$

For $r \neq 0$ we set

$$\gamma = \text{atan2}(u/r, v/r). \tag{3.35}$$

Notice from the definition of the atan2-function ,

$$\gamma = \text{atan2}(u, v). \tag{3.36}$$

Then (again if $r \neq 0$)

$$\begin{aligned} u/r &= \sin(\gamma), \\ v/r &= \cos(\gamma) \end{aligned} \tag{3.37}$$

and thus

$$\begin{aligned} x &= r\sin(\gamma)c_2 + r\cos(\gamma)s_2, \\ z &= -r\sin(\gamma)s_2 + r\cos(\gamma)c_2. \end{aligned} \tag{3.38}$$

By the trigonometric addition formulas this is the same as

$$\begin{aligned} x &= r\sin(\gamma + \theta_2), \\ z &= r\cos(\gamma + \theta_2). \end{aligned} \tag{3.39}$$

Now we have

$$x/r = \sin(\gamma + \theta_2),$$
$$z/r = \cos(\gamma + \theta_2) \tag{3.40}$$

or

$$\gamma + \theta_2 = \text{atan2}(x/r, z/r). \tag{3.41}$$

From this, we see that

$$\theta_2 = \text{atan2}(x/r, z/r) - \gamma \tag{3.42}$$

By the definition of γ, and the definition of the atan2-function, the latter equation reduces to

$$\theta_2 = \text{atan2}(x, z) - \text{atan2}(u, v). \tag{3.43}$$

Remark 3.1

A small detail has been overlooked in our derivation for θ_2. We must be sure that the value r defined in Eq. 3.34 is not zero, since we later divide by this value. A detailed discussion shows that r can only be zero if $a_2 = d_4$ and $\sin(\theta_3) = 0$. This is equivalent to $\mathbf{q}$ coinciding with the origin, which is mechanically impossible for robots with $a_2 \neq d_4$. (See also Exercise 4 at the end of this chapter.)

(End of Remark 3.1)

Remark 3.2

For both θ_1 and θ_3 we each have two solutions. This gives rise to a total of four solutions, which correspond to the four configurations of the robot obtained by choosing values ± 1 for each of the two variables shoulder and elbow.
For θ_2, we have a single solution, which will depend on the configurations chosen via θ_1 and θ_3.

(End of Remark 3.2)

In summary, we obtain the following values for θ_1, θ_2 and θ_3.

$$\theta_1 = \text{atan2}(\text{shoulder} \cdot q_y, \text{shoulder} \cdot q_x) \tag{3.44}$$

If $\cos(\theta_1) \neq 0$

$$\begin{aligned} \theta_2 = {} & \text{atan2}(-\text{shoulder} \cdot \text{elbow} \cdot q_x / \cos(\theta_1), -\text{shoulder} \cdot \text{elbow} \cdot q_z) \\ & - \text{atan2}(-\text{shoulder} \cdot \text{elbow} \cdot u, -\text{shoulder} \cdot \text{elbow} \cdot v) \end{aligned} \tag{3.45}$$

else

$$\begin{aligned} \theta_2 = {} & \text{atan2}(-\text{shoulder} \cdot \text{elbow} \cdot q_y / \sin(\theta_1), -\text{shoulder} \cdot \text{elbow} \cdot q_z) \\ & - \text{atan2}(-\text{shoulder} \cdot \text{elbow} \cdot u, -\text{shoulder} \cdot \text{elbow} \cdot v) \end{aligned} \tag{3.46}$$

where

$$u = a_2 + d_4 s_3 \tag{3.47}$$

and

$$v = d_4 c_3. \tag{3.48}$$

Then

$$s_3 = \frac{||\mathbf{q}||^2 - a_2^2 - d_4^2}{2 a_2 d_4} \tag{3.49}$$

and

$$\theta_3 = \text{atan2}(s_3, -\text{shoulder} \cdot \text{elbow} \cdot \sqrt{1 - s_3^2}). \tag{3.50}$$

We must now solve for the remaining angles θ_4, θ_5 and θ_6. As we shall see, this is much simpler than the case of θ_1, θ_2 and θ_3. All we need here is the technique which we called equation-searching.

Solving for θ_4, θ_5 and θ_6

We start from Eq. 3.20. We rewrite this equation in a shorter form to

$${}^3\mathbf{M}_6 = {}^0\mathbf{M}_3^{-1} \cdot \mathbf{T}. \tag{3.51}$$

Here again, **T** denotes our target matrix as in Eq. 3.1, i.e.

$$\mathbf{T} = \begin{pmatrix} n_x & o_x & a_x & p_x \\ n_y & o_y & a_y & p_y \\ n_z & o_z & a_z & p_z \\ 0 & 0 & 0 & 1 \end{pmatrix}. \tag{3.52}$$

Let **M** denote the matrix on the right hand side of Eq. 3.51. Notice that we can now assume that **M** is constant, since the angles $\theta_1, \theta_2, \theta_3$ are the only variables on the right hand side of Eq. 3.51, and we have already solved for these variables.
We evaluate both sides of Eq. 3.51, by multiplying the matrices.
First, we must compute ${}^3\mathbf{M}_6$:

$${}^3\mathbf{M}_6 = \begin{pmatrix} c_4c_5c_6 - s_4s_6 & -c_4c_5s_6 - s_4c_6 & c_4s_5 & d_6c_4s_5 \\ s_4c_5c_6 + c_4s_6 & -s_4c_5s_6 + c_4c_6 & s_4s_5 & d_6s_4s_5 \\ -s_5c_6 & s_5s_6 & c_5 & d_4 + d_6c_5 \\ 0 & 0 & 0 & 1 \end{pmatrix}. \tag{3.53}$$

Next, we compute ${}^0\mathbf{M}_3^{-1}$:

$${}^0\mathbf{M}_3^{-1} = \begin{pmatrix} c_{23}c_1 & c_{23}s_1 & -s_{23} & -a_2c_3 \\ -s_1 & c_1 & 0 & 0 \\ s_{23}c_1 & s_{23}s_1 & c_{23} & -a_2s_3 \\ 0 & 0 & 0 & 1 \end{pmatrix} \tag{3.54}$$

Finally, we obtain the first and second columns of ${}^0\mathbf{M}_3^{-1}\mathbf{T}$ as follows:

$$\begin{matrix} n_xc_{23}c_1 + n_yc_{23}s_1 - n_zs_{23} & o_xc_{23}c_1 + o_yc_{23}s_1 - o_zs_{23} \\ -n_xs_1 + n_yc_1 & -o_xs_1 + o_yc_1 \\ n_xs_{23}c_1 + n_ys_{23}s_1 + n_zc_{23} & o_xs_{23}c_1 + o_ys_{23}s_1 + o_zc_{23} \\ 0 & 0 \end{matrix} \tag{3.55}$$

Columns three and four of the product ${}^0\mathbf{M}_3^{-1}\mathbf{T}$ are:

$$\begin{array}{cc} a_x c_{23} c_1 + a_y c_{23} s_1 - a_z s_{23} & p_x c_{23} c_1 + p_y c_{23} s_1 - p_z s_{23} - a_2 c_3 \\ -a_x s_1 + a_y c_1 & -p_x s_1 + p_y c_1 \\ a_x s_{23} c_1 + a_y s_{23} s_1 + a_z c_{23} & p_x s_{23} c_1 + p_y s_{23} s_1 + p_z c_{23} - a_2 s_3 \\ 0 & 1 \end{array} \quad (3.56)$$

Looking at Eq. 3.53, we see that we have an equation for c_5 from the element (3,3) of this matrix. Specifically,

$$c_5 = a_x s_{23} c_1 + a_y s_{23} s_1 + a_z c_{23}. \quad (3.57)$$

For any angle θ, we have $\sin^2\theta + \cos^2\theta = 1$. Thus

$$\sin\theta_5 = \pm\sqrt{1-\cos^2\theta_5}, \quad (3.58)$$

and we again apply the atan2-function.
Set

$$v = a_x s_{23} c_1 + a_y s_{23} s_1 + a_z c_{23} \quad (3.59)$$

and

$$u = \pm\sqrt{1-v^2}. \quad (3.60)$$

Given the $\pm$-sign in Eq. 3.60, we have two solutions:

$$\theta_5 = \text{atan2}(\text{hand} \cdot u, v) \quad (3.61)$$

Here the parameter 'hand' represents the two solutions of Eq. 3.58, and the two possible configurations of the hand (see Fig. 3.6). As for the values 'shoulder' and 'elbow', 'hand' is an input value, to be specified by the user.
We return to Eq. 3.51.
We compare the elements (3,1) and (3,2) in this matrix equation, and conclude that

$$\begin{aligned} c_4 s_5 &= m_{13}, \\ s_4 s_5 &= m_{23}; \end{aligned} \quad (3.62)$$

or (assuming $s_5 \neq 0$), that

$$\begin{aligned} c_4 &= m_{13}/s_5, \\ s_4 &= m_{23}/s_5. \end{aligned} \quad (3.63)$$

We consider three cases: s_5 is zero, negative or positive.
We first discuss the cases s_5 being strictly positive or strictly negative. The latter two cases correspond to the two possible configurations of the hand (see Fig. 3.6). Both cases are valid, and we can choose either one.

$$\theta_4 = \text{atan2}(m_{23}, m_{13}) \tag{3.64}$$

or

$$\theta_4 = \text{atan2}(-m_{23}, -m_{13}). \tag{3.65}$$

This is similar to the case of θ_1, and we summarize it to

$$\theta_4 = \text{atan2}(\text{hand} \cdot m_{23}, \text{hand} \cdot m_{13}). \tag{3.66}$$

Recall that the input parameter 'hand' takes the values ± 1.
Using Eq. 3.55, we can resolve this in the following way:
Set

$$\begin{aligned} u_4 &= -a_x s_1 + a_y c_1, \\ v_4 &= a_x c_{23} c_1 + a_y c_{23} s_1 - a_z s_{23}. \end{aligned} \tag{3.67}$$

Then

$$\theta_4 = \text{atan2}(\text{hand} \cdot u_4, \text{hand} \cdot v_4). \tag{3.68}$$

The last remaining case is the case $s_5 = 0$. It will imply $\theta_5 = 0$ since positions $\theta_5 = \pm\pi$ are mechanically unreachable. From the mechanical construction of the robot, we see that for $\theta_5 = 0$, the angles θ_4 and θ_6 can compensate for each other. This means that for $s_5 = 0$, the number of solutions for θ_4 is infinite, and we can, for example, choose $\theta_4 = 0$. Notice, however, that the case $s_5 = 0$ represents an exceptional case, and our choice of $\theta_4 = 0$ is arbitrary. Such exceptional cases do occur in practice. For example the zero position of the robot is such a case.
We will discuss the case $s_5 = 0$ after having stated a solution for θ_6 (see Remark 3.3).

Solving for θ_6

In our matrix in Eq. 3.53, we see that the same method which led to the solution for θ_4 can also give us θ_6. Specifically, the entries m_{31} and m_{32} of the matrix give us:

$$\begin{aligned} -s_5c_6 &= n_x s_{23} c_1 + n_y s_{23} s_1 + n_z c_{23} \\ s_5 s_6 &= o_x s_{23} c_1 + o_y s_{23} s_1 + o_x c_{23} \end{aligned} \tag{3.69}$$

Now, we can set

$$\begin{aligned} u_6 &= o_x s_{23} c_1 + o_y s_{23} s_1 + o_x c_{23}, \\ v_6 &= n_x s_{23} c_1 + n_y s_{23} s_1 + n_z c_{23} \end{aligned} \tag{3.70}$$

and obtain:

$$\theta_6 = \text{atan2}(\text{hand} \cdot u_6, -\text{hand} \cdot v_6). \tag{3.71}$$

Note that we have not yet addressed the case $s_5 = 0$.

Remark 3.3

As noted above, an exception occurs whenever $s_5 = 0$. This implies that θ_5 is zero or an integer multiple of π. From the construction of the robot we see that in this case, joints 4 and 6 can compensate for each other. Due to mechanical joint limits for joint 5, it suffices to look at the case $\theta_5 = 0$. In this case, our matrix ${}^3\mathbf{M}_6$ (see Eq. 3.53) reduces to

$${}^3\mathbf{M}_6 = \begin{pmatrix} c_4c_6 - s_4s_6 & -c_4s_6 - s_4c_6 & 0 & 0 \\ s_4c_6 + c_4s_6 & -s_4s_6 + c_4c_6 & 0 & 0 \\ 0 & 0 & 1 & d_4 + d_6 \\ 0 & 0 & 0 & 1 \end{pmatrix} \tag{3.72}$$

or

$${}^3\mathbf{M}_6 = \begin{pmatrix} c_{46} & -s_{46} & 0 & 0 \\ s_{46} & c_{46} & 0 & 0 \\ 0 & 0 & 1 & d_4 + d_6 \\ 0 & 0 & 0 & 1 \end{pmatrix}. \tag{3.73}$$

We conclude that

$$\theta_4 + \theta_6 = \mathrm{atan2}(-n_x s_1 + n_y c_1, n_x c_{23} c_1 + n_y c_{23} s_1 - n_z s_{23}). \quad (3.74)$$

With other words, in typical situations, first choose an arbitrary value for θ_4, (i.e. set $\theta_4 = 0$). Then θ_6 can be computed from Eq. 3.74. In practice, it is often important to discuss the choice of θ_4 (under $s_5 = 0$, or s_5 close to zero) in more detail, considering mechanical joint limitations, and motion paths for the robot. Thus, $\theta_4 = 0$ may not always be the best choice in Eq. 3.74.

(End of Remark 3.3)

We conclude that solutions for our six-joint robot are unique except for cases with $s_5 = 0$, as long as we provide input values for 'shoulder', 'elbow' and 'hand'. This completes the analysis of the six-joint robot.

3.3 Inverse Solution for the Seven-Joint DLR-Kuka Robot

Surgical robots should be as small as possible, for two reasons. (1) the work space in the operating room is often very limited. (2) smaller robots typically have lower weight. Safety is an important issue, and clearly, bigger robots can cause more damage.
However, if the robot is very small, the range of reachable points becomes small as well. Considering the range of reachable positions, it quickly becomes clear that not so much the reachable positions count here, but much more the positions reachable in arbitrary orientations. Thus, points which can be reached in principle, but where the tool cannot be reoriented freely are not useful.
The range of positions reachable in all orientations is surprisingly small even for large six-joint industrial robots. Therefore, different types of kinematic constructions have been designed. One such design is a light-weight seven-joint serial robot.

Figure 3.10 shows the seven-joint DLR-Kuka robot. The new element is a revolute joint between joints 2 and 3. Figure 3.11 shows the kinematic structure. Following the yaw-pitch-roll-convention for angles (see Chap. 2), horizontal cylinders in the figure correspond to *pitch joints* (P-joints). Vertical cylinders correspond to *roll joints* (R-joints). As a result, we can describe the structure of the robot as an alternating chain of Rs and Ps. The full kinematic chain is thus given by the string *RPRPRPR*. We group this sequence into three parts, i.e. we spell it as

$$R - PRP - RPR. \tag{3.75}$$

The robot's wrist is the same as the wrist of the six-joint robot, i.e. a spherical wrist.
The DH-table of the DLR-Kuka robot is shown in Table 3.1:

The seven-joint robot in Fig. 3.10 can move the elbow in a way similar to the human elbow. This elbow motion (for a fixed position of the hand) is illustrated in Figs. 3.12, 3.13 and 3.14.

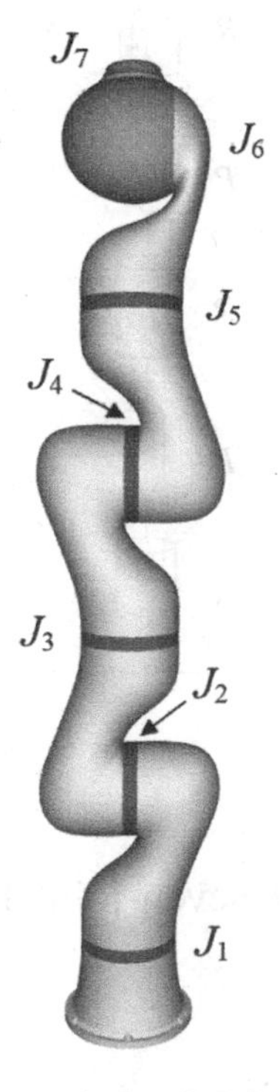

Fig. 3.10: Seven-joint DLR-Kuka robot

Table 3.1: DH-table for the DLR-Kuka robot (Fig. 3.10)

i	α_i	a_i	d_i	θ_i
1	-90	0	d_1	θ_1
2	90	0	0	θ_2
3	-90	0	d_3	θ_3
4	90	0	0	θ_4
5	-90	0	d_5	θ_5
6	90	0	0	θ_6
7	0	0	d_7	θ_7

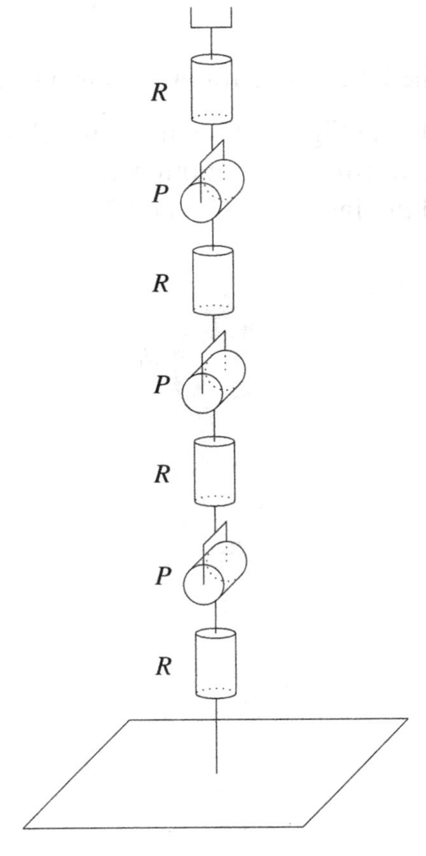

Fig. 3.11: Schematic of the seven-joint DLR-Kuka robot with $R - PRP - RPR$ structure

Remark 3.4

The n angle values of a robot with n joints specify a point in an n-dimensional space. This space is called the configuration space (or joint space) of the robot. For our six-joint robot, the configuration space is a 6D space, and we see that a given target position of the effector will correspond to single isolated points in configuration space. This solution subspace typically consists of more than one point, since we can vary the configurations of the robot (left-shoulder, right-shoulder etc.). Nonetheless, for typical cases, the solution space will still be a set of isolated points. For the seven-joint robot, this solution subspace consists of curves rather than points in configuration space, due to the elbow motion (see also Fig. 3.12). Given a target matrix, we call the curve corresponding to this target matrix the null-space of the robot.

(End of Remark 3.4)

Remark 3.5

In practice the angular ranges for revolute joints are limited. Typical values are $\pm 170°$ for the R-joints and $\pm 120°$ for the P-joints. Taking into account these limitations, the range of the elbow angle (null-space in Fig. 3.12) is limited as well. It turns out that the null-space is fragmented for some positions of the effector, i.e. the null-space consists of several disconnected pieces. This effect is illustrated in Fig. 3.15.

(End of Remark 3.5)

Inverse Solution

We begin with an informal overview of the solution path. We solve for the first joint variable in much the same way as in the case of the six-joint robot. That is, we look at the robot from above, and project the wrist center point $\mathbf{q}$ onto the x-y-plane. As in the case of the six-joint robot, we could then simply find the first joint angle as in Eq. 3.44, i.e.

$$\theta_1 = \text{atan2}(\text{shoulder} \cdot q_y, \text{shoulder} \cdot q_x). \tag{3.76}$$

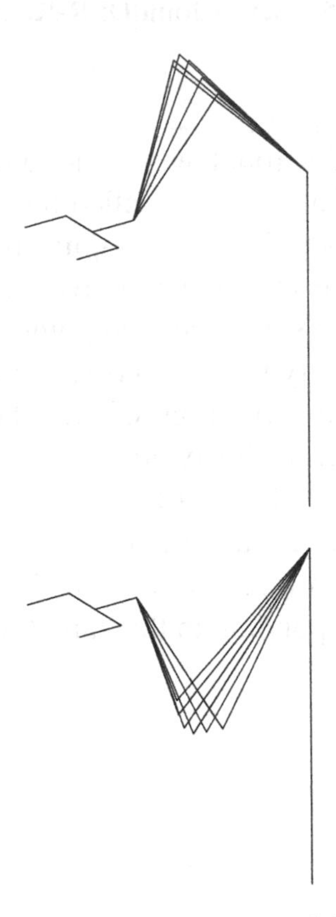

Fig. 3.12: Position-redundancy of the elbow. The end effector remains in the same position and orientation

But this will be not quite the solution for the first joint. Rather, we allow for some extra 'slack' for choosing our first angle value. This is illustrated in Fig. 3.16. The slack is denoted by Δ.
To illustrate the solution path, we compare the seven-joint robot to the six-joint robot under the *R-P*-notation introduced above. For the six-joint robot, we had an *RPPRPR* structure. To find the inverse solution, we grouped the structure into two parts, namely $RPP-RPR$. The robot's wrist has an *RPR*-structure.
If we have assigned a value for the first joint variable (including some slack value Δ), the remainder of the seven-joint robot is an $PRP-RPR$ structure. This is a six-joint robot, but different from the one we analyzed above. The wrist is the same, but the robot's base is a *PRP*-structure. The main observation in the analysis of the seven-joint robot is simple: we set up a matrix equation for a three-joint *PRP*-robot,

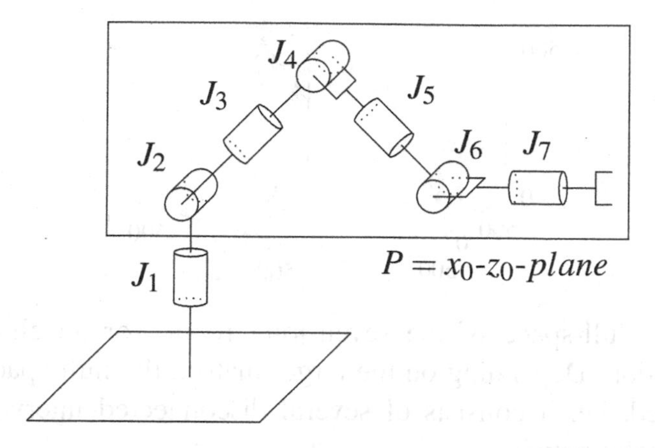

Fig. 3.13: Elbow position redundancy of the seven-joint robot. Center points of joints 2,4,6 are in the x_0-z_0-plane

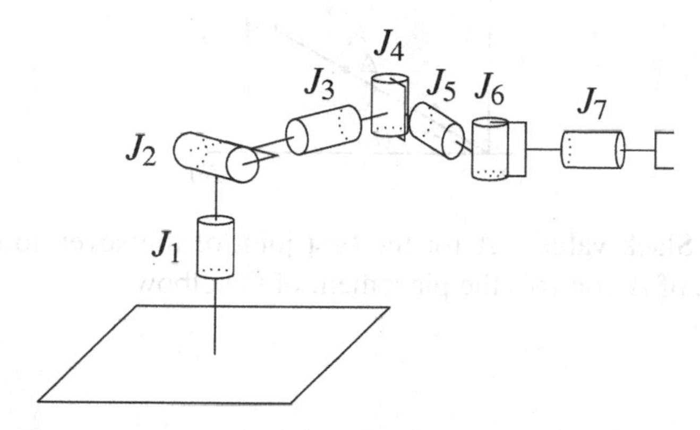

Fig. 3.14: Elbow position redundancy of the seven-joint robot. Center points of joints 2,4,6 are in a plane parallel to the $x_0 - y_0$-plane. The hand is in the same position/orientation as in Fig. 3.13

and extract the angles θ_2, θ_3, θ_4 from this matrix equation. This will be a straightforward exercise, very similar to the analysis of the base for the six-joint robot. Finally, the analysis of the wrist can again be decoupled and is the same as the analysis of the wrist for the six-joint robot.

We will now look at the actual solution. We start from the target matrix $\mathbf{T}$, which is of course a homogeneous 4×4 matrix with

$$\mathbf{T} = \begin{pmatrix} \mathbf{n} & \mathbf{o} & \mathbf{a} & \mathbf{p} \\ 0 & 0 & 0 & 1 \end{pmatrix} \tag{3.77}$$

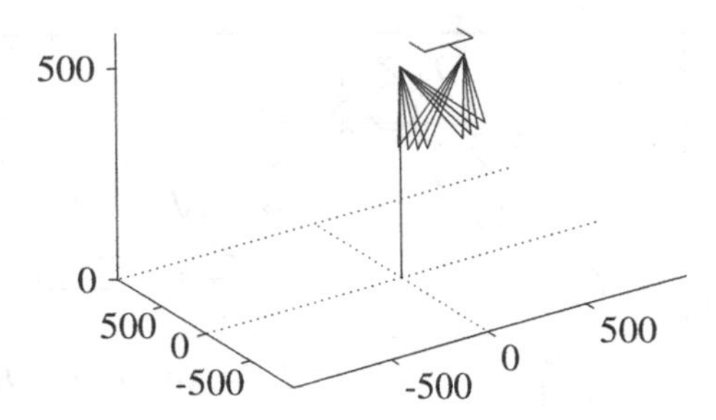

Fig. 3.15: Null-space of the seven-joint robot, for an elbow-down configuration. Depending on the target matrix, the null-space can be fragmented, i.e. it consists of several disconnected intervals, given standard joint ranges

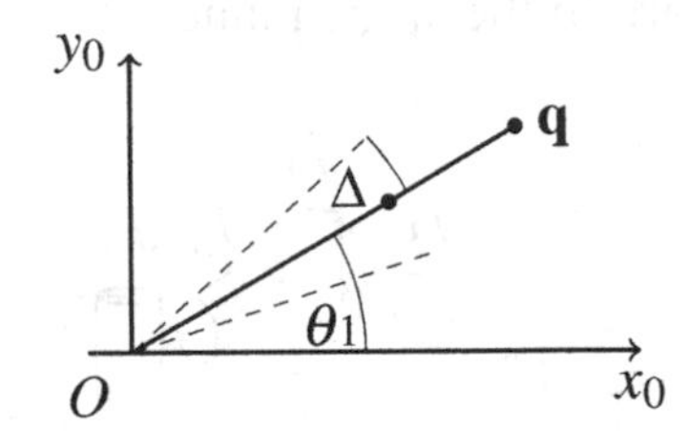

Fig. 3.16: Slack value $\pm\Delta$ for the first joint of the seven-joint robot. The value of Δ controls the placement of the elbow

Set

$$\mathbf{q} = \mathbf{p} - d_7\mathbf{a} \tag{3.78}$$

where

$$\mathbf{q} = (q_x, q_y, q_z)^{\mathrm{T}} \tag{3.79}$$

is again our wrist center point.

Solving for θ_1

Set

$$\theta_1 = \operatorname{atan2}(\text{shoulder} \cdot q_y, \text{shoulder} \cdot q_x) + \Delta \tag{3.80}$$

where $\Delta \in [-\pi, \pi]$.

Solving for $\theta_2, \theta_3, \theta_4$

Let

$$\left({}^1\mathbf{M}_2 \cdot \ldots \cdot {}^5\mathbf{M}_6\right)_{[4]} \tag{3.81}$$

denote the fourth column of the matrix ${}^1\mathbf{M}_2 \cdot \ldots \cdot {}^5\mathbf{M}_6$.
Since $\mathbf{q}$ is our wrist center, we have

$$\left({}^0\mathbf{M}_1 \cdot \ldots \cdot {}^5\mathbf{M}_6\right)_{[4]} = \begin{pmatrix} \mathbf{q} \\ 1 \end{pmatrix} \tag{3.82}$$

or

$$\left({}^1\mathbf{M}_2 \cdot \ldots \cdot {}^5\mathbf{M}_6\right)_{[4]} = ({}^0\mathbf{M}_1)^{-1} \begin{pmatrix} \mathbf{q} \\ 1 \end{pmatrix} \tag{3.83}$$

We have already solved for the angle θ_1, so that the matrix $({}^0\mathbf{M}_1)^{-1}$, and with it the entire right hand side of the last equation is constant.
We define a point $\mathbf{q'}$ by setting

$$({}^0\mathbf{M}_1)^{-1} \begin{pmatrix} \mathbf{q} \\ 1 \end{pmatrix} = \begin{pmatrix} \mathbf{q'} \\ 1 \end{pmatrix} \tag{3.84}$$

For $\mathbf{q'}$, we have

$$\left({}^1\mathbf{M}_2 \cdot \ldots \cdot {}^5\mathbf{M}_6\right)_{[4]} = \begin{pmatrix} \mathbf{q'} \\ 1 \end{pmatrix}. \tag{3.85}$$

We now evaluate the expression

$$\left({}^1\mathbf{M}_2 \cdot \ldots \cdot {}^5\mathbf{M}_6\right)_{[4]}. \tag{3.86}$$

To this end, we need the explicit expressions for the matrices and matrix products. Appendix D lists these matrices and products, as derived from the DH-table.
We find that

$$\left({}^1\mathbf{M}_2 \cdot \ldots \cdot {}^5\mathbf{M}_6\right)_{[4]} = \begin{pmatrix} d_5(c_2c_3s_4 + s_2c_4) + s_2d_3 \\ d_5(s_2c_3s_4 - c_2c_4) - c_2d_3 \\ s_3s_4d_5 \\ 1 \end{pmatrix}. \tag{3.87}$$

As expected, since **q** is indeed the wrist center, this expression does not contain any of the angles $\theta_5, \theta_6, \theta_7$. Our goal is now to extract the angles $\theta_2, \theta_3, \theta_4$ from Eq. 3.87. This will be very similar to the case of the six-joint robot.

Solving for $\theta_2, \theta_3, \theta_4$

Looking at Eq. 3.87, we set

$$\begin{aligned} q'_x &= d_5(c_2c_3s_4 + s_2c_4) + s_2d_3, \\ q'_y &= (s_2c_3s_4 - c_2c_4) - c_2d_3, \\ q'_z &= s_3s_4d_5. \end{aligned} \tag{3.88}$$

Taking the square of **q'**, we obtain

$$\| \mathbf{q'} \|^2 = q'^2_x + q'^2_y + q'^2_z. \tag{3.89}$$

Evaluating the right hand side yields

$$c_4 = \frac{\| \mathbf{q'} \|^2 - d_3^2 - d_5^2}{2d_3d_5}, \tag{3.90}$$

which implies

$$s_4 = \pm\sqrt{1 - c_4^2}, \tag{3.91}$$

and finally

$$\theta_4 = \text{atan2}(s_4, c_4). \tag{3.92}$$

Having solved for θ_4, we can use the last line in Eq. 3.88 to solve for θ_3. If s_4 is not zero, we set

$$s_3 = \frac{q'_z}{s_4d_5} \tag{3.93}$$

and

$$c_3 = \pm\sqrt{1 - s_3^2} \tag{3.94}$$

so that

$$\theta_3 = \text{atan2}(s_3, c_3). \tag{3.95}$$

Otherwise ($s_4 = 0$), we set $s_3 = 0$.
Finally, for the last angle (θ_2), a procedure similar to the case of the six-joint robot applies.
Set

$$\begin{aligned} u &= c_3 s_4 d_5, \\ v &= c_4 d_5 + d_3. \end{aligned} \tag{3.96}$$

Then

$$\begin{aligned} q'_x &= u c_2 + v s_2, \\ q'_y &= u s_2 - v c_2. \end{aligned} \tag{3.97}$$

Define an angle γ by setting

$$\begin{aligned} r &= \sqrt{u^2 + v^2} \\ \gamma &= \text{atan2}\left(\frac{v}{r}, \frac{u}{r}\right) \end{aligned} \tag{3.98}$$

As for the six-joint robot, the case $r = 0$ can be excluded. We thus have

$$\begin{aligned} \frac{v}{r} &= \sin(\gamma), \\ \frac{u}{r} &= \cos(\gamma). \end{aligned} \tag{3.99}$$

Therefore, we can rewrite the expressions for q'_x, q'_y as

$$\begin{aligned} q'_x &= r\cos(\gamma)c_2 + r\sin(\gamma)s_2, \\ q'_y &= r\cos(\gamma)s_2 - r\sin(\gamma)c_2. \end{aligned} \tag{3.100}$$

With the trigonometric addition formulas, we can simplify this to

$$\begin{aligned} q'_x &= r\cos(\gamma + \theta_2), \\ q'_y &= r\sin(\gamma + \theta_2), \end{aligned} \tag{3.101}$$

so that

$$\gamma + \theta_2 = \text{atan2}(q'_y, q'_x) \tag{3.102}$$

or

$$\theta_2 = \text{atan2}(q'_y, q'_x) - \text{atan2}(v, u). \tag{3.103}$$

Solving for $\theta_5, \theta_6, \theta_7$

As a last step, it remains to solve for the three wrist angles $\theta_5, \theta_6, \theta_7$. This is again similar to the case of the six-joint robot.
We start from the matrix ${}^4\mathbf{M}_7$, simply obtained as

$${}^4\mathbf{M}_7 = ({}^0\mathbf{M}_4)^{-1} \cdot \mathbf{T}. \tag{3.104}$$

Evaluating the left side, we find

$${}^4\mathbf{M}_7 = \begin{pmatrix} c_5c_6c_7 - s_5s_7 & -c_7s_5 - c_5c_6s_7 & c_5s_6 & d_7c_5s_6 \\ c_6c_7s_5 + c_5s_7 & c_5c_7 - c_6s_5s_7 & s_5s_6 & d_7s_5s_6 \\ -c_7s_6 & s_6s_7 & c_6 & d_5 + d_7c_6 \\ 0 & 0 & 0 & 1 \end{pmatrix}. \tag{3.105}$$

This matrix is of course the same matrix which we obtained for the wrist of the six-joint arm, the only difference being the names of the angles.
The right side of Eq. 3.104 is constant, and we can evaluate it, since we have already solved for $\theta_1, ..., \theta_3$.
Thus, we can define

$$\begin{aligned} m_{13} &= {}^4\mathbf{M}_{7(1,3)}, \\ m_{23} &= {}^4\mathbf{M}_{7(2,3)}, \\ m_{33} &= {}^4\mathbf{M}_{7(3,3)}, \\ m_{31} &= {}^4\mathbf{M}_{7(3,1)}, \\ m_{32} &= {}^4\mathbf{M}_{7(3,2)}. \end{aligned} \tag{3.106}$$

With these definitions, we can solve for θ_6:

$$\theta_6 = \text{atan2}(\pm\sqrt{1-m_{33}^2}, m_{33}) \tag{3.107}$$

The case $s_6 = 0$ can be addressed in the same way as for the six-joint robot. Assuming $s_6 \neq 0$, we obtain

$$\theta_5 = \text{atan2}(m_{23}, m_{13}) \tag{3.108}$$

and

$$\theta_7 = \text{atan2}(m_{32}, -m_{31}). \tag{3.109}$$

As for the six-joint case, parameters *shoulder*, *elbow* and *hand* with values ± 1 control the robot configuration. With this, we summarize the inverse analysis for the seven-joint robot:

For a given target matrix **T**, DH-constants d_i and configuration parameters *shoulder*, *elbow*, *hand*, Δ with

$$\mathbf{T} = \begin{pmatrix} \mathbf{n}\ \mathbf{o}\ \mathbf{a}\ \mathbf{p} \\ 0\ 0\ 0\ 1 \end{pmatrix} \tag{3.110}$$

define

$$\mathbf{q} = \begin{pmatrix} q_x \\ q_y \\ q_z \end{pmatrix} = \mathbf{p} - d_7\mathbf{a} \tag{3.111}$$

Then

$$\theta_1 = \text{atan2}(\text{shoulder} \cdot q_y, \text{shoulder} \cdot q_x) + \Delta \tag{3.112}$$

The angle θ_1 is contained in ${}^0\mathbf{M}_1$, and we define a point **q'** via

$$\begin{pmatrix} \mathbf{q'} \\ 1 \end{pmatrix} = \begin{pmatrix} q'_x \\ q'_y \\ q'_z \\ 1 \end{pmatrix} = ({}^0\mathbf{M}_1)^{-1} \begin{pmatrix} \mathbf{q} \\ 1 \end{pmatrix}. \tag{3.113}$$

Then

$$\theta_4 = \text{atan2}(\text{shoulder} \cdot \text{elbow} \cdot s_4, c_4) \tag{3.114}$$

where we set

$$c_4 = \frac{\| \mathbf{q'} \|^2 - d_3^2 - d_5^2}{2d_3d_5} \tag{3.115}$$

and

$$s_4 = \sqrt{1 - c_4^2} \tag{3.116}$$

For $s_4 \neq 0$

$$\theta_3 = \operatorname{atan2}(\text{shoulder} \cdot \text{elbow} \cdot s_3, c_3) \tag{3.117}$$

where

$$s_3 = \frac{q'_z}{s_4 d_5} \tag{3.118}$$

and

$$c_3 = \sqrt{1 - s_3^2} \tag{3.119}$$

(Otherwise set $\theta_3 = 0$.)
Then

$$\theta_2 = \operatorname{atan2}(\text{shoulder} \cdot \text{elbow} \cdot q'_y, \text{shoulder} \cdot \text{elbow} \cdot q'_x) - \operatorname{atan2}(\text{shoulder} \cdot \textbf{elbow} \cdot v, u) \tag{3.120}$$

where

$$\begin{aligned} u &= c_3 s_4 d_5 \\ v &= d_5 c_4 + d_3 \end{aligned} \tag{3.121}$$

For

$$\mathbf{M} = {}^4\mathbf{M}_7 = {}^0\mathbf{M}_4{}^{-1}\mathbf{T}, \tag{3.122}$$

we define the entries of $\mathbf{M}$ as m_{ij}. Then

$$\theta_6 = \operatorname{atan2}(hand \cdot \sqrt{1 - m_{33}^2}, m_{33}). \tag{3.123}$$

For $s_6 \neq 0$:

$$\theta_5 = \text{atan2}(hand \cdot m_{23}, hand \cdot m_{13}) \tag{3.124}$$

and

$$\theta_7 = \text{atan2}(hand \cdot m_{32}, -hand \cdot m_{31}). \tag{3.125}$$

(Otherwise set $\theta_5 = \theta_7 = 0$.)
The DH-matrices ${}^0\mathbf{M}_1, \ldots, {}^6\mathbf{M}_7$ for the seven-joint robot (and matrix products needed here) are shown in Appendix D.

3.4 Eight-Joint Robot

We now consider the following eight-joint robot: Take a small robot with only two joints. Assume this little robot has the same joints 1 and 2 as our six-joint robot before. At the end of the second link, we place

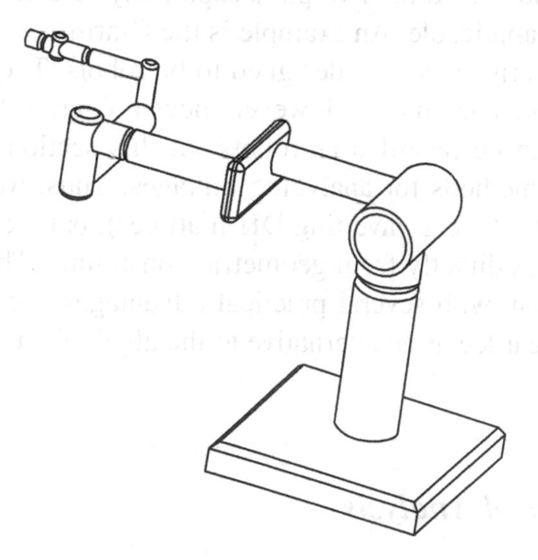

Fig. 3.17: Eight-joint robot

a base plate, and call that the tool flange. Call this 2-joint robot $\mathbf{R_1}$. Now we mount a copy of our six-joint robot to this flange. Call this robot $\mathbf{R_2}$ (Fig. 3.17).
The kinematic analysis of this new eight-joint robot is very simple, and we have already done most of the work: We are given our target matrix $\mathbf{T}$ from Eq. 3.52. We use $\mathbf{R_1}$ as a positioning unit, and choose a target position for $\mathbf{R_1}$ with a heuristic scheme. For example, this heuristic scheme can be based on an analysis of the obstacles in the surrounding workspace. The second robot $\mathbf{R_2}$ provides the transformation between the tool flange and the target. This transformation is a 4×4-matrix, and we already have the complete kinematic solution for this transformation.

3.5 C-Arm

For the analysis of the six-joint robot and the seven-joint robot we applied a useful method: We partitioned the joint set into two parts (base and wrist), and solved the two parts separately. Clearly, this strategy is not always applicable. An example is the C-arm.
Originally, C-arms were not designed to be robots. They were meant to be positioned by hand. However, newer C-arms have actuated joints, and can be regarded as robots. In this section we will look at *geometric* methods for analyzing linkages. Thus, we will not use our standard tools (e.g. inverting DH-matrices), but we will compute the joint angles directly from geometric constraints. This results in a simple solution, with several practical advantages. Geometric methods can be regarded as an alternative to the algebraic methods presented before.

3.5.1 Forward Analysis

We have introduced C-arms in the preceding chapters (see e.g. Fig. 1.9). Figure 3.18 shows the first two coordinate systems for the C-arm. The point O_5 is the mid-point between the source and the detector. Notice that O_5 is not the center of rotation of the C-arm's C. Rather, the center of rotation is the point O_4. The offset between O_4 and O_5 complicates the inverse analysis. The orbital rotation of the C is indicated by its axis (dotted line) and its angle (θ_5). The so-called angulation of the C is also marked in the figure (angle θ_4).

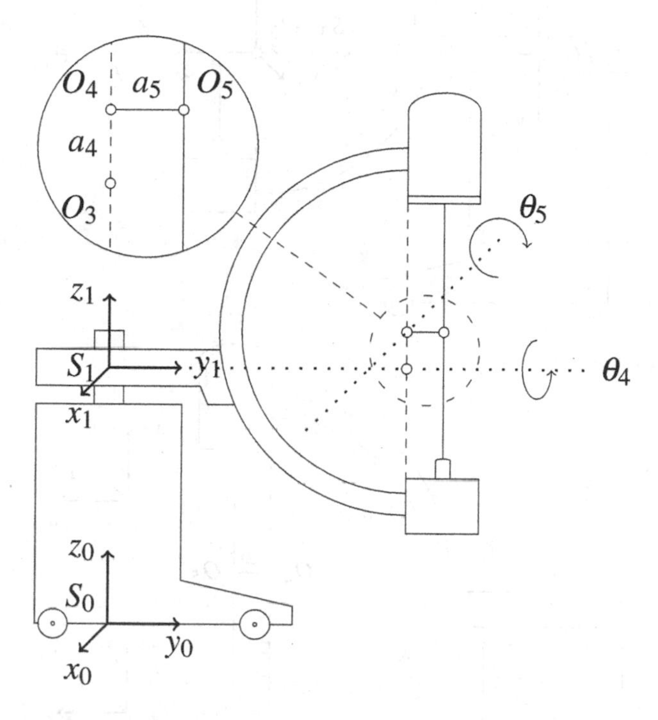

Fig. 3.18: The first two coordinate systems S_0, S_1 and the origins O_3 to O_5 for the forward kinematic analysis of a C-arm

The distance between O_4 and O_5 is called a_5. Likewise, a_4 is the distance between O_3 and O_4. Notice also that the point O_5 rotates on a circle around O_4 when θ_5 changes. Figure 3.19 shows the remaining coordinate systems S_2, S_3, S_4, S_5.
Given the coordinate systems, we can set up the DH-table for the C-arm (see Table 3.2). Recall that the first line in the table describes the transition from the coordinate system S_0 to system S_1 (Fig. 3.18).

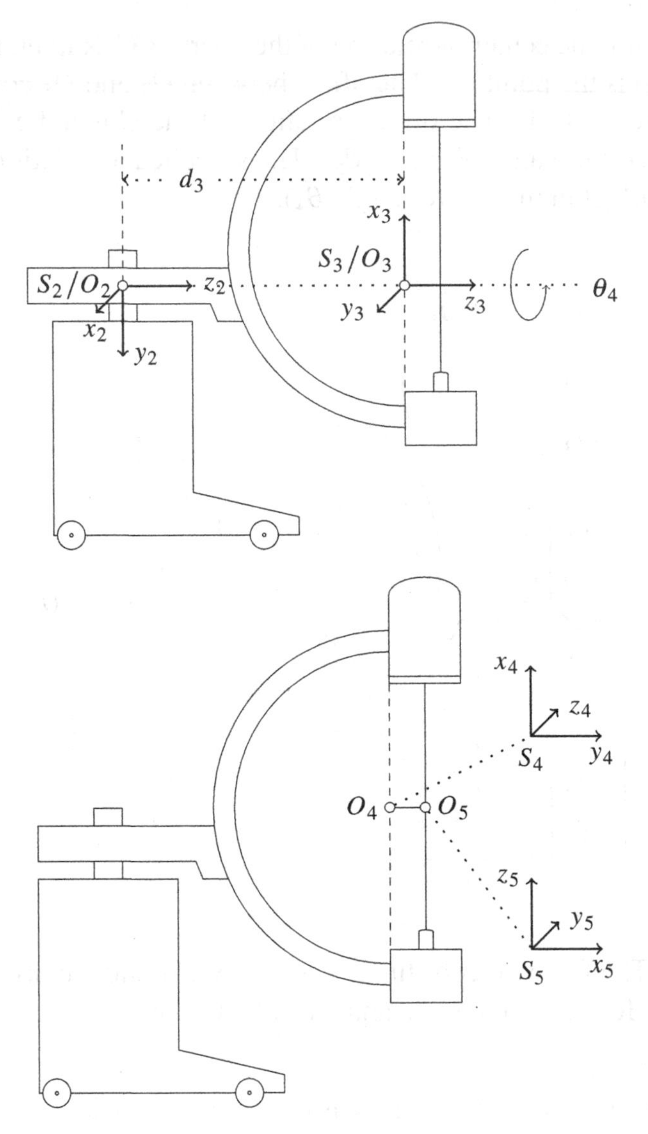

Fig. 3.19: Coordinate systems S_2, S_3, S_4, S_5. Notice that O_4 is the center of rotation of the C. a_4 is the distance between O_3 and O_4

From the table, we derive the matrices for the forward transformation.

$$
{}^0\mathbf{M}_1 = \begin{pmatrix} 1 & 0 & 0 & 0 \\ 0 & 1 & 0 & 0 \\ 0 & 0 & 1 & d_1 \\ 0 & 0 & 0 & 1 \end{pmatrix} \quad {}^1\mathbf{M}_2 = \begin{pmatrix} c_2 & 0 & -s_2 & 0 \\ s_2 & 0 & c_2 & 0 \\ 0 & -1 & 0 & 0 \\ 0 & 0 & 0 & 1 \end{pmatrix}
$$

Table 3.2: DH-Parameters for the C-arm

i	α_i	a_i	d_i	θ_i
1	0	0	d_1	0
2	-90	0	0	θ_2
3	0	0	d_3	-90
4	90	a_4	0	θ_4
5	90	a_5	0	$\theta_5 + 90$

$$
{}^{2}\mathbf{M}_3 = \begin{pmatrix} 0 & 1 & 0 & 0 \\ -1 & 0 & 0 & 0 \\ 0 & 0 & 1 & d_3 \\ 0 & 0 & 0 & 1 \end{pmatrix} \quad {}^{3}\mathbf{M}_4 = \begin{pmatrix} c_4 & 0 & s_4 & a_4c_4 \\ s_4 & 0 & -c_4 & a_4s_4 \\ 0 & 1 & 0 & 0 \\ 0 & 0 & 0 & 1 \end{pmatrix}
$$

$$
{}^{4}\mathbf{M}_5 = \begin{pmatrix} -s_5 & 0 & c_5 & -a_5s_5 \\ c_5 & 0 & s_5 & a_5c_5 \\ 0 & 1 & 0 & 0 \\ 0 & 0 & 0 & 1 \end{pmatrix}
$$

We multiply the matrices just derived for the C-arm and obtain:

$$
{}^{0}\mathbf{M}_5[1] = \begin{pmatrix} -c_2s_4s_5 - s_2c_5 \\ -s_2s_4s_5 + c_2c_5 \\ -c_4s_5 \\ 0 \end{pmatrix}
$$

$$
{}^{0}\mathbf{M}_5[2] = \begin{pmatrix} -c_2c_4 \\ -s_2c_4 \\ s_4 \\ 0 \end{pmatrix}
$$

$$^0\mathbf{M}_5[3] = \begin{pmatrix} c_2s_4c_5 - s_2s_5 \\ s_2s_4c_5 + c_2s_5 \\ c_4c_5 \\ 0 \end{pmatrix}$$

$$^0\mathbf{M}_5[4] = \begin{pmatrix} -a_5c_2s_4s_5 - a_5s_2c_5 + a_4c_2s_4 - s_2d_3 \\ -a_5s_2s_4s_5 + a_5c_2c_5 + a_4s_2s_4 + c_2d_3 \\ -a_5c_4s_5 + a_4c_4 + d_1 \\ 1 \end{pmatrix} \tag{3.126}$$

Here, $^0\mathbf{M}_5[1], \ldots, ^0\mathbf{M}_5[4]$ denote the four columns of $^0\mathbf{M}_5$.

3.5.2 Inverse Analysis

For some C-arms, we do have $a_4 = a_5 = 0$. Such C-arms are called isocentric C-arms. In general, $a_4, a_5 \neq 0$, and we must take these offsets into account (Fig. 3.20).

Above we saw two basic ideas for solving inverse kinematic equations. The first idea was equation searching (applied for the three-joint robot), the second was joint set partitioning with decoupling.

None of these ideas will work here. We cannot decouple rotation from translation. Also, there are no pairs of equations of the form $\sin(\theta_i) = a$, and $\cos(\theta_i) = b$ in Eq. 3.126.

Furthermore, we do not have a full 4-by-4 matrix to start from. Rather, our target is given as a direction from which to image, and a point on the beam's central axis.

Thus, we assume we only have a point $\mathbf{p}$ and a unit vector $\mathbf{u}$ with

$$\mathbf{p} = \begin{pmatrix} p_x \\ p_y \\ p_z \end{pmatrix} \quad \text{and} \quad \mathbf{u} = \begin{pmatrix} u_x \\ u_y \\ u_z \end{pmatrix}, \tag{3.127}$$

rather than the full 4×4 target matrix.

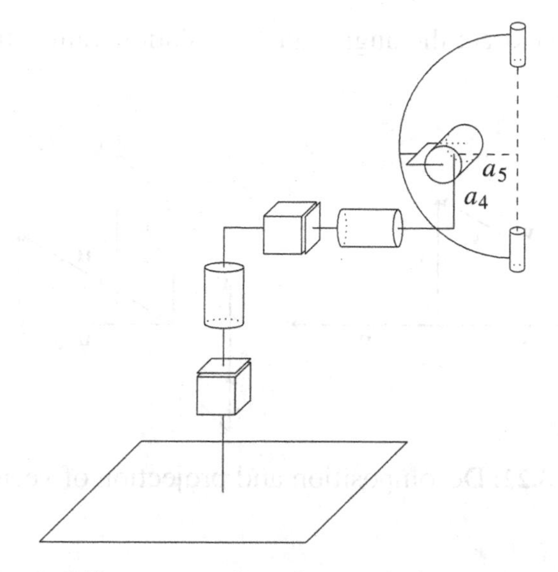

Fig. 3.20: Offsets a_4 and a_5 for a non-isocentric C-arm

Here **p** is our target position of the point O_5, and **u** is the axis of the X-ray beam. Recall that O_5 is the origin of S_5. O_4 is the center of rotation of the C-arm's C. The vector **u** is the z-vector of the last coordinate frame. The inputs for the inverse analysis are shown in Fig. 3.21.

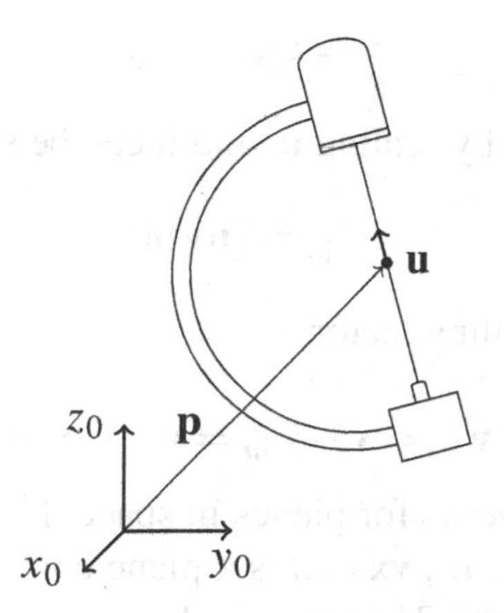

Fig. 3.21: Target position and orientation for the inverse analysis of the C-arm

Our goal is to extract the angles and translation values from **p** and **u** alone.

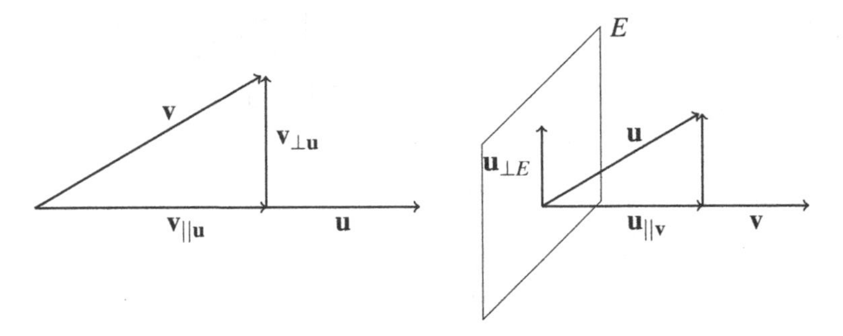

Fig. 3.22: Decomposition and projection of vectors

3.5.2.1 Geometric Preliminaries

We will need two definitions from analytic geometry. Let **u**, **v** be vectors. We split **v** into two components, one orthogonal to **u** and one parallel to **u** (Fig. 3.22). Let $\mathbf{v}_{||\mathbf{u}}$ denote the parallel component, and $\mathbf{v}_{\perp\mathbf{u}}$ be the orthogonal component of **v**.
Then from Fig. 3.22 we see that

$$\mathbf{v} = \mathbf{v}_{||\mathbf{u}} + \mathbf{v}_{\perp\mathbf{u}} \tag{3.128}$$

Here $\mathbf{v}_{||\mathbf{u}}$ is obtained by scaling **u**, and it can be shown that

$$\mathbf{v}_{||\mathbf{u}} = (\mathbf{u}\mathbf{v})\mathbf{u} \tag{3.129}$$

where $(\mathbf{u}\mathbf{v})$ is the scaling factor.
Thus,

$$\mathbf{v}_{\perp\mathbf{u}} = \mathbf{v} - \mathbf{v}_{||\mathbf{u}} = \mathbf{v} - (\mathbf{u}\mathbf{v})\mathbf{u} \tag{3.130}$$

The same notation works for planes in space. Let $\mathbf{v}\mathbf{x} = 0$ be the equation of a plane E, i.e. $E : \mathbf{v}\mathbf{x} = 0$ is a plane containing the origin, and having normal vector **v**. Then $\mathbf{u}_{\perp E}$ is defined as $\mathbf{u}_{\perp E} = \mathbf{u} - (\mathbf{u}\mathbf{v})\mathbf{v}$.

For the inverse analysis, we start from point O_5. As noted above, our target is not a homogeneous matrix, but rather the position of O_5 and

a direction vector **u** pointing along this central axis. We assume **u** is a unit vector. Also, by **p** we denoted the coordinate vector for the point O_5.
We place a line g along the z_2-axis (see Fig. 3.19). Notice in the figure, that the axis z_2 will always coincide with axis z_3. Our line g has a direction vector, which we will call **v**.
The second joint of the C-arm is a revolute joint with axis z_1 and joint angle θ_2. We will now assume that we have already solved for this angle θ_2. Hence our line g and its direction vector **v** is fixed from now on. From Figs. 3.18 and 3.19, we see that the coordinates of **v** can be calculated explicitly, as $\mathbf{v} = (-\sin\theta_2, \cos\theta_2, 0)^T$.
Our strategy will be the following: we solve for the open variables $d_1, d_3, \theta_4, \theta_5$, based on the assumption that we already have a value for θ_2. Thus we will have equations for the values of $d_1, d_3, \theta_4, \theta_5$ as functions of θ_2.

Solving for θ_4

The analysis is based on the two direction vectors **u** and **v**.

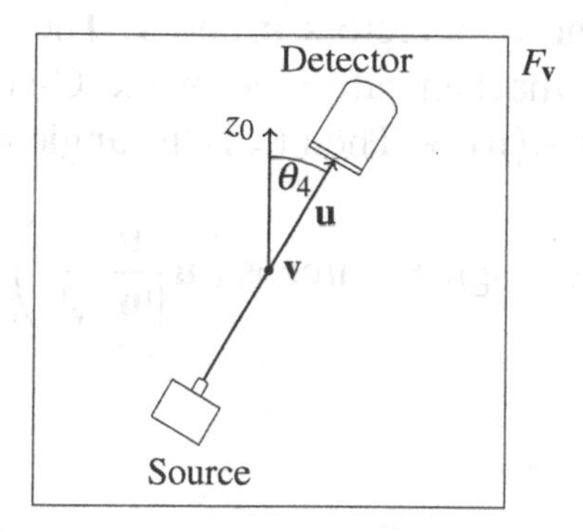

Fig. 3.23: Calculation of θ_4. **v** is the normal vector of the plane $F_\mathbf{v}$ (drawing plane). We project **u** onto this plane. The projection is $\mathbf{u}_{\perp F_\mathbf{v}}$, and we have calculated it above. Then θ_4 is the angle between $\mathbf{u}_{\perp F_\mathbf{v}}$ and z_0

Figure 3.23 shows the situation from which we set out to find a solution for θ_4. Our vector **v** defines a plane in space (called $F_\mathbf{v}$), i.e. **v** is the normal vector of this plane $F_{\mathbf{v}} : \mathbf{vx} = 0$. The z-vector of our base coordinate system (z_0) is contained in this plane. We project the vector $\mathbf{u}$ onto $F_{\mathbf{v}}$. According to the notation in Fig. 3.22 we can obtain this projection by setting

$$\mathbf{u}_{\perp F_{\mathbf{v}}} = \mathbf{u} - (\mathbf{uv})\mathbf{v}. \tag{3.131}$$

Although $\mathbf{u}$ has unit length, the projected vector $\mathbf{u}_{\perp F_{\mathbf{v}}}$ may not be a unit vector, so we normalize it. Then the angle between z_0 and this projection is simply the inverse cosine of the product.
Thus we set

$$\theta_4 = \mathrm{sgn}(\theta_4) \arccos\left(z_0 \frac{\mathbf{u}_{\perp F_{\mathbf{v}}}}{||\mathbf{u}_{\perp F_{\mathbf{v}}}||} \right). \tag{3.132}$$

We must define the sign of this angle by hand, since the arccos-function alone will return only positive values for arguments from $(-1,1)$. Set $\mathrm{sgn}(\theta_4) = 1$, if $\mathbf{u}(\mathbf{v} \times z_0) > 0$ and $\mathrm{sgn}(\theta_4) = -1$ otherwise.

Solving for θ_5

We again look at the two vectors $\mathbf{u}$ and $\mathbf{v}$. The two vectors span a plane, which is the mechanical plane of the C-arm's C. The vector $\mathbf{u}_{\perp \mathbf{v}}$ is obtained as $\mathbf{u} - (\mathbf{uv})\mathbf{v}$. Then θ_5 is the angle between $\mathbf{u}$ and $\mathbf{u}_{\perp \mathbf{v}}$, hence we set

$$\theta_5 = \mathrm{sgn}(\theta_5) \arccos\left(\mathbf{u} \frac{\mathbf{u}_{\perp \mathbf{v}}}{||\mathbf{u}_{\perp \mathbf{v}}||} \right). \tag{3.133}$$

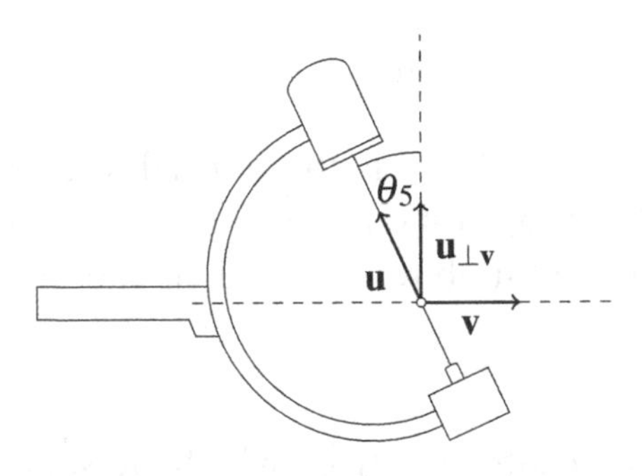

Fig. 3.24: Computing θ_5

Figure 3.24 illustrates the situation.
Again, we must compute the sign of θ_5 from the vectors **u** and **v**. Set $\mathrm{sgn}(\theta_5) = 1$ if $\mathbf{uv} > 0$ and $\mathrm{sgn}(\theta_5) = -1$ otherwise.

Solving for d_1

Having computed θ_4 and θ_5, we can directly find d_1 from the forward equation in Eq. 3.126. From the last entry of the third row in the matrix, we find that

$$p_z = -a_5 c_4 s_5 + a_4 c_4 + d_1. \tag{3.134}$$

Thus, $d_1 = p_z + a_5 c_4 s_5 - a_4 c_4$.

Solving for d_3

The points O_3, O_4 and O_5 span a plane. This plane contains the vectors **u** and **v** defined above. The situation is illustrated in Fig. 3.25.

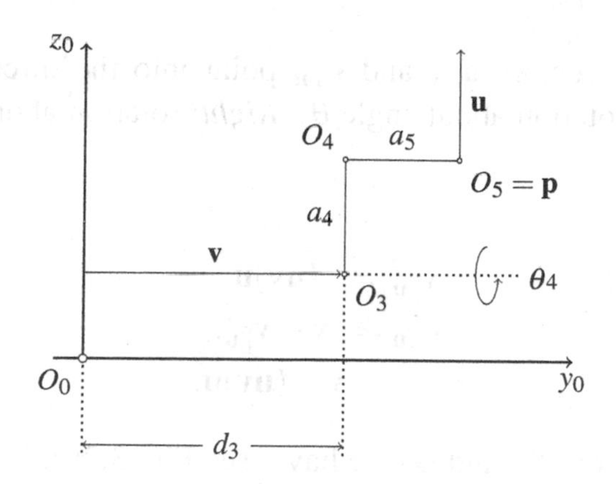

Fig. 3.25: Computing d_3

Notice that the lengths of the offsets are a_4 and a_5, while the vectors $\mathbf{u}_{\perp\mathbf{v}}$ and $\mathbf{v}_{\perp\mathbf{u}}$ point into the directions of these offsets (Fig. 3.26).

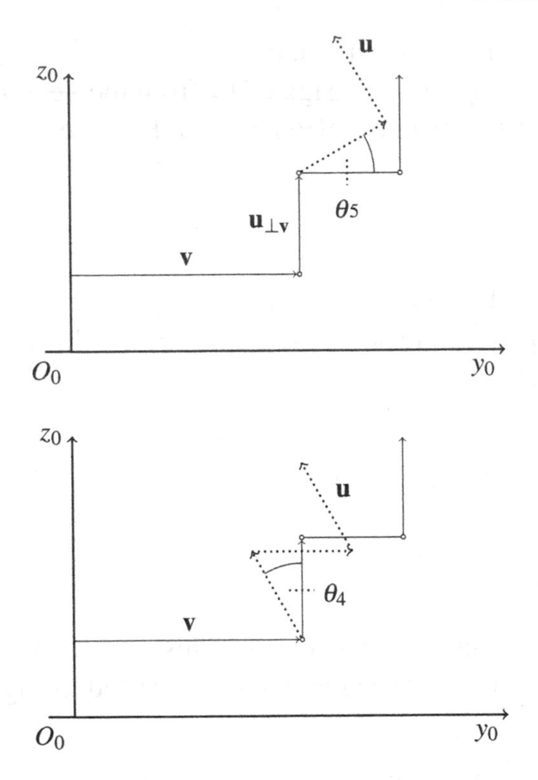

Fig. 3.26: The vectors $\mathbf{u}_{\perp\mathbf{v}}$ and $\mathbf{v}_{\perp\mathbf{u}}$ point into the directions of the offsets. *Left*: rotation about angle θ_5. *Right*: rotation about angle θ_4

We have

$$\begin{aligned} \mathbf{v}_{||\mathbf{u}} = & \ (\mathbf{uv})\mathbf{u}, \\ \mathbf{v}_{\perp\mathbf{u}} = & \ \mathbf{v} - \mathbf{v}_{||\mathbf{u}}, \\ & \ \mathbf{v} - (\mathbf{uv})\mathbf{u}. \end{aligned} \tag{3.135}$$

For the points O_4, O_5 and O_3 we have (see Fig. 3.26):

$$O_4 = O_5 - \frac{\mathbf{v}_{\perp\mathbf{u}}}{||\mathbf{v}_{\perp\mathbf{u}}||} a_5 \tag{3.136}$$

$$O_3 = O_4 - \frac{\mathbf{u}_{\perp\mathbf{v}}}{||\mathbf{u}_{\perp\mathbf{v}}||} a_4 \tag{3.137}$$

Thus,

$$O_3 = O_5 - \frac{\mathbf{v}_{\perp\mathbf{u}}}{||\mathbf{v}_{\perp\mathbf{u}}||} a_5 - \frac{\mathbf{u}_{\perp\mathbf{v}}}{||\mathbf{u}_{\perp\mathbf{v}}||} a_4 \tag{3.138}$$

Since we have already computed $\mathbf{u}_{\perp \mathbf{v}}$, and we also know that

$$O_5 = \mathbf{p}, \tag{3.139}$$

where $\mathbf{p}$ is one of our inputs, we have all the ingredients in Eq. 3.138. Our unknown d_3 is the distance between O_2 and O_3, i.e.

$$d_3 = ||O_2 - O_3|| \tag{3.140}$$

and

$$O_2 = (0, 0, d_1)^{\mathrm{T}}. \tag{3.141}$$

Solving for θ_2

Our solution for the remaining angle θ_2 is very pragmatic. First, we fix the value for θ_2 by setting it to zero. We input this value, together with the values for $d_1, d_3, \theta_4, \theta_5$ (as computed above) into the forward equation. From this forward transformation, we obtain a value $\mathbf{u}_0$ and a value $\mathbf{p}_0$ as an estimate. But this is only an estimate based on the assumption $\theta_2 = 0$. We define an error term: subtract the input vector $\mathbf{u}$ from $\mathbf{u}_0$ and $\mathbf{p}$ from $\mathbf{p}_0$. We now minimize the error term $e = (\mathbf{u}_0 - \mathbf{u})^2 + (\mathbf{p}_0 - \mathbf{p})^2$ via grid search and/or bisection. The range of the angle θ_2 is very small for C-arms. Typically, it is $\pm 10°$. Thus, bisection or grid search is adequate for finding θ_2. This completes our inverse kinematic analysis of the C-arm.

3.5.3 Applications

Given the forward and inverse kinematic solution for the C-arm, we can obtain several interesting applications of robotic C-arms.

1. image stitching
2. intraoperative 3D reconstruction and CT imaging
3. 4D imaging
4. cartesian control

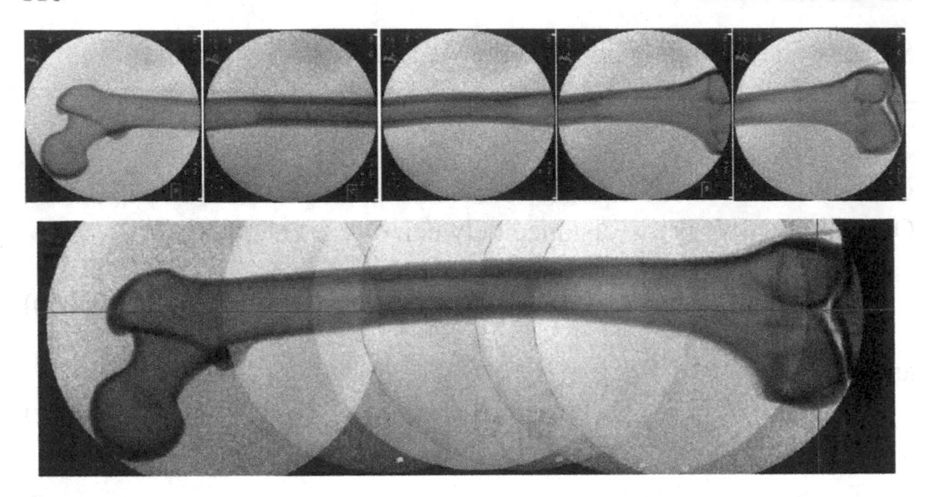

Fig. 3.27: Image stitching (without registration) for a femur bone

In the first application, we paste several images to obtain a panorama image, e.g. of a long bone or full leg (see Fig. 3.27). For the second application, we move joint five, to obtain images from a large number of angles, and reconstruct them for a full intra-operative CT image. If we tilt joint four, we can obtain CT images from non-standard angles. By taking a series of 3D images with the C-arm, each from a different respiratory or cardiac phase, we obtain a 4D CT.
It is often difficult to center an image, while remaining in the image plane. Thus, suppose we take an image of a femur head. After taking the image, the femur head is not in the center of the image, and important structures are poorly visible. Based on our inverse analysis we can compute new joint settings, such that a new image will be centered appropriately.
The above list is not yet complete. A further application is described in the following example. This example combines navigation and kinematics, and we obtain a method for registration-less navigation.

Example 3.1

Assume we have acquired a CT with the robotic C-arm. Assume also we have placed a laser beam pointing along the central axis of C-arm's X-ray beam. Then the surgeon can mark a line in the CT image. The

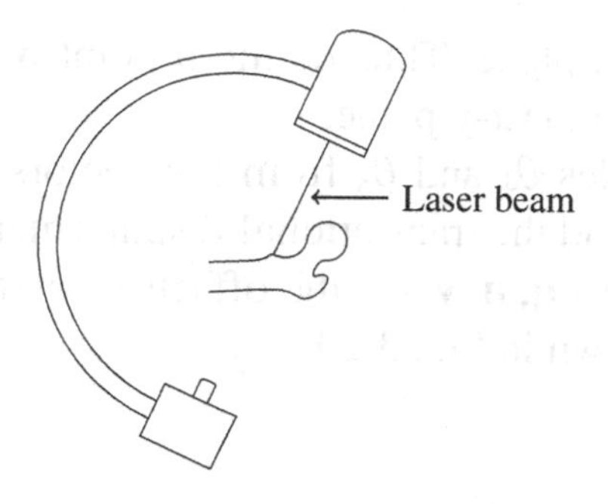

Fig. 3.28: Registration-less navigation with the C-arm

C-arm can then mark this line in space with the built-in laser beam (Fig. 3.28).
The advantage of this procedure is the following. The C-arm serves both as pointing device and CT-imaging device. Thus the spatial referencing between the two devices (imaging and navigation) is automatically given after appropriate calibration. We can navigate without image registration. This advantage is very significant in practice. It simplifies the procedure, while increasing its accuracy and reliability.
Commercial C-arms only have four motorized axes. This excludes the second axis (θ_2). The so-called wig-wag motion of the C-arm (joint 2) is difficult to motorize for mechanical reasons. But notice that four axes is all we need: mathematically, four parameters suffice to specify a line in space. Our goal is to move four joints in such a way, that our central axis coincides with a predefined line in space. (If you are unclear about the mathematics behind this argument, think of the following: We saw that six parameters specify a coordinate system with respect to a fixed base coordinate system. But for a line, two of those six parameters are not needed. One first parameter is lost, since we can rotate the line about itself without changing its position. The second parameter vanishes, because we can translate the line along itself. Thus four parameters suffice, and we only need four motorized axes.)
The four parameters are $d_1, d_3, \theta_4, \theta_5$
We have marked a line on the CT image stack. Call this line h. As above, $\mathbf{u}$ is its direction vector. We assume h is not horizontal, i.e. not

parallel to the x_0-y_0-plane. Thus define a point $\mathbf{q}$ as the intersection point between h and the x-y-plane.
We extract the angles θ_4 and θ_5 from the vectors $\mathbf{u}$ and $\mathbf{v}$ as above. It thus remains to find the translational displacement values d_1 and d_3 from the given inputs $\mathbf{q}$, $\mathbf{u}$, $\mathbf{v}$ and the offsets a_4 and a_5.
The situation is shown in Fig. 3.29.

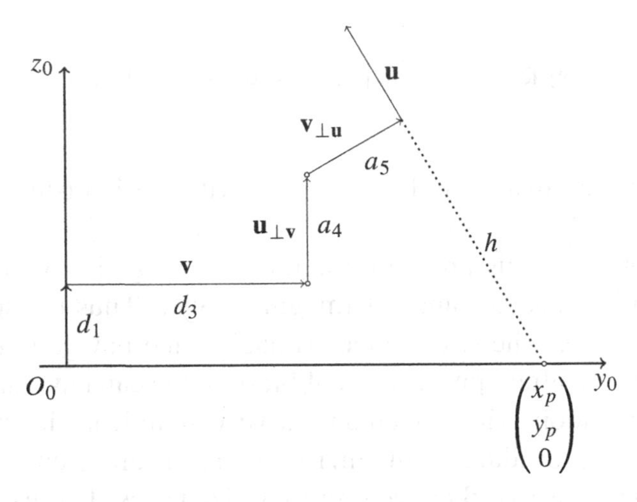

Fig. 3.29: Vector chain for the linear equation system in Eq. 3.142

From the figure, we see that a chain of vectors leads from the origin to the point $\mathbf{q} = (x_p, y_p, 0)^{\mathrm{T}}$. In this chain there are three variables: d_1, d_3 and λ (scale factor of the direction vector for h). Thus, if h is in general position, then d_1 and d_3 will occur as solutions of the following linear equation system:

$$d_1 \begin{pmatrix} 0 \\ 0 \\ 1 \end{pmatrix} + d_3 \begin{pmatrix} v_x \\ v_y \\ v_z \end{pmatrix} + a_4 \frac{\mathbf{u}_{\perp \mathbf{v}}}{||\mathbf{u}_{\perp \mathbf{v}}||} + a_5 \frac{\mathbf{v}_{\perp \mathbf{u}}}{||\mathbf{v}_{\perp \mathbf{u}}||} + \lambda \begin{pmatrix} u_x \\ u_y \\ u_z \end{pmatrix} = \begin{pmatrix} x_p \\ y_p \\ 0 \end{pmatrix} \tag{3.142}$$

Exercise 3.6 at the end of this chapter discusses a short program for solving the four-axes problem for C-arms.

(End of Example 3.1)

3.6 Center-of-Arc Kinematics

We saw that the methods for kinematic analysis not only apply for revolute joints, but also for translational joints. The C-arm is one such example, as it consists of several translational and revolute joints. Many medical devices are based on a so-called center-of-arc kinematic construction. This means that a rotation about the patient's head or body is the basic motion type built into the system. The effector is thus mounted to an arc in space. This arc is frequently mounted to a base, which itself can be rotated. Examples for devices following this general convention are: neurosurgical frames for stereotaxis, angiography systems and radiation therapy machines.
Figure 3.30 shows an example of a particularly simple center-of-arc construction. This robotic construction is used in functional neurosurgery. There are four translational axes (t_1, t_2, t_3, t_4) and two revolute axes r_1, r_2. The two revolute axes intersect in space.

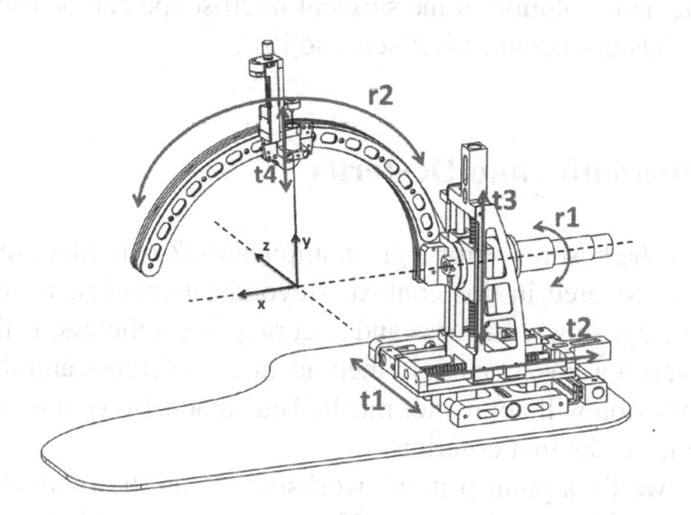

Fig. 3.30: Center-of-arc kinematic construction

It turns out that the inverse analysis for the center-of-arc mechanism in Fig. 3.30 is much simpler than the analysis of the C-arm and the six-joint robot, and is left as an exercise.

3.7 Surgical Microscopes

All robots considered so far were chains of joints, with a hand or tool at the end of this chain. Let us assume we attach the hand to the ground. The base joint also remains attached to the ground. Then both ends of the chain are grounded. Now the robot can still move, as long as there are enough joints. We call such a robot a parallel robot. What can we do with parallel robots? Surprisingly, such robots have a number of practical advantages, e.g. stiffness and safety. The mechanical construction of the surgical microscope in Fig. 1.22 is a parallel robot.
The basic structure of the microscope is a linkage with both ends attached to the same base plate. Thus, we can follow a trace from the base of the device to the tip and then return to the base along a second path. (Notice that the two paths will cross.) The overall structure consists of two parallelograms. This illustrates the name 'parallel robot'. The kinematic solution of the surgical microscope can be found with the methods discussed above (see also [5]).

3.8 Kinematics and Dexterity

Which is the best robot for a given application? A number of criteria can be considered in this context. Beyond kinematics, we can look at forces, dynamics, stiffness and accuracy. Nonetheless, if the robot cannot reach a given position, then accuracy, stiffness and dynamics at this position will not matter much. Thus reachability, and with that, kinematics is the first criterion.
Assume we fix a point $\mathbf{p}$ in the workspace. Can the robot reach this point $\mathbf{p}$ in arbitrary orientation? If not, can we quantify the range of reachable orientations at $\mathbf{p}$? The *solid angle* is a measure for dexterity at $\mathbf{p}$. To compute the solid angle, we plot the range of reachable orientations at $\mathbf{p}$ as points on a unit sphere, and measure the reachable sub-surface. A straightforward way to evaluate the solid angle at $\mathbf{p}$ is to discretize the orientational range, i.e. place a large number of grid points on the unit sphere, interpret each grid point as an orientation,

and check whether the robot can reach **p** under this orientation. The last step can be implemented by a routine for inverse kinematics.
An alternative is to require a full sphere be reachable at **p**, and then plot all points **p** in the work space, admissible under this measure. We can then compare different constructions, and we will do this in the following example.

Example 3.2

Above we looked at the seven-joint DLR-Kuka robot. Clearly, we would expect the seven-joint arm to have better dexterity properties than a standard six-joint elbow manipulator. But how much do we gain by adding a seventh joint?
To answer this question, we compute the volume of points **p** reachable in arbitrary orientation. We compare a seven-joint robot to a six-joint robot. To obtain a six-joint version of the seven-joint robot, we set the slack value Δ in Eq. 3.80 to zero. As a result, we will always have $\theta_3 = 0$, so that we obtain a six-joint version of the seven-joint robot. To be specific with respect to the link parameters and joint ranges we use the values in Table 3.3.

Table 3.3: Link parameters (in mm) and joint ranges the seven-joint robot in the example

i	α_i	a_i	d_i	joint range
1	−90	0	340	−170...+170
2	90	0	0	−120...+120
3	−90	0	400	−170...+170
4	90	0	0	−120...+120
5	−90	0	400	−170...+170
6	90	0	0	−120...+120
7	0	0	111	−170...+170

Figures 3.31 and 3.32 show the results for the six-joint version compared to the seven-joint version. As expected, the seven-joint robot does have a larger range of points reachable in arbitrary orientation. But what is the influence of the joint ranges? In other words, can we

increase the joint ranges of the six-joint version in such a way that it matches (or outperforms) the seven-joint version?
To answer this second question, we increase the joint ranges of the six-joint version from

$$R\text{-joints: } -170 \ldots +170 \qquad P\text{-joints: } -120 \ldots +120 \tag{3.143}$$

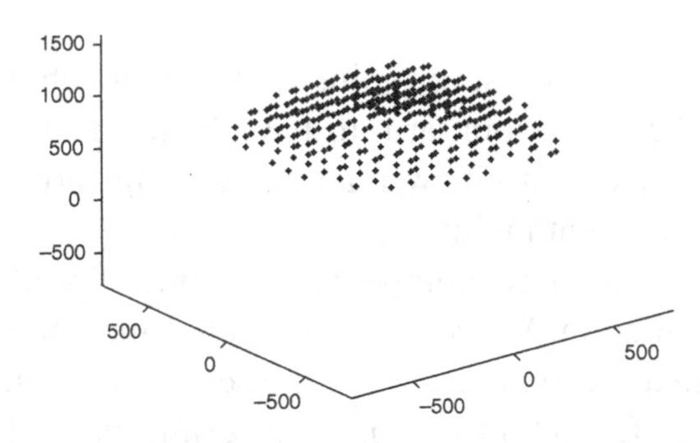

Fig. 3.31: Dexterity volume for the six-joint version of the seven-joint robot. Grid points marked in black are reachable in arbitrary orientation (full sphere). The grid points **p** have a grid distance of 100 mm

to

$$R\text{-joints: } -170 \ldots +170 \qquad P\text{-joints: } -150 \ldots +150 \tag{3.144}$$

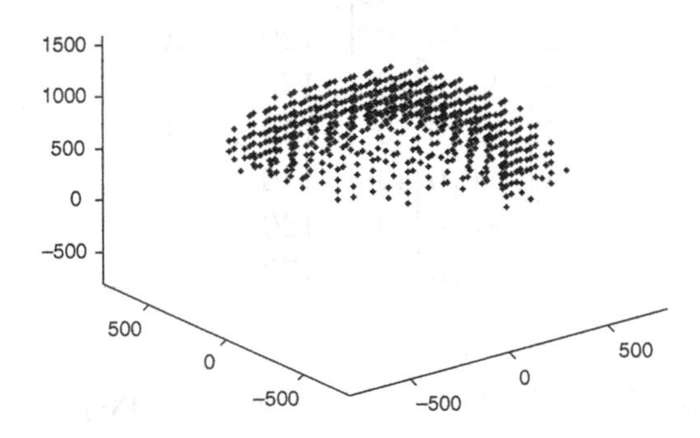

Fig. 3.32: Dexterity volume for the seven-joint robot

and recompute the dexterity map. The result is shown in Fig. 3.33.

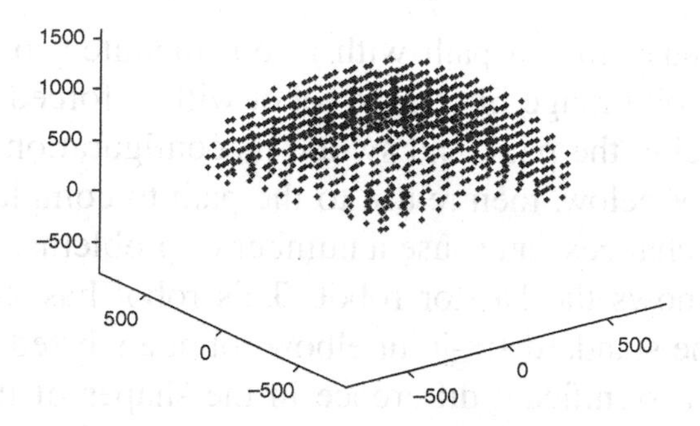

Fig. 3.33: Dexterity volume for the six-joint robot, with joint ranges enhanced to $-150°, \ldots, +150°$ for the P-joints

We see that the enhanced version of the six-joint robot (enhancement with respect to joint ranges) clearly outperforms the seven-joint version with the standard ranges.

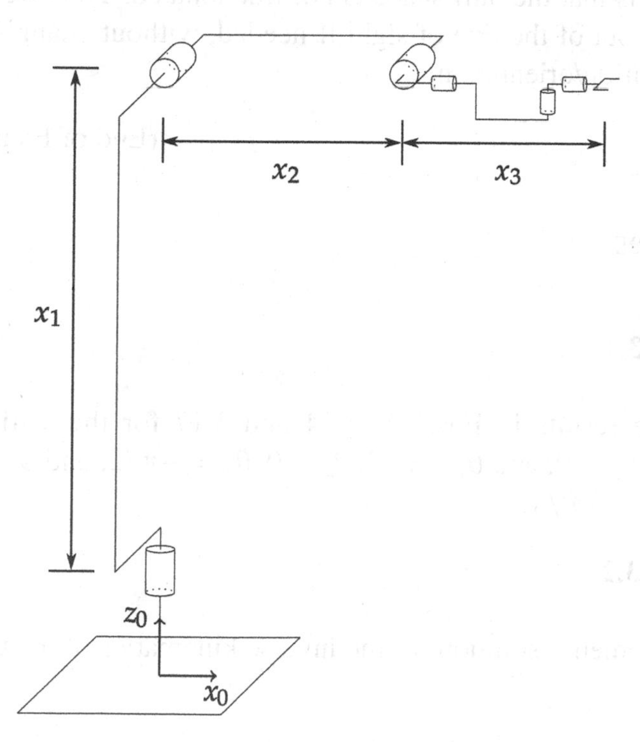

Fig. 3.34: Six-joint Dextor robot with unlimited joint ranges. Self-collisions are mechanically excluded

Assume we must trace a path with a tool mounted to a robot arm. Often, due to joint range limits, the robot will be forced to retract the arm while tracing the path, and switch its configuration from elbow-above to elbow-below, then return to the path to complete it. Cleary, configuration changes can cause a number of problems.
Figure 3.34 shows the Dextor robot. This robot has the same DH-structure as the standard six-joint elbow robot analyzed above. However, there is a significant difference in the shapes of the arm links. The links are u-shaped, so that self-collisions can be excluded. Thus, the joint ranges are unlimited. This leads to an interesting property: the robot can trace any path within the workspace without having to switch configurations along the path. This comes at a cost, however: the Dextor robot will have to be relatively large since the conditions $x_1 \geq x_2 + x_3$ and $x_2 \geq x_3$ have to hold.
Figure 3.35 shows a seven-joint version of Dextor. The advantage of this robot is that the null-space is not fractionated. Thus we can push the elbow out of the line of sight if needed, without changing the effector position/orientation.

(End of Example 3.2)

Exercises

Exercise 3.1

Verify the results in Eqs. 3.5, 3.14 and 3.17 for the settings $\theta_1 = 0, \theta_2 = 0, \theta_3 = 0$, and $\theta_1 = \pi/2, \theta_2 = 0, \theta_3 = -\pi/2$, and $\theta_1 = 0, \theta_2 = -\pi/4, \theta_3 = -\pi/4$.

Exercise 3.2

Find a geometric solution for the inverse kinematics of the three-joint robot.

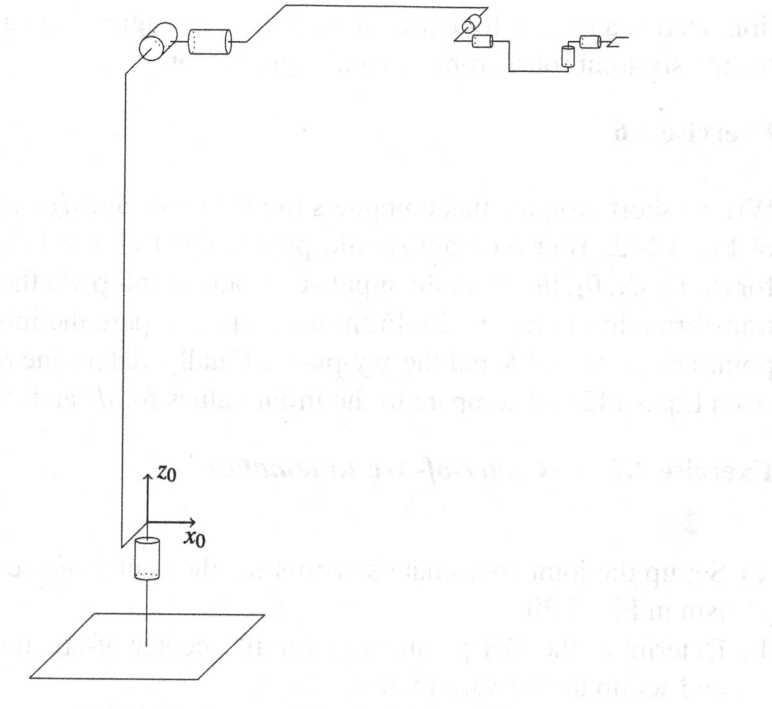

Fig. 3.35: Seven-joint version of Dextor

Exercise 3.3

Show that the value r defined in Eq. 3.34 is not zero, unless $a_2 = d_4$ and $\sin\theta_3 = 0$.

Exercise 3.4

Implement the kinematic solution for the six-joint robot. Inputs: target matrix $\mathbf{T}$ and configuration parameters shoulder, elbow and hand. Extract angles $\theta_1, ..., \theta_6$, and resubstitute these values into the forward kinematic equation, giving a 4×4 matrix. Compare to the input matrix $\mathbf{T}$.

Exercise 3.5

Set up a small routine which tests whether a given angle vector $(\theta_1, ..., \theta_6)^{\mathrm{T}}$ corresponds to an elbow-up or an elbow-down configuration. Derive a routine for extracting all three configuration parameters for the six-joint robot from a given angle vector.

Exercise 3.6

Write a short program that computes the values d_1 and d_3 as solutions of Eq. 3.142. Your program should proceed as follows: Input values for $d_1, \theta_2, d_3, \theta_4, \theta_5$. From the inputs compute **u** and **p** via the forward transformation in Eq. 3.126. From **u** and **p**, compute the intersection point $(x_p, y_p, 0)^{\mathrm{T}}$ of h and the x-y-plane. Finally, determine d_1 and d_3 from Eq. 3.142 and compare to the input values for d_1 and d_3.

Exercise 3.7 ***Center-of-Arc Kinematics***

a) Set up the joint coordinate systems for the center-of-arc mechanism in Fig. 3.30
b) Determine the DH-parameters for the center-of-arc mechanism and set up the forward matrix.
c) Solve the forward matrix for the parameters r_1, r_2 (rotational variables) and t_1, t_2, t_3 (translational variables), assuming t_4 is a constant, such that the tool tip is at the center of the arc.

Summary

Forward kinematic analysis follows standardized rules, and is applicable to most given linkages without modification. By contrast, inverse analysis requires more mathematical intuition. We saw several examples for the inverse analysis of robots. The examples illustrate two different methods. The first method is algebraic. In this case, we directly solve a matrix equation, i.e. the result of the forward analysis. With the atan2-function we solve equations of the form $\sin\theta_i = a$ and $\cos\theta_i = b$, with constants a, b. If such a pair of equations can be found in the forward matrix equation, then we can solve for θ_i. In some cases, after having found a solution for one angle, we can solve for next angles in much the same way. Here it can be useful to simplify

the matrix equation by multiplying with the matrix inverse ${}^{i-1}\mathbf{M}_i$. We solve a six-joint (elbow manipulator) and a seven-joint robot (DLR Kuka robot) with the algebraic method. Both robots are standard robots. The solution for the seven-joint robot is based on the analysis of the six-joint robot.
The second method for inverse kinematic analysis is geometric. The geometric approach also relies on the forward matrix equation, but starts from a detailed geometric analysis of the construction. In the most simple cases, two or more rotation axes intersect and remain fixed with respect to each other. For surgical C-arms, the rotation axes θ_4 and θ_5 do intersect, but the relative angle of the two axes does not remain fixed. Geometric solutions can be found for isocentric and non-isocentric C-arms.

Notes

A number of text books on robotics present different versions of inverse solutions for six-joint elbow robots (see e.g. [4, 6, 8]). A purely geometric solution for joints 1–3 of the six-joint robot is discussed in [9]. A geometric solution of the C-arm is discussed in [1–3]. An algebraic solution for the C-arm is also possible [7].

References

[1] N. Binder. *Realisierung eines robotischen Röntgen C-Bogens-Technische Umsetzung und Applikationen.* Dissertation, Technisch-Naturwissenschaftliche Fakultät der Universität zu Lübeck, 2007. http://d-nb.info/986548871.

[2] N. Binder, L. Matthäus, R. Burgkart, and A. Schweikard. The inverse kinematics of fluoroscopic C-arms. In *3. Jahrestagung der deutschen Gesellschaft für Computer- und Roboterassistierte Chirugie (CURAC)*, München, 2004. CURAC, pages 1–5.

[3] N. Binder, L. Matthäus, R. Burgkart, and A. Schweikard. A robotic C-arm fluoroscope. *International Journal of Medical Robotics and Computer Assisted Surgery*, **1**(3):108–116, 2005. DOI 10.1002/rcs.34.

[4] J. J. Craig. *Introduction to Robotics: Mechanics and Control*. Prentice Hall, 3rd edition, 2005.

[5] M. Finke and A. Schweikard. Motorization of a surgical microscope for intra-operative navigation and intuitive control. *International Journal of Medical Robotics and Computer Assisted Surgery*, **6**(3):269–280, 2010. DOI 10.1002/rcs.314.

[6] O. Khatib and B. Siciliano, editors. *Springer Handbook of Robotics*, volume 9 of *Springer Handbooks*. Springer, Berlin Heidelberg, 2008.

[7] L. Matthäus, N. Binder, C. Bodensteiner, and A. Schweikard. Closed-form inverse kinematic solution for fluoroscopic C-arms. *Advanced Robotics*, **21**(8):869–886, 2007. DOI 10.1163/156855307780851957.

[8] R. P. Paul. *Robot Manipulators: Mathematics, Programming, and Control*. MIT Press, Cambridge, MA, USA, 1982.

[9] H. J. Siegert and S. Bocionek. *Robotik: Programmierung intelligenter Roboter*. Springer, Berlin, 1996.

Chapter 4
Joint Velocities and Jacobi-Matrices

In the previous chapter we discussed the relationship between joint angles and tool positions. We started from given positions for our tool, and computed the joint angles. Suppose now, we wish to trace out a curve in space with our tool. In the most simple case, the curve is a line. Thus, we are given a robot with revolute joints, and we wish to move the gripper along a line segment.
Consider the planar two-joint robot in Fig. 4.1.

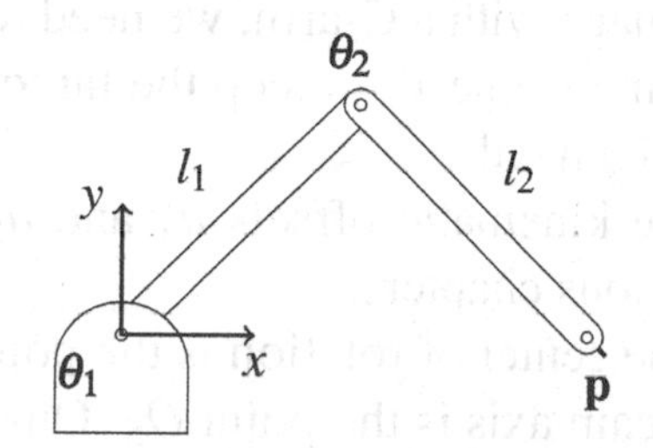

Fig. 4.1: Two link manipulator

This robot has two revolute joints. How do we move the joints, in order to produce a motion of the point $\mathbf{p}$ along the x-axis? As a first guess, assume we move the two joints with constant and equal velocities, ignoring all necessary accelerations. The two links have equal lengths (i.e. $l_1 = l_2$), and we hope to produce our linear motion in this way. Unfortunately, a quick simulation will show that this will not work. Instead, our tool will move along a circular arc. If we modify

A. Schweikard, F. Ernst, *Medical Robotics*,
DOI 10.1007/978-3-319-22891-4_4

our input parameters, the arc will become bigger or smaller, or it will be deformed. But, alas, it will be difficult to deform the arc into a line. What now, if we not only need a line motion, but we also require that the velocity of the tool remains constant throughout the motion? Hence, even if we succeed to produce a line, we may not traverse this line with a very even velocity. As an example, we again look at Fig. 4.1. Assume, the tool is very near the furthest point reachable by the linkage along the x-axis. As we move the joints to stretch out the arm even further, the tool will move more and more slowly, until the velocity will become zero, for the arm fully stretched.

We started the above discussion for the case of a line motion. However, there is an even simpler case for velocities. This most simple case arises when we require to move our joints, but to keep the tool in a fixed position. It will be discussed in the first section of this chapter.

4.1 C-Arm

When taking a CT image with a C-arm, we need to rotate the C-arm's C, but at the same time we need to keep the target point (i.e. the mid point of the beam axis) fixed.
Figure 4.2 shows the kinematic offsets a_4 and a_5 for the C-arm, as discussed in the previous chapters.
Due to the offsets, the center of rotation is the point O_4. However, the center point of the beam axis is the point O_5. Our goal is to move the two prismatic joints in such a way that the C rotates in the drawing plane, and at the same time, O_5 remains in place. Recall that the two prismatic joints have the joint parameters d_1, d_3. Figure 4.3 illustrates the compensating motion of joints 1 and 3 necessary for keeping O_5 fixed.
To capture the motion velocities of the joints, we will now write our joint values as functions of time.
Thus instead of the joint value d_1, we now have a function of a time parameter t, i.e. $d_1(t)$. Likewise, the remaining joint values are written as functions of the same time parameter t. We assume that t moves

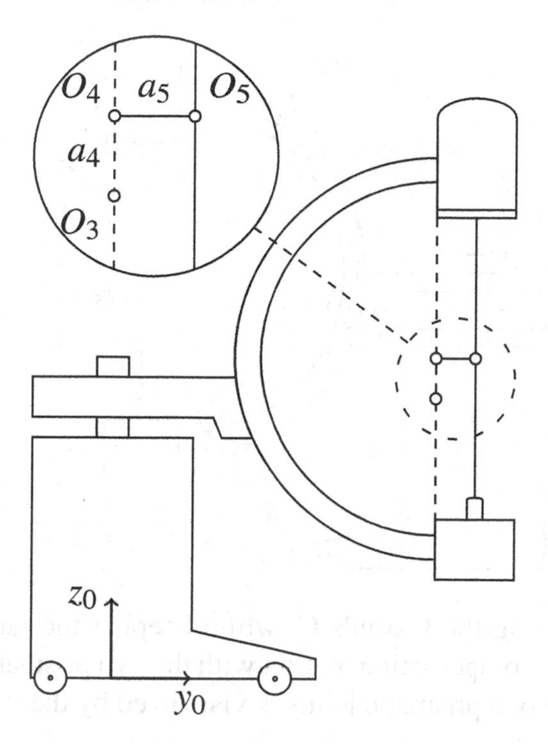

Fig. 4.2: The point O_4 is the center of rotation of the C-arm's C. a_4 and a_5 are the offsets. To obtain a CT image from C-arm X-ray images, we rotate the C in the drawing plane

within the interval $[0, 2\pi]$. It may seem odd to choose this interval for a prismatic joint, but the reason will soon become clear.
We insert the functions of t thus defined into the forward kinematic matrix, and obtain a matrix, representing tool orientation and tool position as a function of time.
Can we state explicit time functions for $d_1(t)$ and $d_3(t)$ which will keep the point O_5 static during orbital rotation of the C-arm's C?
First, note that in practice our orbital rotation should have constant velocity. Hence, the derivative $\theta_5'(t)$ should be constant, or, to be more specific, we set

$$\theta_5(t) = t \tag{4.1}$$

Here θ_5 runs from 0 to 2π, and this is why we chose the same range for t. A full rotation of 2π is unrealistic for mechanical reasons, but we will ignore this for now.

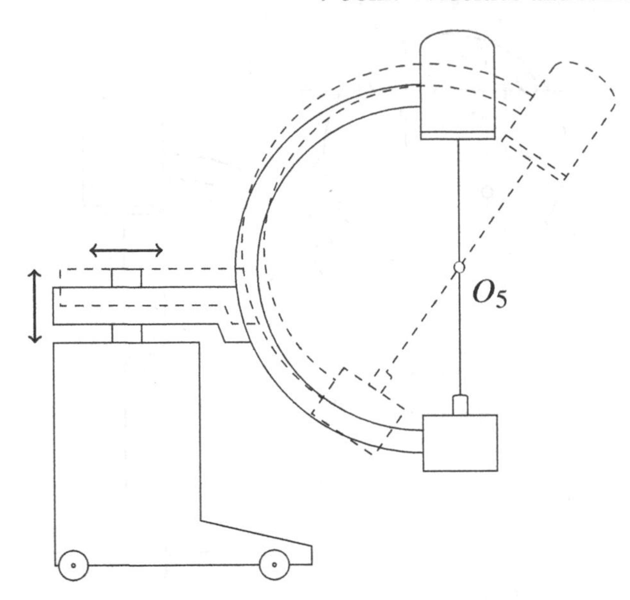

Fig. 4.3: Rotating the C-arm's C, while keeping the target point O_5 static requires compensating motion with the two prismatic joints. The motion of the two prismatic joints is visualized by the two arrows

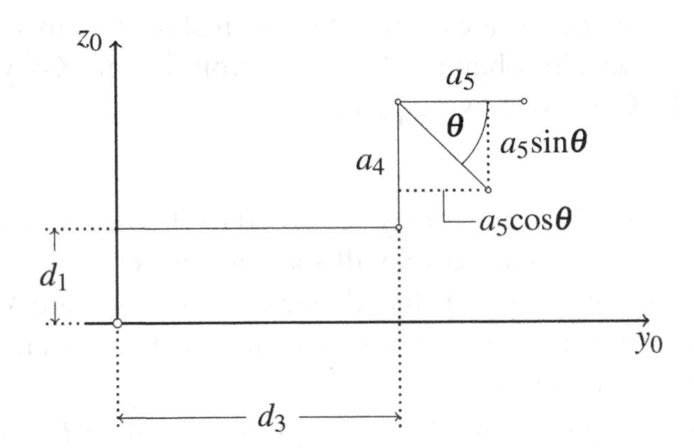

Fig. 4.4: Deriving explicit joint velocity functions $d_1(t)$ and $d_3(t)$

Figure 4.4 shows how to obtain explicit joint motion functions for $d_1(t)$ and $d_3(t)$. We see that the displacement required for d_3 amounts to $-a_5 \cos(\theta)$, where θ is the angle marked in the figure. Likewise, we find that the displacement for d_1 over time is $a_5 \sin(\theta)$.

Subtracting the kinematic offset a_4 (see Fig. 4.2), we obtain the following motion functions

$$\begin{aligned} d_1(t) &= a_5 \sin(t) - a_4 + z_p \\ d_3(t) &= -a_5 \cos(t) + y_p \end{aligned} \tag{4.2}$$

Here the constants y_p and z_p denote the target position for O_5. Having found the motion functions for the joints, we can obtain the velocities for the prismatic joints by taking derivatives.
By $\dot{d}_1$ we denote the joint velocity $d_1'(t)$. With this notation, we obtain

$$\begin{aligned} \dot{d}_1 &= a_5 \cos(t) \\ \dot{d}_3 &= a_5 \sin(t) \end{aligned} \tag{4.3}$$

Non-vertical CT Image Acquisition

Above, we have assumed that the C-arm is in vertical position, (i.e. $\theta_4 = 0$). Moving $\theta_4 = 0$ to a non-zero value, we obtain a tilted position, i.e. the C moves out of the drawing plane (see Fig. 4.2). We can incorporate the angle θ_4 of the C-arm, to obtain non-vertical CT images. Again, the required joint velocities of the prismatic joints ($d_1(t)$ and $d_3(t)$) can be computed explicitly, based on an elementary geometric analysis. Here θ_4 of the C-arm remains fixed, i.e. $\theta_4(t) = \alpha$ for a fixed angle α. We obtain:

$$\begin{aligned} d_1(t) &= cos\alpha(a_5 \sin(t) - a_4) + z_p \\ d_3(t) &= -a_5 \cos(t) + y_p \end{aligned} \tag{4.4}$$

We have thus derived explicit motion functions and velocities for the joints, which correspond to a specific tool motion.

Velocities and Discretized Motions

In practice, explicit joint motion functions are not always needed. Instead, we can discretize the required motion. For example, to move the tip of a linkage from a point $\mathbf{p}$ to a point $\mathbf{q}$ along a straight line, we simply place intermediate points $\mathbf{p}_1, \mathbf{p}_2, \ldots, \mathbf{p}_n$ along the line segment

p to **q**. But now suppose we prescribe a new orientation at point **q**. That is, the 3×3 orientation matrices at **p** and **q** are different. How do we interpolate between two 3×3 orientation matrices? As an example, we would like to go from the orientation **O** to **O**′, where

$$\mathbf{O} = \begin{pmatrix} 0 & 0 & -1 \\ 0 & 1 & 0 \\ 1 & 0 & 0 \end{pmatrix} \tag{4.5}$$

and

$$\mathbf{O}' = \begin{pmatrix} 0 & -1 & 0 \\ 1 & 0 & 0 \\ 0 & 0 & 1 \end{pmatrix} \tag{4.6}$$

A straightforward method for finding such intermediate orientations is described in the following example.

Example 4.1

Assume we are given two arbitrary orientation matrices, such as the matrices in Eqs. 4.5 and 4.6. Our goal is to interpolate between these matrices, i.e. find a series of matrices $\mathbf{O}_1, ..., \mathbf{O}_n$, interpolating for the corresponding orientations.
We first extract the yaw-pitch-roll angles from **O** and also from and **O**′. A method for doing this is described in Exercise 2.5. This method converts a 3×3 matrix to yaw-pitch-roll angles.
We obtain a triple (α, β, γ), extracted from **O**. Likewise $(\alpha', \beta', \gamma')$ are obtained from **O**′. Now we can regard both triples as points in a three-dimensional space. We connect the two points by a line segment, and obtain an angle interpolation, i.e. a series of triples $(\alpha_1, \beta_1, \gamma_1), ..., (\alpha_n, \beta_n, \gamma_n)$. For each interpolating point, we reassemble the orientation matrix. To assemble an orientation matrix from three angles α, β, γ, simply multiply the three elementary rotation matrices $\mathbf{R}(z, \gamma), \mathbf{R}(y, \beta), \mathbf{R}(x, \alpha)$.
Note, however, that this will most likely not be the ideal way for interpolating orientations. Using the concept of representing the orientation by a quaternion (see Sect. 2.7), a much more natural interpolation of orientation is possible. Refer to [1] for more details.

(End of Example 4.1)

Given the interpolating points $\mathbf{p}_1, ..., \mathbf{p}_n$ as well as the interpolating orientation matrices $\mathbf{O}_1, ..., \mathbf{O}_n$, we can apply the inverse kinematic equations for the linkage, and find a series of joint angle placements for following the given path.
We can then obtain approximations for the local velocities along the path. We simply divide the path increments by the time increments, when moving from point $\mathbf{p}_i$ to $\mathbf{p}_{i+1}$. Here, we can obtain both the joint velocities and the tool velocities.
This straightforward method requires inverse kinematics. In the next section we will discuss an alternative way to follow a given path, where no explicit inverse kinematic solution is needed. This alternative relies on the so-called Jacobi-matrix.

4.2 Jacobi-Matrices

Suppose we have interpolation points along a given path, and we wish to follow these interpolation points with our tool. If we have a large number of such interpolation points, then the angle increments will be small, and we can work with approximations. As a typical figure, our increments are given as time increments, and one increment corresponds to 4 ms.
We now pick a fixed position and orientation along the path. We have both the current values for all joint angles, and we also have the tool position and orientation. The tool position and orientation are given as a 4×4 matrix. We refer to this matrix as the current tool position and orientation. Let

$$\begin{pmatrix} \mathbf{n}\,\mathbf{o}\,\mathbf{a}\,\mathbf{p} \\ 0\,0\,0\,1 \end{pmatrix} \tag{4.7}$$

be this matrix, hence the matrix has constant entries, and

$$\begin{pmatrix} \mathbf{n}\,\mathbf{o}\,\mathbf{a} \end{pmatrix} \tag{4.8}$$

is a 3×3 orientation matrix, i.e. $\mathbf{n} = (n_x, n_y, n_z)^{\mathrm{T}}$.
To be specific, we assume our robot is a six-joint robot. The forward kinematic equation of our robot is a matrix equation, where the left side is given by the constant matrix in Eq. 4.7 and the right side is a matrix containing the six angles $\theta_1, ..., \theta_6$ as variables.

This matrix equation consists of 12 individual equations, since we have 4×4 matrices, where we can ignore the last matrix line. Each equation has a constant on the left side, and variables θ_i on the right side.
We take partial derivatives of these 12 equations with respect to the 6 variables. This works as follows: assume the current position of our robot is known and given both in terms of the joint variables and in terms of the tool matrix. When taking the partial derivative of one such equation with respect to, say, θ_1, we insert the constant values for all other joint variables $\theta_2, ..., \theta_6$ into the equation, and obtain an equation of a single variable (here variable θ_1). We can now take the derivative of this single-variable equation. To see why we have the joint angle values for all joints, at the current position, we look at the following argument: We step through the sequence of points $\mathbf{p}_1, ..., \mathbf{p}_n$, and we can assume that we have the joint angles corresponding to $\mathbf{p}_i$, when we compute the joint angles for $\mathbf{p}_{i+1}$. This argument holds for $\mathbf{p}_1$, since here we can read the encoders of our joints.
For the six-joint robot, we obtain a matrix of the form

$$\mathbf{J} = \begin{pmatrix} \frac{\partial m_{11}}{\partial \theta_1} \cdots \frac{\partial m_{11}}{\partial \theta_6} \\ \frac{\partial m_{21}}{\partial \theta_1} \cdots \frac{\partial m_{21}}{\partial \theta_6} \\ \vdots \\ \frac{\partial m_{34}}{\partial \theta_1} \cdots \frac{\partial m_{34}}{\partial \theta_6} \end{pmatrix}. \tag{4.9}$$

$\mathbf{J}$ is called the Jacobi-matrix for our robot, or the Jacobian, for short. We can now set up an equation, relating joint increments to path increments:

$$\begin{pmatrix} dn_x \\ dn_y \\ \vdots \\ dp_z \end{pmatrix} = \mathbf{J} \begin{pmatrix} d\theta_1 \\ \vdots \\ d\theta_6 \end{pmatrix}. \tag{4.10}$$

Notice that the equation gives an approximation. Thus, we require the increments to be small.
Now $\mathbf{J}$ is a matrix of partial derivatives. Each matrix entry is a function of a single variable θ_i. We fill all such variables with the joint value

for the current position (recall that the joint angles for $\mathbf{p}_i$ are known, and that the joint angles for $\mathbf{p}_{i+1}$ are yet unknown, and we compute them in the process). Then $\mathbf{J}$ becomes a constant matrix. Furthermore, Eq. 4.10 is a linear system of equations, where the unknown values are the joint angle increments $d\theta_1, ..., d\theta_6$, leading from $\mathbf{p}_i$ to $\mathbf{p}_{i+1}$.
However, Eq. 4.10 is not yet complete, i.e. we do not have all ingredients yet. Specifically, the increments on the left hand side are not all known. What we do know are the position increments dp_x, dp_y, dp_z. Thus, we know three values out of twelve. The matrix increments $dn_x, ..., da_z$ are yet unknown.
A simple case arises when the orientations at $\mathbf{p}_1$ and $\mathbf{p}_n$ are the same. Then we would have $dn_x = ... = da_z = 0$. However, this will not always be the case. So first note we can obtain a series of intermediate orientations from the technique in Example 4.2. Subtracting matrix $\mathbf{O}_i$ from $\mathbf{O}_{i+1}$ will give us the required matrix increments $dn_x, ..., da_z$.
An alternative way out (i.e. a second method for finding $dn_x, ..., da_z$) will be described next. This alternative relies on so-called skew-symmetric matrices, which are related to Jacobi-matrices.
Here the scenario is slightly different. We start from given angular increments $d\alpha, d\beta, d\gamma$, referring to the axes of the base coordinate system. Our goal is to find matrix increments $d\mathbf{n}, d\mathbf{o}, d\mathbf{a}$, such that

$$\begin{pmatrix} \mathbf{n} + d\mathbf{n} & \mathbf{o} + d\mathbf{o} & \mathbf{a} + d\mathbf{a} \end{pmatrix} \tag{4.11}$$

describes the next orientation along the path. Here again,

$$\begin{pmatrix} \mathbf{n} & \mathbf{o} & \mathbf{a} \end{pmatrix} \tag{4.12}$$

is the current (known) orientation.
We assume our angular increments $d\alpha$, $d\beta$, $d\gamma$ refer to the x-, y- and z-axes respectively. Hence, we can set up a matrix with these increments.
The matrix is obtained by multiplying the elementary rotations, i.e.

$$R(z, d\gamma)R(y, d\beta)R(x, d\alpha) =$$

$$\begin{pmatrix} c_{d\gamma} & -s_{d\gamma} & 0 \\ s_{d\gamma} & c_{d\gamma} & 0 \\ 0 & 0 & 1 \end{pmatrix} \begin{pmatrix} c_{d\beta} & 0 & s_{d\beta} \\ 0 & 1 & 0 \\ -s_{d\beta} & 0 & c_{d\beta} \end{pmatrix} \begin{pmatrix} 1 & 0 & 0 \\ 0 & c_{d\alpha} & -s_{d\alpha} \\ 0 & s_{d\alpha} & c_{d\alpha} \end{pmatrix}. \tag{4.13}$$

We now evaluate the matrix product in Eq. 4.13. To do this we will use two simplifications, both arising from the fact that our angles are small. Firstly, we set the cosine of each angle to 1. Thus we set $c_{d\alpha} = c_{d\beta} = c_{d\gamma} = 1$. Likewise, we use the approximation

$$s_{d\alpha} = d_\alpha \tag{4.14}$$

for small angles. Furthermore, we set any products of *two* small angles to zero.
Then, after multiplying, we obtain the approximation matrix **D**, approximating the matrix in Eq. 4.13, where

$$\mathbf{D} = \begin{pmatrix} 1 & -d\gamma & d\beta \\ d\gamma & 1 & -d\alpha \\ -d\beta & d\alpha & 1 \end{pmatrix}. \tag{4.15}$$

To compute the unknown matrix increments $d\mathbf{n}$, $d\mathbf{o}$, $d\mathbf{a}$ we now proceed as follows. Set

$$\mathbf{D} \cdot (\mathbf{n} \;\; \mathbf{o} \;\; \mathbf{a}) = (\mathbf{n} + d\mathbf{n} \;\; \mathbf{o} + d\mathbf{o} \;\; \mathbf{a} + d\mathbf{a}). \tag{4.16}$$

We rewrite this equation:

$$(\mathbf{D} - \mathbf{I}) \cdot (\mathbf{n} \;\; \mathbf{o} \;\; \mathbf{a}) = (d\mathbf{n} \;\; d\mathbf{o} \;\; d\mathbf{a}). \tag{4.17}$$

where **I** is the 3-by-3 unit matrix.
This gives

$$\begin{pmatrix} 0 & -d\gamma & d\beta \\ d\gamma & 0 & -d\alpha \\ -d\beta & d\alpha & 0 \end{pmatrix} \begin{pmatrix} n_x & o_x & a_x \\ n_y & o_y & a_y \\ n_z & o_z & a_z \end{pmatrix} = \begin{pmatrix} dn_x & do_x & da_x \\ dn_y & do_y & da_y \\ dn_z & do_z & da_z \end{pmatrix}. \tag{4.18}$$

All matrix entries on the left side of Eq. 4.18 are known. We can thus compute the unknowns on the right hand side, simply by multiplying the two matrices on the left side.

Remark 4.1

The matrix

$$\mathbf{S} = \begin{pmatrix} 0 & -d\gamma & d\beta \\ d\gamma & 0 & -d\alpha \\ -d\beta & d\alpha & 0 \end{pmatrix} \tag{4.19}$$

is obtained as $\mathbf{S} = \mathbf{D} - \mathbf{I}$, and has a special property, namely

$$\mathbf{S} + \mathbf{S}^{\mathrm{T}} = 0 \tag{4.20}$$

Matrices with this property are called skew-symmetric. Notice that $\mathbf{S}$ is not orthogonal, and does not represent a rotation.

(End of Remark 4.1)

After having found all constant values, Eq. 4.10 is a linear equation system, and we can solve for the variables $d\theta_1, ..., d\theta_6$.

Remark 4.2

The approach described in this section also provides a straightforward method for inverse kinematics: given a 4×4 matrix, denoting a desired goal position and orientation for our tool, we can move to this goal incrementally. To this end, we simply place a line segment connecting the current position and the goal position. We then follow the line segment with the above interpolation scheme. The Jacobi-matrix defined above is not symmetric, nor does it have an inverse or a determinant. In the form in Eq. 4.9, a Jacobi-matrix is simply obtained by taking component-wise derivatives of a kinematic matrix. However, the concept of component-wise derivatives can be extended. In the next section, we will see such extensions. This will help us to find explicit velocity functions for the joints in a more systematic way.

(End of Remark 4.2)

4.3 Jacobi-Matrices and Velocity Functions

When looking at the six-joint robot in Fig. 3.1 or even the eight-joint robot in Fig. 3.17 we see that the most important element is the recurrent two-link sub-assembly with parallel joint axes. We have discussed this two-link sub-assembly in several examples throughout the preceding chapters and also in the introduction of this chapter (Fig. 4.1).

Why is this element the most important element? We have already observed that our six-joint robot consists of two three-joint sub-assemblies. In the kinematic analysis, we separated these two sub-assemblies.
We now look at the first of these sub-assemblies. It is the well-known three-joint robot from Chap. 2. Here, the base joint determines a coarse pre-positioning in the work space. Recall that the kinematic analysis for this joint was particularly simple, and we were able to decouple it from the entire rest of the robot. Now the next two joints (joints 2 and 3 for the six-joint robot) do the actual manipulation at the target, while all remaining joints only provide hand orientation. Thus, roughly speaking, joints 2 and 3 provide the main elements of the robot, when it comes to handling and manipulation. We give a name to the corresponding sub-assembly, and refer to it as the (planar) two-link manipulator.
We compute the forward matrix for a planar two-link manipulator. We obtain

$$
{}^{0}\mathbf{M}_2 = \begin{pmatrix} c_{12} & -s_{12} & 0 & l_2c_{12}+l_1c_1 \\ s_{12} & c_{12} & 0 & l_2s_{12}+l_1s_1 \\ 0 & 0 & 1 & 0 \\ 0 & 0 & 0 & 1 \end{pmatrix}. \tag{4.21}
$$

Notice that here we refer to the two joints of our two-link manipulator as joint 1 and joint 2, ignoring the fact that the two-link manipulator may be part of a larger robot with more joints.
Our goal is to find explicit velocity functions for the two-link manipulator. We have already done this for the case of a C-arm, in the introduction of this chapter, but this was a particularly simple case, and we did not need any dedicated methods.
We consider the elements (1,4) and (2,4) of the matrix in Eq. 4.21. These two elements give the x- and y-positions of our tool.
Hence, we have

$$
\begin{aligned}
x &= l_2c_{12}+l_1c_1, \\
y &= l_2s_{12}+l_1s_1.
\end{aligned} \tag{4.22}
$$

Restating these equations as functions of time, as the joints move, we obtain

$$x(t) = l_2 \cos(\theta_1(t) + \theta_2(t)) + l_1 \cos(\theta_1(t)),$$
$$y(t) = l_2 \sin(\theta_1(t) + \theta_2(t)) + l_1 \sin(\theta_1(t)). \quad (4.23)$$

Here $\theta_1(t)$ and $\theta_2(t)$ are two separate functions, describing the motions of the two joints over time.
We differentiate these two functions with respect to the time parameter t. This gives

$$x'(t) = -l_1 \sin(\theta_1(t)) \cdot \theta_1'(t) - l_2 \sin(\theta_1(t) + \theta_2(t)) \cdot (\theta_1'(t) + \theta_2'(t)),$$
$$y'(t) = l_1 \cos(\theta_1(t)) \cdot \theta_1'(t) + l_2 \cos(\theta_1(t) + \theta_2(t)) \cdot (\theta_1'(t) + \theta_2'(t)). \quad (4.24)$$

We recall the notation from Eq. 4.3. With this notation (replace $\theta_i'(t)$ by $\dot{\theta}_i$) and the familiar short forms $s_i = \sin(\theta_i)$ we rewrite Eq. 4.24 to

$$\dot{x} = -l_1 s_1 \cdot \dot{\theta}_1 - l_2 s_{12} \cdot (\dot{\theta}_1 + \dot{\theta}_2)$$
$$\dot{y} = l_1 c_1 \cdot \dot{\theta}_1 + l_2 c_{12} \cdot (\dot{\theta}_1 + \dot{\theta}_2) \quad (4.25)$$

We now assemble the two functions into a matrix. This is done in a purely symbolic way!
We set

$$\mathbf{p} = \begin{pmatrix} x \\ y \end{pmatrix}, \qquad \dot{\theta} = \begin{pmatrix} \dot{\theta}_1 \\ \dot{\theta}_2 \end{pmatrix}. \quad (4.26)$$

Define a matrix $\mathbf{J}$ by setting

$$\mathbf{J} = \begin{pmatrix} -l_1 s_1 - l_2 s_{12} & -l_2 s_{12} \\ l_1 c_1 + l_2 c_{12} & l_2 c_{12} \end{pmatrix}. \quad (4.27)$$

Now $\mathbf{J}$ is arranged in such a way that it allows for writing Eq. 4.25 in a shorter form, namely

$$\dot{\mathbf{p}} = \mathbf{J}\dot{\theta}. \quad (4.28)$$

You may wish to take a minute to multiply the product $\mathbf{J}\dot{\theta}$ and see that this will indeed result in the right hand side of Eq. 4.25.
The matrix $\mathbf{J}$ is a 2-by-2 matrix, and has an interesting property: we can invert it! Thus we can write

$$\dot{\theta} = \mathbf{J}^{-1}\dot{\mathbf{p}}. \quad (4.29)$$

Now, let us compute the inverse of $\mathbf{J}$ explicitly.

We recall that the inverse of an arbitrary 2-by-2 matrix $\mathbf{A}$ with

$$\mathbf{A} = \begin{pmatrix} a & b \\ c & d \end{pmatrix} \tag{4.30}$$

is given by

$$\mathbf{A}^{-1} = \frac{1}{ad - bc} \begin{pmatrix} d & -b \\ -c & a \end{pmatrix}. \tag{4.31}$$

Thus

$$\mathbf{J}^{-1} = \frac{1}{l_1 l_2 s_2} \begin{pmatrix} l_2 c_{12} & l_2 s_{12} \\ -l_1 c_1 - l_2 c_{12} & -l_1 s_1 - l_2 s_{12} \end{pmatrix}. \tag{4.32}$$

Now we can derive explicit velocity functions for the joints of our two-link manipulator.
Suppose we wish to move the tool along the x-axis. Thus we set the velocity along the x-axis to 1 and the velocity along the y-axis to 0.
Then

$$\dot{\mathbf{p}} = \begin{pmatrix} 1 \\ 0 \end{pmatrix}. \tag{4.33}$$

Multiplying, we obtain

$$\dot{\theta} = \mathbf{J}^{-1}\dot{\mathbf{p}} = \begin{pmatrix} \frac{c_{12}}{l_1 s_2} \\ -\frac{c_1}{l_2 s_2} - \frac{c_{12}}{l_1 s_2} \end{pmatrix}. \tag{4.34}$$

This shows that the velocity will tend to infinity as our angle θ_2 tends to 0, i.e. as the arm stretches.
In Eq. 4.34 we have explicitly stated the non-linear joint velocity functions which will move the tip along a straight line.

Remark 4.3

From Eq. 4.31 we see that we cannot invert the matrix $\mathbf{A}$ in Eq. 4.30 if $ad - bc = 0$. In this case the inverse $\mathbf{A}^{-1}$ does not exist, and $\mathbf{A}$ is called singular. We apply this to Eq. 4.32. Here, $\mathbf{J}$ has no inverse, whenever $s_2 = 0$. This means that $\mathbf{J}$ is singular if $\theta_2 = 0$ or $\theta_2 = \pi/2$. Looking at the robot, we see that such a configuration occurs, when the two links are aligned, i.e. the arm is stretched.

(End of Remark 4.3)

4.4 Geometric Jacobi-Matrix

In literature, the matrix $\mathbf{J}$ defined in Eq. 4.27 is also called the Jacobian, although it is somewhat different from the matrix defined in Eq. 4.9. In the process of obtaining Eq. 4.9, we differentiated with respect to all six joint angles. When deriving Eq. 4.27, we differentiated with respect to a single variable, namely the time parameter t. Notice that the 2-by-2 matrix in Eq. 4.27 is invertible, and has a determinant. The matrix in Eq. 4.9 is a 6-by-12 matrix, hence has no inverse, nor determinant.

But a further difference between the two Jacobians should be mentioned. This regards the process of setting up the matrix $\mathbf{J}$ in order to arrive at the shorter form $\dot{\mathbf{p}} = \mathbf{J}\dot{\theta}$ of the equations in Eq. 4.25. This process did not involve taking partial derivatives. It is not immediately clear how this process would generalize to the case of other robots, with more joints.

Hence, we saw two versions of Jacobi-matrices. With the second version, we were able to derive explicit functions for the joint velocities. Our goal is now to derive a standardized version of the Jacobi-matrix. This standardized version will also be called the geometric Jacobian. To obtain a standard version, it is necessary to specify the goals of the standardization. Our goal will be to find two $3 \times n$ matrices, which we will call $\mathbf{J}_v$ and $\mathbf{J}_\omega$. (n is again the number of joints.) The two matrices will then relate the joint velocities $\theta_1'(t), \ldots \theta_n'(t)$ to the velocity of the effector. We again write $\dot{\theta}_i$ as a shorthand for the time derivate $\theta_i'(t)$, and likewise, in vector notation,

$$\dot{\theta} = \begin{pmatrix} \dot{\theta}_1 \\ \vdots \\ \dot{\theta}_n \end{pmatrix}. \tag{4.35}$$

To describe the velocity of the effector, we will be somewhat more specific than above. In particular, we will distinguish two types of velocities, namely *linear velocity* and *angular velocity*. We next define the latter two terms.

Suppose we have a coordinate frame S rotating within the base frame. The axis of rotation is a (unit) vector $\mathbf{a}$, given in the base frame. Also, assume S has its origin at the origin of the base frame. We define the *angular velocity* of the rotating frame as follows.

$$\omega = \dot{\theta}\mathbf{a} \tag{4.36}$$

Here $\dot{\theta}$ is a scalar function of time. Thus, the angular velocity ω is simply a vector, the length of which gives the magnitude of the velocity, and the direction gives the axis of the rotation (here unit vector $\mathbf{a}$). Now suppose we have a point $\mathbf{p}$ which is given in the coordinates of the frame S, and rotates with S. We define the *linear velocity* of $\mathbf{p}$ as

$$\mathbf{v} = \omega \times \mathbf{p}. \tag{4.37}$$

This definition may seem odd, and we visualize the effects of the latter definition for the case of a small example.

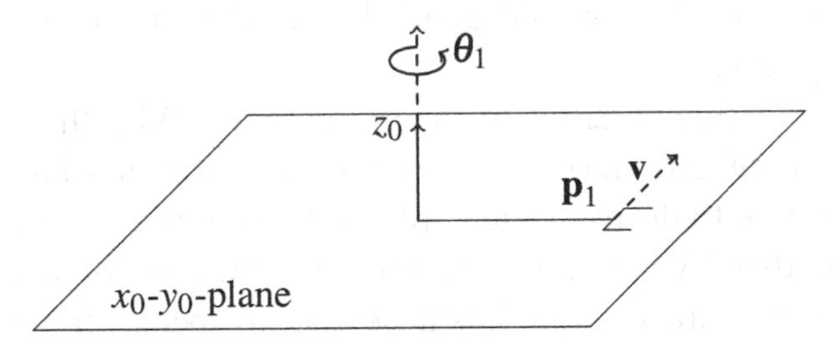

Fig. 4.5: Linear velocity $\mathbf{v}$ resulting from an angular velocity ω. Notice that $\mathbf{v}$ is a vector in the x_0-y_0-plane. $\mathbf{v}$ is the cross-product of $\dot{\theta}_1 z_0$ and $\mathbf{p}_1$

Example 4.2

Figure 4.5 shows a one-joint robot, which moves in the x_0-y_0-plane. The robot rotates about the z_0-axis. The joint angle is θ_1. The position of the end effector is given by the point $\mathbf{p}_1$ in the center of the gripper. Now we move the only joint. The angular velocity is the scaling factor $\dot{\theta}_1$ of the vector z_0. The linear velocity of $\mathbf{p}_1$ is $\mathbf{v}$. This linear velocity $\mathbf{v}$ is the cross-product of $\dot{\theta}_1 z_0$ and $\mathbf{p}_1$. We see that an increase of the link length of the robot, or an increase of $\dot{\theta}_1$ will increase the linear velocity. By contrast, an increase in link length will not increase angular velocity.

Thus, our linear velocity is in fact a linear velocity resulting from an angular velocity, and it is an *instantaneous* velocity. Notice that the vector $\mathbf{v}$ in Fig. 4.5 changes direction as the robot moves.

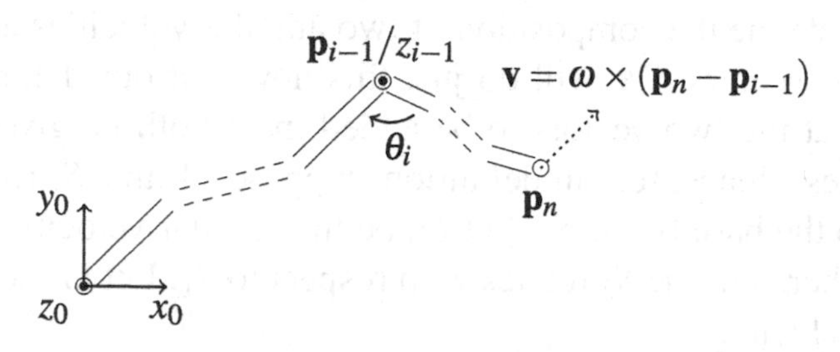

Fig. 4.6: Linear velocity $\mathbf{v}$ of the point $\mathbf{p}_n$, resulting from the motion of a single joint (here joint i, with axis z_{i-1}). The axes z_0 and z_{i-1} are orthogonal to the drawing plane, and are indicated by *circles with dots*

In Fig. 4.6 we see a planar robot with several revolute joints, again moving in the x_0-y_0-plane. Suppose now only a single joint of this robot is moving, namely joint i. According to the DH-rules, the joint axis is the axis z_{i-1}. Here z_{i-1} is again orthogonal to our drawing plane, and parallel to z_0, the z-axis of the base frame. The vectors $\mathbf{p}_i$ and $\mathbf{p}_n$ give the coordinates of the origins of the DH-frames i and n, respectively. Then the angular velocity of the DH-frame i is given by

$$\omega = \dot{\theta}_i z_{i-1}. \tag{4.38}$$

The linear velocity $\mathbf{v}$ of the point $\mathbf{p}_n$, resulting from the rotation at joint i, is then

$$\mathbf{v} = \omega \times (\mathbf{p}_n - \mathbf{p}_{i-1}) = z_{i-1} \times (\mathbf{p}_n - \mathbf{p}_{i-1})\dot{\theta}_i. \tag{4.39}$$

Notice now, that although the example in Fig. 4.6 is planar, the same holds for the three-dimensional case, i.e. when the axis z_{i-1} is no longer parallel to z_0.

(End of Example 4.2)

We should also note that the angular velocity, according to the above definition, is a property of a frame, while the linear velocity is a property of a point.

Composition of Angular Velocities

Above, we have defined an angular velocity as a vector. We have not yet defined a composition for two angular velocities. It would seem natural to define the composition of two angular velocities as the sum of the two vectors. We will do just this now, but our definition will require that the two vectors to be added must both be given in base coordinates. Hence, for our definition, suppose a frame S_1 rotates with respect to the base frame S_0. Let ω_0 be the angular velocity.
Then further, a frame S_2 rotates with respect to S_1. Let ω_1 be the latter angular velocity.
We assume that S_1 and S_2 have their origin at the origin of the base frame S_0.
Then we express the position of S_1 with respect to S_0 by a matrix ${}^0\mathbf{R}_1$. ${}^0\mathbf{R}_1$ is a 3×3-matrix depending on the parameter θ. Hence, we will write ${}^0\mathbf{R}_1(\theta)$.
We now define the combined angular velocity as

$$\omega = \omega_0 + {}^0\mathbf{R}_1(\theta)\omega_1. \tag{4.40}$$

Then ω is again a vector, given with respect to the base frame, so that we can iterate the definition, for more (revolute) joints.
Here we have simply defined the composite angular velocity by a vector addition. We must now confirm that this definition is in agreement with our intuitive understanding of a combined rotation of two coordinate frames. This will be done in the following example. The example will also illustrate the application of angular velocities.

Example 4.3

We are given a robot with four revolute joints. The four joints form a kinematic chain, as in typical robots. Now suppose the four rotations are the following:

1. Rotation about the z-axis of the base frame S_0 (angle α)
2. Rotation about the x-axis of the new coordinate system S_1 (angle β)
3. Rotation about the x-axis of S_2 (angle $-\beta$)
4. Rotation about the z-axis of S_3 (angle $-\alpha$)

Assume also that

$$\alpha(t) = t,$$
$$\beta(t) = t. \tag{4.41}$$

Hence,

$$-\alpha(t) = -t,$$
$$-\beta(t) = -t. \tag{4.42}$$

Then we have

$$\omega_0 = \begin{pmatrix} 0 \\ 0 \\ 1 \end{pmatrix}, \qquad \omega_1 = \begin{pmatrix} 1 \\ 0 \\ 0 \end{pmatrix}, \tag{4.43}$$

and

$$\omega_2 = \begin{pmatrix} -1 \\ 0 \\ 0 \end{pmatrix}, \qquad \omega_3 = \begin{pmatrix} 0 \\ 0 \\ -1 \end{pmatrix}. \tag{4.44}$$

From Chap. 3 we know that the combined rotation is simply given by the matrix product

$$\mathbf{R}(z, \alpha(t))\mathbf{R}(x, \beta(t))\mathbf{R}(x, -\beta(t))\mathbf{R}(z, -\alpha(t))). \tag{4.45}$$

Multiplying these matrices, we obtain

$$\mathbf{R}(z, \alpha(t))\mathbf{R}(x, \beta(t))\mathbf{R}(x, -\beta(t))\mathbf{R}(z, -\alpha(t))) = \begin{pmatrix} 1 & 0 & 0 \\ 0 & 1 & 0 \\ 0 & 0 & 1 \end{pmatrix} \tag{4.46}$$

i.e. a zero rotation. But we are not supposed to know this yet. Instead we would like to apply the composition rule for angular velocities. We should then obtain a total angular velocity of zero.
Recall that we must express all angular velocities in the common base frame. Now ω_0 is already given in base coordinates.
To express ω_1 in base coordinates, we simply multiply with the matrix

$${}^0\mathbf{R}_1 = \mathbf{R}(z, \alpha(t)). \tag{4.47}$$

Thus, the angular velocity of S_2 with respect to S_1, given in base coordinates is

$$\mathbf{R}(z, \alpha(t))\omega_1. \tag{4.48}$$

Likewise, ω_2 is base coordinates is

$$\mathbf{R}(z, \alpha(t))\mathbf{R}(x, \beta(t))\omega_2. \tag{4.49}$$

Finally, ω_3 in base coordinates is

$$\mathbf{R}(z, \alpha(t))\mathbf{R}(x, \beta(t))\mathbf{R}(x, -\beta(t))\omega_3 = \mathbf{R}(z, \alpha(t))\omega_3. \tag{4.50}$$

Adding and evaluating, we obtain

$$\omega_0 + \mathbf{R}(z, \alpha(t))\omega_1 + \mathbf{R}(z, \alpha(t))\mathbf{R}(x, \beta(t))\omega_2 + \mathbf{R}(z, \alpha(t))\omega_3 =$$

$$\begin{pmatrix} 0 \\ 0 \\ 1 \end{pmatrix} + \begin{pmatrix} c_\alpha & -s_\alpha & 0 \\ s_\alpha & c_\alpha & 0 \\ 0 & 0 & 1 \end{pmatrix} \begin{pmatrix} 1 \\ 0 \\ 0 \end{pmatrix} + \begin{pmatrix} c_\alpha & -s_\alpha & 0 \\ s_\alpha & c_\alpha & 0 \\ 0 & 0 & 1 \end{pmatrix} \begin{pmatrix} 1 & 0 & 0 \\ 0 & c_\beta & -s_\beta \\ 0 & s_\beta & c_\beta \end{pmatrix} \begin{pmatrix} -1 \\ 0 \\ 0 \end{pmatrix}$$

$$+ \begin{pmatrix} c_\alpha & -s_\alpha & 0 \\ s_\alpha & c_\alpha & 0 \\ 0 & 0 & 1 \end{pmatrix} \begin{pmatrix} 0 \\ 0 \\ -1 \end{pmatrix} = \begin{pmatrix} 0 \\ 0 \\ 0 \end{pmatrix}. \tag{4.51}$$

(End of Example 4.3)

With the definitions of angular and linear velocity, we can specify our goals with respect to the geometric Jacobian. Our goal is thus to find two $3 \times n$ matrices $\mathbf{J}_v$ and $\mathbf{J}_\omega$, such that the linear velocity $\mathbf{v}$ and the angular velocity ω of the end effector can be expressed in terms of the joint velocity vector $\dot{\theta}$ as

$$\begin{aligned} \mathbf{v} &= \mathbf{J}_v \dot{\theta}, \\ \omega &= \mathbf{J}_\omega \dot{\theta}. \end{aligned} \tag{4.52}$$

The two parts $\mathbf{J}_v$ and $\mathbf{J}_\omega$ of the geometric Jacobian will then be assembled into a single matrix

$$\mathbf{J} = \begin{pmatrix} \mathbf{J}_v \\ \mathbf{J}_\omega \end{pmatrix}. \tag{4.53}$$

We then have

$$\begin{pmatrix} \mathbf{v} \\ \omega \end{pmatrix} = \mathbf{J}\dot{\theta}. \tag{4.54}$$

This is a direct extension of Eq. 4.28. Notice again that in this equation, both the angular and the linear velocity (of our effector) are given in terms of the base frame.

Theorem 4.1:

For a robot with n revolute joints, the geometric Jacobian is given by

$$\mathbf{J} = \begin{pmatrix} \mathbf{J}_v \\ \mathbf{J}_\omega \end{pmatrix} = \begin{pmatrix} \mathbf{z}_0 \times (\mathbf{p}_n - \mathbf{p}_0) & \mathbf{z}_1 \times (\mathbf{p}_n - \mathbf{p}_1) & \dots & \mathbf{z}_{n-1} \times (\mathbf{p}_n - \mathbf{p}_{n-1}) \\ \mathbf{z}_0 & \mathbf{z}_1 & \dots & \mathbf{z}_{n-1} \end{pmatrix}. \tag{4.55}$$

Here again, $\mathbf{p}_i$ denotes the position of the origin of the i-th DH-frame, and can be read from the last column of the DH-matrix ${}^0\mathbf{M}_i$ (see Chap. 3). Likewise, $\mathbf{z}_i$ is short for

$${}^0\mathbf{R}_i \begin{pmatrix} 0 \\ 0 \\ 1 \end{pmatrix}, \tag{4.56}$$

where ${}^0\mathbf{R}_i$ is the 3×3 rotational part of ${}^0\mathbf{M}_i$. Clearly, both $\mathbf{p}_i$ and $\mathbf{z}_i$ can be computed with the forward analysis methods from Chap. 3. Notice that the theorem requires robots with revolute joints. In case joint i is a prismatic joint, we replace the column

$$\begin{pmatrix} \mathbf{z}_{i-1} \times (\mathbf{p}_n - \mathbf{p}_{i-1}) \\ \mathbf{z}_{i-1} \end{pmatrix} \tag{4.57}$$

by the column

$$\begin{pmatrix} \mathbf{z}_{i-1} \\ 0 \end{pmatrix}. \tag{4.58}$$

Before we prove the theorem, we will look at two examples.

Example 4.4

We begin with the one-joint robot from Fig. 4.5. Here, we have

$$\mathbf{p}_n = \mathbf{p}_1 = \begin{pmatrix} c_1 \\ s_1 \\ 0 \end{pmatrix}. \tag{4.59}$$

Also,

$$z_0 = \begin{pmatrix} 0 \\ 0 \\ 1 \end{pmatrix}. \tag{4.60}$$

Thus

$$z_0 \times (\mathbf{p}_1 - \mathbf{p}_0) = z_0 \times \mathbf{p}_1 = \begin{pmatrix} 0 \\ 0 \\ 1 \end{pmatrix} \times \begin{pmatrix} c_1 \\ s_1 \\ 0 \end{pmatrix} = \begin{pmatrix} -s_1 \\ c_1 \\ 0 \end{pmatrix}. \tag{4.61}$$

This gives $\mathbf{J}_{v1}$.
Moving joint 1 with a magnitude of $\dot{\theta}_1$ will hence result in a linear velocity of $\mathbf{p}_1$ of

$$\dot{\theta}_1 \begin{pmatrix} -s_1 \\ c_1 \\ 0 \end{pmatrix}. \tag{4.62}$$

We see that this is consistent with the linear velocity $\mathbf{v}$ in our definition, which we had looked at in Example 4.2 (see Eq. 4.39).
For $\mathbf{J}_{\omega_1}$, we have

$$\mathbf{J}_{\omega 1} = z_0 = \begin{pmatrix} 0 \\ 0 \\ 1 \end{pmatrix}. \tag{4.63}$$

Thus the angular velocity (again joint 1 moving at magnitude $\dot{\theta}_1$) is

$$\begin{pmatrix} 0 \\ 0 \\ \dot{\theta}_1 \end{pmatrix}. \tag{4.64}$$

Therefore the full geometric Jacobian is

$$\begin{pmatrix} \mathbf{J}_v \\ \mathbf{J}_\omega \end{pmatrix} = \begin{pmatrix} -s_1 \\ c_1 \\ 0 \\ 0 \\ 0 \\ 1 \end{pmatrix}. \tag{4.65}$$

Very similarly, for the two-link manipulator (see Fig. 4.1), we obtain

$$\mathbf{J} = \begin{pmatrix} \mathbf{J}_v \\ \mathbf{J}_\omega \end{pmatrix} = \begin{pmatrix} -l_1 s_1 - l_2 s_{12} & -l_2 s_{12} \\ l_1 c_1 + l_2 c_{12} & +l_2 c_{12} \\ 0 & 0 \\ 0 & 0 \\ 0 & 0 \\ 1 & 1 \end{pmatrix}. \tag{4.66}$$

We compare to the matrix derived in Eq. 4.27. Clearly, the first two lines are the same. The third line in Eq. 4.66 has only zeros. This is simply due to the fact that we now look at the Jacobi-matrix for a full three-dimensional robot, and our planar two-link manipulator can never leave the plane. Finally, the three lines at the bottom of Eq. 4.66 describe angular velocity, and we see that we add the angular velocity from the two joints.

Finally, we look at an extension of the two-link manipulator. We add a third revolute joint at the end of the two-link manipulator. The entire mechanism can only move in the plane. The length of the third link is l_3.

In this case, we obtain the geometric Jacobi-matrix

$$\mathbf{J} = \begin{pmatrix} -l_1 s_1 - l_2 s_{12} - l_3 s_{123} & -l_2 s_{12} - l_3 s_{123} & -l_3 s_{123} \\ l_1 c_1 + l_2 c_{12} + l_3 c_{123} & l_2 c_{12} + l_3 c_{123} & l_3 c_{123} \\ 0 & 0 & 0 \\ 0 & 0 & 0 \\ 0 & 0 & 0 \\ 1 & 1 & 1 \end{pmatrix}. \tag{4.67}$$

(End of Example 4.4)

We now turn to the proof of Theorem 4.1, for revolute joints.

Proof of Theorem 4.1 (Revolute Joints)

The matrix in Eq. 4.55 consists of two lines. We will first consider the second line.
We will see that it follows directly from the composition rule for angular velocities.
We must show (compare Eq. 4.54) that

$$\omega = \mathbf{J}_\omega \begin{pmatrix} \dot{\theta}_1 \\ \vdots \\ \dot{\theta}_n \end{pmatrix}. \tag{4.68}$$

Given the definition of J in Eq. 4.55, we have

$$\mathbf{J}_\omega = \left(\mathbf{z}_0\ \mathbf{z}_1\ \ldots\ \mathbf{z}_{n-1},\right) \tag{4.69}$$

and we must show that

$$\omega = \mathbf{z}_0\dot{\theta}_1 + \mathbf{z}_1\dot{\theta}_2 + \ldots + \mathbf{z}_{n-1}\dot{\theta}_n. \tag{4.70}$$

From the composition rule (Eq. 4.40), we have

$$\omega = \omega_0 + {}^0\mathbf{R}_1\omega_1 + \ldots + {}^0\mathbf{R}_{n-1}\omega_{n-1}. \tag{4.71}$$

Each individual rotation is a rotation about the z-axis of a DH-frame, hence (written in coordinates of DH-frame S_i) we have

$$\omega_i = \begin{pmatrix} 0 \\ 0 \\ 1 \end{pmatrix} \dot{\theta}_{i+1} \tag{4.72}$$

for $0 \le i < n$.
We insert this into Eq. 4.71, and obtain

$$\omega = \begin{pmatrix} 0 \\ 0 \\ 1 \end{pmatrix} \dot{\theta}_1 + {}^0\mathbf{R}_1 \begin{pmatrix} 0 \\ 0 \\ 1 \end{pmatrix} \dot{\theta}_2 + \ldots + {}^0\mathbf{R}_{n-1} \begin{pmatrix} 0 \\ 0 \\ 1 \end{pmatrix} \dot{\theta}_n. \tag{4.73}$$

But by the definition in Eq. 4.56,

$$\begin{pmatrix}0\\0\\1\end{pmatrix} = \mathbf{z}_0 \tag{4.74}$$

and

$${}^0\mathbf{R}_i \begin{pmatrix}0\\0\\1\end{pmatrix} = \mathbf{z}_i. \tag{4.75}$$

Comparing to Eq. 4.56 gives the desired result for the second matrix line.

We now turn to linear velocities, i.e. the first line of the matrix in the theorem.

We must show

$$\mathbf{v} = \mathbf{z}_0 \times (\mathbf{p}_n - \mathbf{p}_0)\dot{\theta}_1 + \mathbf{z}_1 \times (\mathbf{p}_n - \mathbf{p}_1)\dot{\theta}_2 + \ldots + \mathbf{z}_{n-1} \times (\mathbf{p}_n - \mathbf{p}_{n-1})\dot{\theta}_n \tag{4.76}$$

We first assume, only a single joint, namely joint i, is moving. All other joints do not move. We observe that in this case, we already have a proof of the result. If we move only a single joint, then what we must show simply reduces to Eq. 4.39.

The case of multiple moving joints will now directly follow from the composition rule for angular velocities. Recall that we defined the linear velocity $\mathbf{v}$ of a point $\mathbf{p}$ (resulting from an angular velocity) in Eq. 4.37. i.e. $\mathbf{v} = \omega \times \mathbf{p}$.

Assume now we have two linear velocities $\mathbf{v}_1$ and $\mathbf{v}_2$ both acting on a point $\mathbf{p}$.

Further assume $\mathbf{v}_1$ and $\mathbf{v}_2$ stem from angular velocities ω_1 and ω_2 respectively, so that

$$\mathbf{v}_1 = \omega_1 \times \mathbf{p}, \tag{4.77}$$

$$\mathbf{v}_2 = \omega_2 \times \mathbf{p}. \tag{4.78}$$

$$\tag{4.79}$$

But then $\mathbf{v}_1$ and $\mathbf{v}_2$ are vectors, and we can add them:

$$\mathbf{v}_1 + \mathbf{v}_2 = \omega_1 \times \mathbf{p} + \omega_2 \times \mathbf{p} \tag{4.80}$$

By linearity, the right hand side of the last equation reduces to

$$\omega_1 \times \mathbf{p} + \omega_2 \times \mathbf{p} = (\omega_1 + \omega_2) \times \mathbf{p}. \tag{4.81}$$

We see that the vector $\mathbf{v}_1 + \mathbf{v}_2$ also represents a linear velocity, acting on the same point $\mathbf{p}$. But this new linear velocity stems from an angular velocity ω, for which we have

$$\omega_1 + \omega_2 = \omega. \tag{4.82}$$

Similar to the composition rule for angular velocities, we thus obtain a composition rule for linear velocities (stemming from angular velocities), which holds whenever the vectors are defined within the same base frame. But now the desired result in Eq. 4.76 follows from the fact that all vectors $\mathbf{z}_i$ and $\mathbf{p}_i$ are given with respect to the base frame.

(End of Proof)

In the following example we will set up the geometric Jacobian for a C-arm.

Example 4.5

In Eq. 4.3 we derived explicit velocity functions for CT-imaging with the C-arm. Recall that we rotate the orbital axis of a C-arm such that the center point of the beam axis (point $\mathbf{p}$) remains at the same position. We saw that we must compensate with the two prismatic joints. The derivation in Eq. 4.3 was elementary, and we did not use Jacobi-matrices.
We will now set up the geometric Jacobian for CT-imaging with the C-arm. We can simplify the construction. As discussed in the introduction of this chapter, only three joints are needed in this case. Thus, we set the joint angles θ_2 and θ_4 to zero. Figure 4.7 shows the null position and the coordinate systems.
We obtain the DH-parameters shown in the following table.

i	α_i	a_i	d_i	θ_i
1	-90	0	d_1	0
2	90	a_4	d_3	-90
3	90	a_5	0	$\theta_5 + 90$

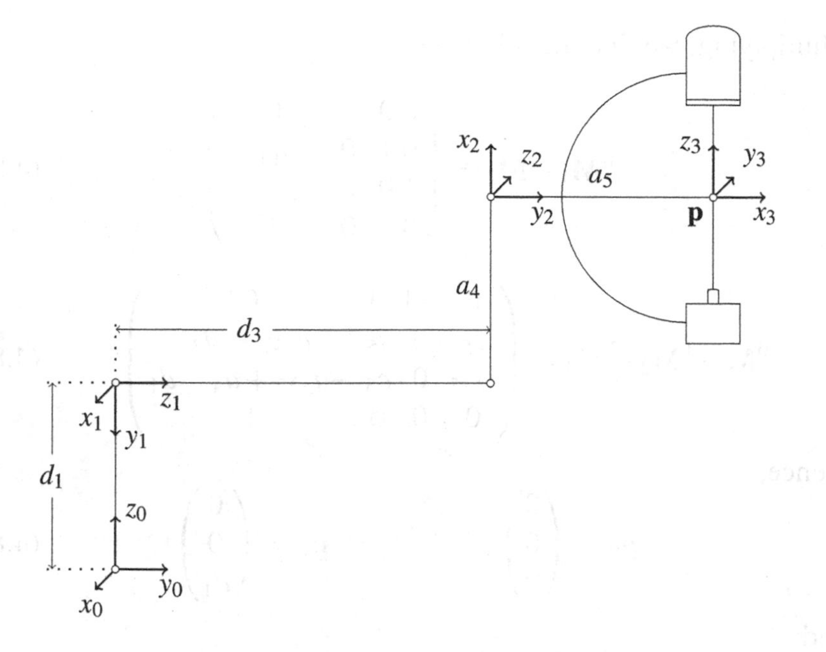

Fig. 4.7: Null position and coordinate systems for **CT** imaging with the C-arm

From the DH-parameters, we obtain the matrices

$$^{0}\mathbf{M}_1 = \begin{pmatrix} 1 & 0 & 0 & 0 \\ 0 & 0 & 1 & 0 \\ 0 & -1 & 0 & d_1 \\ 0 & 0 & 0 & 1 \end{pmatrix}, \tag{4.83}$$

$$^{1}\mathbf{M}_2 = \begin{pmatrix} 0 & 0 & -1 & 0 \\ -1 & 0 & 0 & -a_4 \\ 0 & 1 & 0 & d_3 \\ 0 & 0 & 0 & 1 \end{pmatrix}, \tag{4.84}$$

$$^{2}\mathbf{M}_3 = \begin{pmatrix} -s_5 & 0 & c_5 & -a_5 s_5 \\ c_5 & 0 & s_5 & a_5 c_5 \\ 0 & 1 & 0 & 0 \\ 0 & 0 & 0 & 1 \end{pmatrix}. \tag{4.85}$$

Multiplying, we find the following:

$$ {}^{0}\mathbf{M}_1 \cdot {}^{1}\mathbf{M}_2 = \begin{pmatrix} 0 & 0 & -1 & 0 \\ 0 & 1 & 0 & d_3 \\ 1 & 0 & 0 & a_4 + d_1 \\ 0 & 0 & 0 & 1 \end{pmatrix} \tag{4.86} $$

$$ {}^{0}\mathbf{M}_1 \cdot {}^{1}\mathbf{M}_2 \cdot {}^{2}\mathbf{M}_3 = \begin{pmatrix} 0 & -1 & 0 & 0 \\ c_5 & 0 & s_5 & a_5 c_5 + d_3 \\ -s_5 & 0 & c_5 & -a_5 s_5 + a_4 + d_1 \\ 0 & 0 & 0 & 1 \end{pmatrix} \tag{4.87} $$

Hence,

$$ \mathbf{p}_0 = \begin{pmatrix} 0 \\ 0 \\ 0 \end{pmatrix}, \qquad \mathbf{p}_1 = \begin{pmatrix} 0 \\ 0 \\ d_1 \end{pmatrix} \tag{4.88} $$

and

$$ \mathbf{p}_2 = \begin{pmatrix} 0 \\ d_3 \\ a_4 + d_1 \end{pmatrix}, \qquad \mathbf{p}_3 = \begin{pmatrix} 0 \\ a_5 c_5 + d_3 \\ -a_5 s_5 + a_4 + d_1 \end{pmatrix}. \tag{4.89} $$

Finally,

$$ \mathbf{z}_0 = \begin{pmatrix} 0 \\ 0 \\ 1 \end{pmatrix}, \qquad \mathbf{z}_1 = \begin{pmatrix} 0 \\ 1 \\ 0 \end{pmatrix} \tag{4.90} $$

and

$$ \mathbf{z}_2 = \begin{pmatrix} -1 \\ 0 \\ 0 \end{pmatrix}, \qquad \mathbf{z}_3 = \begin{pmatrix} 0 \\ s_5 \\ c_5 \end{pmatrix}. \tag{4.91} $$

The first two joints are prismatic. Thus

$$ \mathbf{J}_v = \left(\mathbf{z}_0 \; \mathbf{z}_1 \; \mathbf{z}_2 \times (\mathbf{p}_3 - \mathbf{p}_2) \right). \tag{4.92} $$

Evaluating, we obtain

$$ \mathbf{J}_v = \begin{pmatrix} 0 & 0 & 0 \\ 0 & 1 & -a_5 s_5 \\ 1 & 0 & -a_5 c_5 \end{pmatrix}. \tag{4.93} $$

We have

$$\dot{\mathbf{p}} = \mathbf{J}_v \dot{\theta}. \tag{4.94}$$

Since we require $\mathbf{p}$ to remain fixed, we have

$$\dot{\mathbf{p}} = \begin{pmatrix} 0 \\ 0 \\ 0 \end{pmatrix}. \tag{4.95}$$

Inserting this into Eq. 4.94, we obtain

$$\begin{pmatrix} 0 \\ 0 \\ 0 \end{pmatrix} = \begin{pmatrix} 0 & 0 & 0 \\ 0 & 1 & -a_5 s_5 \\ 1 & 0 & -a_5 c_5 \end{pmatrix} \begin{pmatrix} \dot{d}_1 \\ \dot{d}_3 \\ \dot{\theta}_5 \end{pmatrix}. \tag{4.96}$$

Furthermore, we move the orbital joint (joint 5) with constant velocity during CT-imaging. Therefore, we can assume that

$$\dot{\theta}_5 = \theta_5'(t) = 1. \tag{4.97}$$

Hence, the last two matrix lines of Eq. 4.96 show that

$$\begin{aligned} \dot{d}_1 - a_5 \cos(t) &= 0, \\ \dot{d}_3 - a_5 \sin(t) &= 0 \end{aligned} \tag{4.98}$$

or that

$$\begin{aligned} \dot{d}_1 &= a_5 \cos(t), \\ \dot{d}_3 &= a_5 \sin(t). \end{aligned} \tag{4.99}$$

We have thus confirmed the result in Eq. 4.3 using the geometric Jacobian. The approach taken in Eq. 4.3 was elementary. We see that the geometric Jacobian is a general tool for finding velocity functions. We will see other applications of the geometric Jacobian in later chapters. Specifically, the geometric Jacobian will be helpful when analyzing forces and joint torques.

(End of Example 4.5)

Example 4.6

Appendix C lists the DH-matrices for the six-joint elbow manipulator and also for the Kuka-DLR seven-joint robot discussed in Chap. 3. From the DH-matrices we derive the geometric Jacobians for both robots.

(End of Example 4.6)

4.5 Singularities and Dexterity

An $n \times n$-matrix $\mathbf{J}$ is called regular if the inverse $\mathbf{J}^{-1}$ exists. Otherwise, $\mathbf{J}$ is called singular. In Remark 4.3 we saw that the Jacobian matrix of a given robot can be singular or regular, depending on the robot configuration. We will call a robot configuration *singular* if the Jacobian for this configuration is singular. Singular configurations will also be called singularities, for short.
We saw above that the Jacobian is not always an $n \times n$-matrix. Rather, for the case of the three-joint robot we obtained a 6×3-matrix (see Eq. 4.67). In this case, ($n \times m$-matrix, $m < n$) we would also like to define singularities, in much the same way. Here, a singularity is a configuration in which the Jacobian has rank less than m.
Extending this approach, we can look at products of the form $\mathbf{J}^{\mathrm{T}}\mathbf{J}$. Assume $\mathbf{J}$ is a 6×3-matrix. Then $\mathbf{J}^{\mathrm{T}}\mathbf{J}$ is a 3×3-matrix. We now use the value d defined in the following equation as a measure for the dexterity of the robot at a given configuration:

$$d = \sqrt{|\det(\mathbf{J}^{\mathrm{T}}\mathbf{J})|} \tag{4.100}$$

Clearly, this definition will work not just for 6×3-matrices, but for general $n \times m$-matrices.
Comparing to the dexterity measures defined in Chap. 3, we see that computing the solid angle requires evaluating orientations in a large grid, while the measure d gives an analytic description of the local dexterity.

Exercises

Exercise 4.1 *Velocity Kinematics*

Insert the functions from Eqs. 4.1 and 4.2 into the forward 4×4-matrix for the C-arm, and verify that the target point O_5 remains fixed while moving t from 0 to 2π.

Exercise 4.2 *Linearized Rotation Matrix*

Derive the matrix $\mathbf{D}$ in Eq. 4.15.

Exercise 4.3 *Interpolating Matrixes*

Given two orientation matrices, such as the matrices $\mathbf{O}$ and $\mathbf{O}'$ in Eqs. 4.5 and 4.6, find a series of interpolation matrices, and visualize the result in a small program.

Exercise 4.4 *Joint Velocities*

Write a short program for verifying the result in Eq. 4.34. Your result should look like the image in Fig. 4.8.

Exercise 4.5 *Analytic Jacobians*

Consider the two-link manipulator in Fig. 4.1. Assume the two link lengths are equal to 1. For this robot, the position of the tool tip is given by the equation

$$\begin{pmatrix} p_x \\ p_y \end{pmatrix} = \begin{pmatrix} c_1 + c_{12} \\ s_1 + s_{12} \end{pmatrix}. \tag{4.101}$$

We now assume our current position is given by $\theta_1 = \pi/2$ and $\theta_2 = -\pi/2$. This is the position shown in Fig. 4.9.
For this position of the robot, we evaluate the matrix equation

$$\begin{pmatrix} dx \\ dy \end{pmatrix} = \begin{pmatrix} \frac{\partial p_x}{\partial \theta_1} & \frac{\partial p_x}{\partial \theta_2} \\ \frac{\partial p_y}{\partial \theta_1} & \frac{\partial p_y}{\partial \theta_2} \end{pmatrix} \begin{pmatrix} d\theta_1 \\ d\theta_2 \end{pmatrix}. \tag{4.102}$$

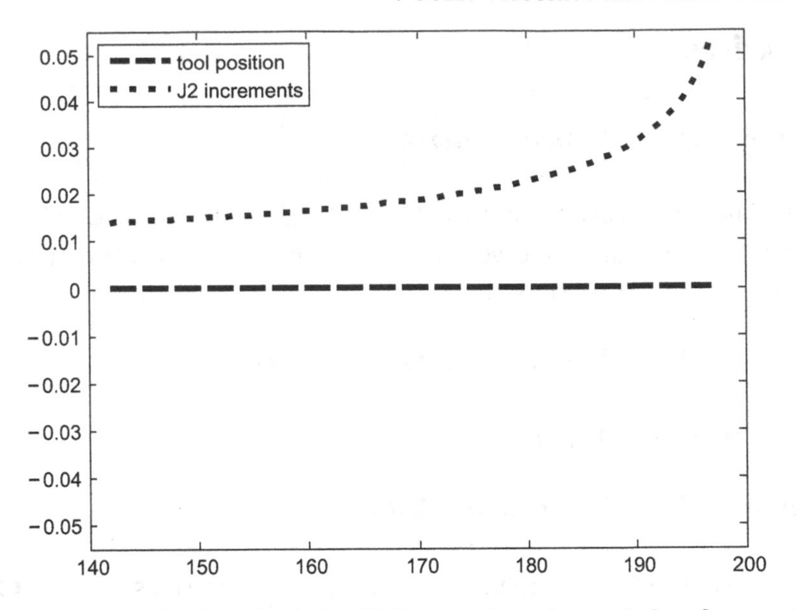

Fig. 4.8: Joint velocity (for joint 2) for moving the tool tip of a two-link manipulator along a line segment, see Eq. 4.34

Show that at the current position the matrix

$$\begin{pmatrix} \frac{\partial p_x}{\partial \theta_1} & \frac{\partial p_x}{\partial \theta_2} \\ \frac{\partial p_y}{\partial \theta_1} & \frac{\partial p_y}{\partial \theta_2} \end{pmatrix} \tag{4.103}$$

evaluates to

$$\begin{pmatrix} -1 & 0 \\ 1 & 1 \end{pmatrix}. \tag{4.104}$$

We thus have

$$\begin{aligned} dx &= -d\theta_1, \\ dy &= d\theta_1 + d\theta_2. \end{aligned} \tag{4.105}$$

Solving this for $d\theta_1$ and $d\theta_2$, we obtain

$$\begin{aligned} d\theta_1 &= -dx, \\ d\theta_2 &= dx + dy. \end{aligned} \tag{4.106}$$

Visualize this result by moving the robot tip to four positions in the vicinity of the current tip position.

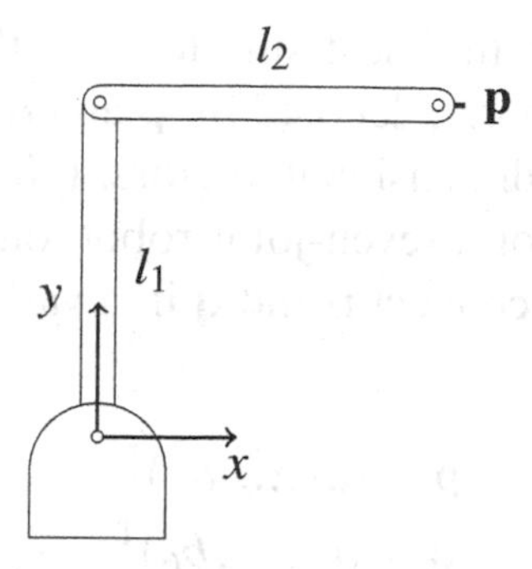

Fig. 4.9: Two link manipulator for position $\theta_1 = \pi/2$ and $\theta_2 = -\pi/2$

Exercise 4.6 ***Geometric Jacobians***

Verify the results in Eqs. 4.66 and 4.67 by direct calculation.

Exercise 4.7 ***Velocity Kinematics for the C-Arm***

The C-arm has five joints. We fix two of these joints, namely joints 2 and 4, and set the joint angles for these two joints to zero. Then the remaining mechanism has three joints. For non-vertical imaging, we include the angulation axis, i.e. joint 4. Set up the upper part of the geometric Jacobian matrix $\mathbf{J}_v$ for arbitrary non-vertical positions. Derive the explicit velocity functions for non-vertical CT-acquisition based on the Jacobian. Compare to the result from Sect. 4.1.

Exercise 4.8 ***Trajectories***

Suppose we have a six-joint robot with revolute joints. The so-called *joint space* of the robot is a six-dimensional space. Each coordinate corresponds to one joint angle. Thus, a position of the robot (given angle values for all joints) can be represented by a point $\mathbf{p} = (a_1, ..., a_6)^{\mathrm{T}}$ in joint space. Likewise, a curve in joint space represents a motion of the robot.
It is often necessary to specify a robot motion by a set of via-points. The via-points are points in joint space. Our goal is now to connect the via-points by a continuous path. We assume the total time for the

motion is 1 second. In the most simple case, the only via-points are the start and the goal point, denoted by $\mathbf{p}$ and $\mathbf{q}$.
Both $\mathbf{p}$ and $\mathbf{q}$ are six-dimensional vectors. (Notice we still assume a six-joint robot here. For a seven-joint robot, our joint space is seven-dimensional.) We can connect $\mathbf{p}$ and $\mathbf{q}$ in a variety of ways.
Let

$$\begin{aligned} \mathbf{p} &= (a_1, ..., a_6)^{\mathrm{T}}, \\ \mathbf{q} &= (b_1, ..., b_6)^{\mathrm{T}}. \end{aligned} \tag{4.107}$$

We look at the path of a single angle, e.g. the first one. Then we must move $\theta = \theta_1$, i.e. the first angle, from a_1 to b_1.
Furthermore, we can constrain the velocity of the joint during the motion. It is useful to require $\theta'(0) = 0$ and $\theta'(1) = 0$, i.e. the velocity at the two end points of the motion should be zero. We thus have four constraints on the trajectory (for the first joint).
Thus

$$\begin{aligned} \theta(0) &= a_1, \\ \theta(1) &= b_1, \\ \theta'(0) &= 0, \\ \theta'(1) &= 0. \end{aligned} \tag{4.108}$$

A cubic polynomial is a polynomial of the form

$$\theta(t) = c_0 + c_1 t + c_2 t^2 + c_3 t^3. \tag{4.109}$$

a) Compute values for the coefficients c_i of the polynomial such that the constraints in Eq. 4.108 are satisfied.
Hint: from the constraints, you can derive four linear equations with the variables c_i.
b) Above we had assumed the total time for the path to be 1s. Generalize to the case of arbitrary total time.
c) Generalize the result from part a) to the case of n via-points.
Hint: assume we specify a non-zero velocity u at the start point of the trajectory. Likewise, v denotes the velocity at the end point.

We first generalize the equations derived in a) to this case. Then a path with several via points is simply obtained by requiring zero velocities at the start and end point, and appropriate non-zero velocities at the intermediate points. Two consecutive segments share the velocity value at the common point.

Summary

Similar to the forward analysis of a manipulator via the DH-rules, the Jacobi-matrix in Eq. 4.27 can be derived in a systematic way, for arbitrary kinematic linkages. The Jacobi-matrix is given by

$$\mathbf{J} = \begin{pmatrix} \mathbf{z}_0 \times (\mathbf{p}_n - \mathbf{p}_0) & \mathbf{z}_1 \times (\mathbf{p}_n - \mathbf{p}_1) & \dots & \mathbf{z}_{n-1} \times (\mathbf{p}_n - \mathbf{p}_{n-1}) \\ \mathbf{z}_0 & \mathbf{z}_1 & \dots & \mathbf{z}_{n-1} \end{pmatrix}. \tag{4.110}$$

With the Jacobi-matrix, we can express the angular and linear velocities of the end effector as functions of the joint velocities. In appropriate cases, the Jacobi-matrix is invertible. By inverting the Jacobi-matrix, we can do the opposite, namely derive explicit functions for the joint motions needed to produce a given velocity at the effector.

The Jacobi-matrix is useful for many other applications. Thus, we can characterize singular configurations of the robot. As a further application, in Chap. 9 we will derive expressions for the force applied by the end effector, given joint torques.

Notes

The text book by Spong, Hutchinson and Vidyasagar [3] gives a detailed analytical derivation of the geometric Jacobi-matrix (including prismatic joints), together with an analysis of singularities and manipulability for many robot constructions. This includes an analytical proof for the composition rule for angular velocity, based on algebraic properties of skew-symmetric matrices. A similar approach is taken in the text book by John Craig [2]. Our description summarizes the results from [3] and [2].

References

[1] A. H. Barr, B. Currin, S. Gabriel, and J. F. Hughes. Smooth interpolation of orientations with angular velocity constraints using quaternions. *SIGGRAPH Computer Graphics*, **26**(2):313–320, 1992. DOI 10.1145/142920.134086.

[2] J. J. Craig. *Introduction to Robotics: Mechanics and Control.* Prentice Hall, 3rd edition, 2005.

[3] M. W. Spong, S. Hutchinson, and M. Vidyasagar. *Robot Modeling and Control.* John Wiley & Sons, Inc., New York, 1st edition, 2005.

Chapter 5
Navigation and Registration

In the preceding chapters we discussed mathematical methods for analyzing robot motion. We will now see how a robot can interact with its environment in a medical application.

Typical medical navigation systems rely on medical imaging. Medical imaging is a vast field of its own, but here we only need a basic connection to robotics. The main elements for establishing this connection are image registration and calibration.

We saw two examples for navigation methods in the introduction (Chap. 1). The examples were: stereotaxic navigation and radiologic navigation. In both cases registration was needed.

Registration brings structures into alignment (Fig. 5.1). In the most simple case, we register two images showing the same object, e.g. a femur bone.

Assume the two images are given as data files. Since the two images are different, the bone will show up in two different positions. We place the second image on top of the first, and manually rotate/translate the top image in the graphical user interface until alignment is reached. We then output the rotation angle θ, as well as the translational displacement (Δx, Δy) in x- and y-directions (Fig. 5.1).

In this example, the registration is done manually. We now consider a more complex example (Fig. 5.2). This example illustrates the connection between navigation and registration. Here, the goal is to register the position of a femur bone in space, during surgery.

A. Schweikard, F. Ernst, *Medical Robotics*,
DOI 10.1007/978-3-319-22891-4_5

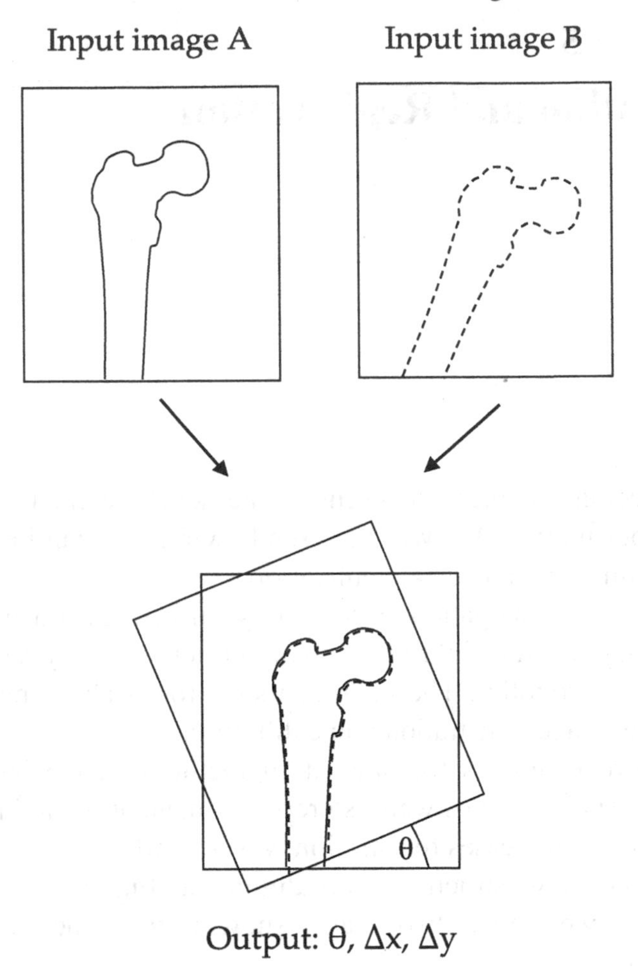

Fig. 5.1: Registration

We first observe that the head of a femur bone has a spherical shape. Thus we can proceed as follows. We take two X-ray images of the femur head from two different angles with a C-arm. We record the position of the C-arm for each of the two images, via markers attached to the C-arm. In each X-ray image, we mark the femur head by drawing a circle onto the image. The software then constructs two cones. The cones are defined by the C-arm's source points (in two distinct positions for the two cones) and the circles delineating the femur head. By intersecting the two cones, we obtain a sphere in space, which corresponds to the current position of the femur head.

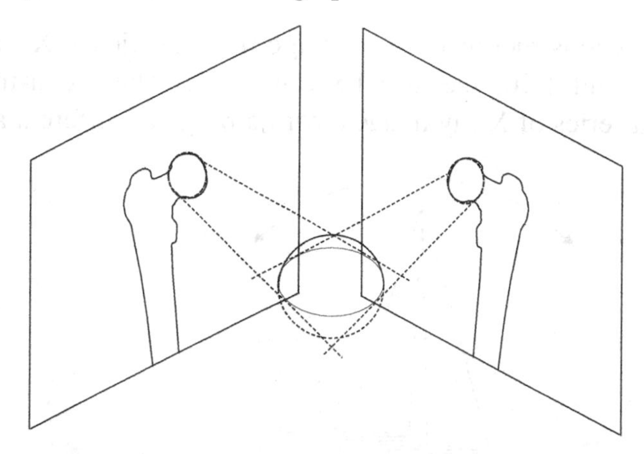

Fig. 5.2: Registration of a femur head with C-arm X-ray images (2D-3D registration)

This example (Fig. 5.2) illustrates several basic concepts. Firstly, we have an example of stereo X-ray imaging as a basis for navigation. Secondly, we have an example of a 2D-3D registration. The two images (X-ray) are two dimensional, and the structure to be registered is three-dimensional. Strictly speaking, we do not register two images in this example. Instead, we register a pair of images (X-ray images) to a model of an anatomical target. This model is a sphere.
Notice that the general problem of registration has a much larger range of applications than just navigation. However, surgical navigation relies on dedicated registration methods. We will focus on this type of registration in this chapter.
Several different types of registration methods are frequently used: landmark-based registration, point-based registration, contour-based registration, intensity-based registration and elastic registration. We will see examples for each type in this chapter.

5.1 Digitally Reconstructed Radiographs

We now consider digitally reconstructed radiographs (DRRs). They form the basis for a widely used 2D-3D registration method.

Recall the reconstruction of a CT image from a series of X-ray images (Figs. 1.19 and 1.20, see also Exercise 1.2). The reconstruction is based on a series of X-ray images from a range of different angles.

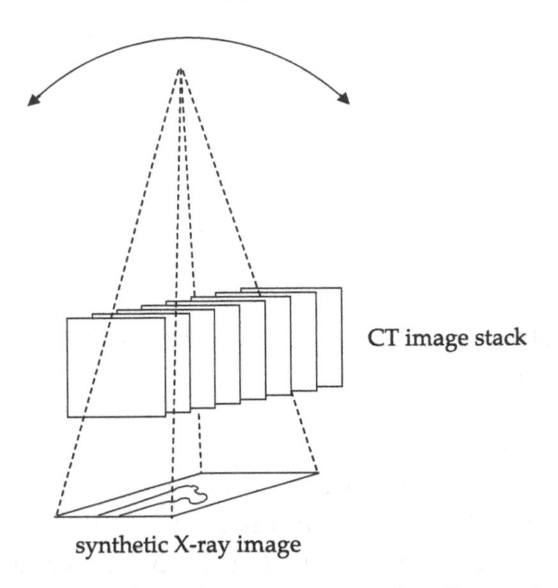

Fig. 5.3: Digitally reconstructed radiographs

Now we invert the reconstruction process. We take the CT data set, and project it onto a two-dimensional surface (Fig. 5.3). We project along a fixed direction in space. This resembles the process of taking an X-ray image, but now our X-ray image is synthetic. We repeat the projection for a large number of distinct directions. Thus we obtain a set of digitally reconstructed X-ray images (or radiographs), in which each image corresponds to one direction.
To apply DRRs in registration we proceed as follows. We compute the DRRs for the anatomical region before the intervention, and then take stereo X-ray images during the intervention (Fig. 5.4). The interoperative X-rays are called live images. To find an alignment position, we search for the pair of DRRs which matches the live images. The matching step simply consists of subtracting the synthetic images from the live images, which gives the result of our registration.
The subtraction proceeds pixel by pixel. This gives an error signal and we determine the DRR pair giving the minimal error signal. Since DRRs were computed from different directions, we can then extract the registration information (angles and translational displacements) for the live images.

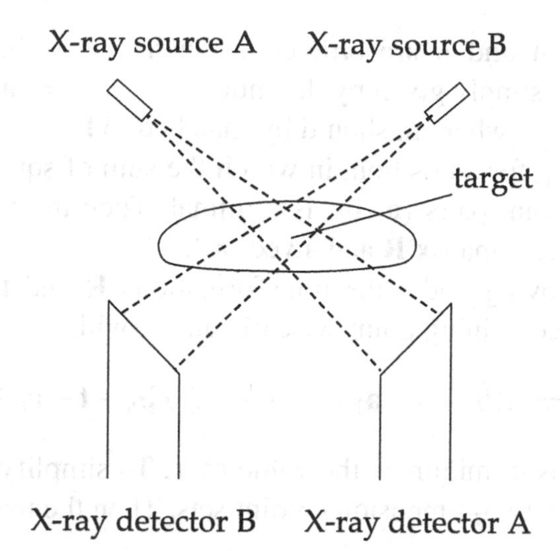

Fig. 5.4: Stereo X-ray imaging. Two fixed X-ray sources and two fixed detectors

One typical application of DRR-registration is the registration of the human skull for treating brain tumors. Here fixed X-ray sources and detectors are used, and typically 400–600 pairs of DRRs are matched to intra-operative live shots.

5.2 Points and Landmarks

Assume we have two clouds of points in space. Call the clouds A and B. Our goal is to bring the two clouds into registration. This means we must move cloud B in such a way that the two clouds match. We allow the point cloud B to move under rotation and translation, but we do not allow B to deform. Thus our goal is to compute a translation vector t and a 3×3 orientation matrix $\mathbf{R}$ such that the set of points $\mathbf{R}\mathbf{b} + \mathbf{t}$ with points $\mathbf{b}$ from B will match A. We will also call B the floating point set, and A the fixed point set.
For simplicity we will first assume that the number of points in both clouds is the same, and that we know in advance which point $\mathbf{b}$ from B should be matched to which point $\mathbf{a}$ from A. With other words, we know the correspondence between the two sets. We thus assume

the points in A and B are ordered in such a way that the correspondences are simply given by the indexing, i.e. $A = (\mathbf{a}_1, \ldots, \mathbf{a}_n)$ and $B = (\mathbf{b}_1, \ldots, \mathbf{b}_n)$, where $\mathbf{a}_i$ should by matched to $\mathbf{b}_i$.
We are looking for a position, in which the sum of squared distances between the point pairs $(\mathbf{a}_i, \mathbf{b}_i)$ is minimal. Then the following approach computes a matrix $\mathbf{R}$ and a vector $\mathbf{t}$.
Since B is moving under the transformations $\mathbf{R}$ and $\mathbf{t}$, we have an expression f containing point-wise distances, with

$$f = \| \mathbf{R}\mathbf{b}_1 + \mathbf{t} - \mathbf{a}_1 \|^2 + \cdots + \| \mathbf{R}\mathbf{b}_n + \mathbf{t} - \mathbf{a}_n \|^2, \tag{5.1}$$

and our goal is to minimize the value of f. To simplify the problem, we first look at two-dimensional point sets. Then the matrix R has the form

$$\mathbf{R} = \begin{pmatrix} \cos\theta & -\sin\theta \\ \sin\theta & \cos\theta \end{pmatrix}. \tag{5.2}$$

The minimization function f has three parameters θ, t_x, t_y where θ is the angle in the matrix $\mathbf{R}$ and t_x, t_y are the coordinates of the vector $\mathbf{t}$:

$$f(\theta, t_x, t_y) = \| \mathbf{R}\mathbf{b}_1 + \mathbf{t} - \mathbf{a}_1 \|^2 + \cdots + \| \mathbf{R}\mathbf{b}_n + \mathbf{t} - \mathbf{a}_n \|^2 \tag{5.3}$$

For small angles, we can replace the expressions $\sin\theta$ and $\cos\theta$ (occurring in $\mathbf{R}$) by linear approximations: Set $\cos\theta$ to 1 and $\sin\theta$ to θ. We thus replace $\mathbf{R}$ from Eq. 5.2 by

$$\begin{pmatrix} 1 & -\theta \\ \theta & 1 \end{pmatrix}. \tag{5.4}$$

The function f is now a quadratic function in the three parameters t_x, t_y and θ. Notice that the coordinates of the points $\mathbf{a}_i, \mathbf{b}_i$ are constants here.
Taking the derivatives with respect to t_x, then with respect to t_y and with respect to θ gives three linear expressions. We set these three linear expressions to zero and obtain a system of three linear equations with three variables. The solution of this system gives an approximation for the desired parameters t_x, t_y and θ.
In the three-dimensional case, we can use the same method with one minor difference. Here the matrix $\mathbf{R}$ depends on three angles α, β, γ. We can linearize this matrix in the following way. Replace $\mathbf{R}$ by

$$\mathbf{D} = \begin{pmatrix} 1 & -\gamma & \beta \\ \gamma & 1 & -\alpha \\ -\beta & \alpha & 1 \end{pmatrix}. \tag{5.5}$$

We see that the matrix $\mathbf{D}$ is the matrix from Eq. 4.15. Thus, recall that $\mathbf{D} - \mathbf{I}$ is a skew-symmetric matrix. The derivation of the matrix $\mathbf{D}$ is not difficult, and is given in Chap. 4.
We again obtain a linear system of equations after taking derivatives. In this case we have a linear system of six equations in the six variables $t_x, t_y, t_z, \alpha, \beta, \gamma$.

Example 5.1

Suppose we wish to register the head of a patient to preoperative MR-data. This means, we have MR images of the patient. During the operation, we must move an instrument to a position marked on this MR image.

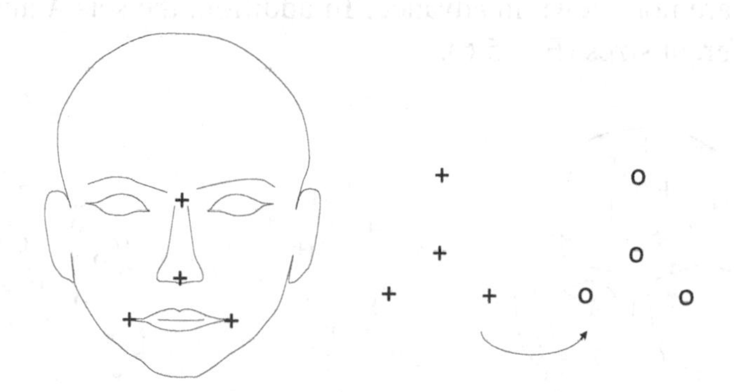

Fig. 5.5: Registration with landmarks

Figure 5.5 illustrates registration with landmarks, based on point cloud matching.
To register patient data during the intervention, we proceed as follows. We mark four landmark points on the head in the MR image data set (see figure). Additionally, we delineate the target in the brain on one or more of the MR slices. During the intervention, we touch the same four points (in the same order!) with the pointer of a tracking system, and record the positions (points marked as small circles in the figure).

We can then infer the position of the internal target point in the brain from the current position of the marker points.
In this example we consider the robotic system for transcranial magnetic stimulation in Fig. 1.16. A magnetic coil is held by a robot arm. The coil generates a short magnetic pulse, and acts as a stimulator for small regions on the cortex. The surgeon delineates a target on an MR image of the brain. The registration then provides a way to move the coil to the target. Repeated registration then allows for keeping the coil in the planned position during small involuntary motions of the patient.

(End of Example 5.1)

5.2.1 Iterative Closest Points

In many applications, point-to-point correspondences between the sets A and B are not known in advance. In addition, the sets A and B may have different sizes (Fig. 5.6).

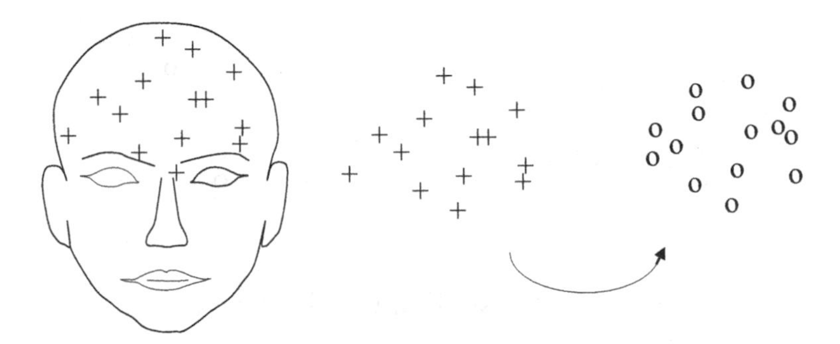

Fig. 5.6: Registration with surface points

Here the points are on the head surface, automatically extracted from an MR data set. A second cloud of points is acquired later, and our goal is to register the two point sets. In this case, an additional procedure must iteratively compute the best set of correspondences. Only heuristic methods are known for this problem, since the number

of possible pairwise correspondences for two sets of n points is $n!$. The iterative-closest-point method (ICP method) is an approximation method for this purpose.
ICP proceeds as follows. We again have two point sets A and B, but now the number of points in the two sets does not necessarily have to be the same. ICP alternates between a matching step and a moving step. The matching step determines a set of correspondences between points in A and B. The moving step computes a rotation matrix $\mathbf{R}$ and a translation vector $\mathbf{t}$.
Set $\mathbf{R} = \mathbf{I}$ (the identity matrix), $\mathbf{t} = 0$ and a random matching m_{new} between points A and B.
Repeat

1. Set $m_{old} = m_{new}$
2. Moving step: Given this matching m_{new}, compute $\mathbf{R}$ and $\mathbf{t}$.
3. Matching step: Compute a new matching m_{new} between the point sets after having moved the points in B by $\mathbf{R}$ and $\mathbf{t}$.

Until $m_{new} = m_{old}$
The stopping criterion can be modified, depending on the application. The moving step has been discussed above. For the matching step, proceed as follows. For each $\mathbf{a}$ in A, take the closest point in B, and add this match to the set of correspondences. Obviously, since the sizes of the sets A and B may be different, this will typically not result in a one-to-one matching. In this case, we can simply stop adding correspondences whenever one of the two sets has been exhausted.
For the matching step, we compute the nearest neighbors of the points by k-d-trees (see Exercise 5.2 at the end of this chapter).

5.3 Contour-Based Registration

Contour-based registration is a direct extension of the above point-based registration method. Instead of registering points in a set A to points in a set B, we now have contours in one or both sets. Suppose we are given a surface model of a bone reconstructed from CT data and projected bone contours from an X-ray image. Our goal is to estimate the spatial position of the bone.

To this end we want to place the surface model in such a way that the 2D bone contours match optimally.
Contour-based methods need contours, and hence segmented images to start from. Let us first assume the entire problem was two-dimensional. This 2D version of the problem does not have much practical value. But the discussion can be simplified quite substantially. Thus, we assume we have a 2D object and take images of this object from two camera positions C and C' (Fig. 5.7).
In the 2D case the projected object contours each consist of two points and there are four tangents $l_a, l_b, l_{a'}, l_{b'}$ to the object. We can determine these four tangents, since C and C' are known (Fig. 5.7).
We manually place the bone model in an approximate position over the X-ray images. This gives us an initial estimate for the bone position. Of course, this initial placement is not optimal and needs to be refined. In many cases, CT images are taken in standard positions, and X-ray images are also taken from standard angles, so that this estimate for the pose of the model is already known, and the step of manually placing the model is not needed.

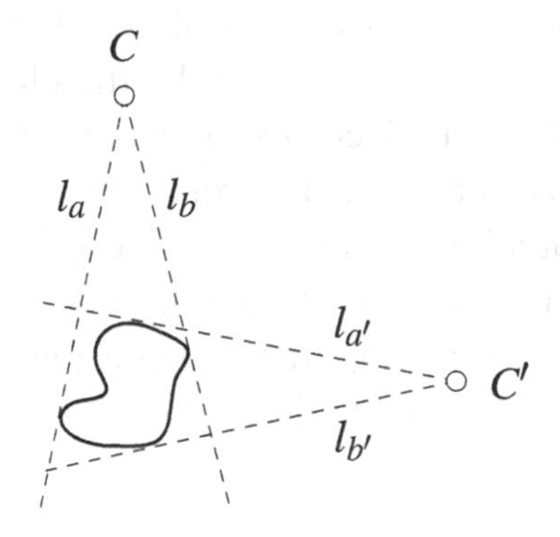

Fig. 5.7: Two-dimensional illustration of contour-based registration. Known camera positions C, C'. Tangents touch the contour of the object

After having obtained the initial estimate, we can extract four points $\mathbf{a}, \mathbf{b}, \mathbf{a}', \mathbf{b}'$ on the bone model in the following way: We extract a second set of four tangents, but now these tangents touch the bone model (in the estimated pose) (Fig. 5.8).

We then minimize the point-line-distances between the original tangents $l_a, l_b, l_{a'}, l_{b'}$ and the surface points $\mathbf{a}, \mathbf{b}, \mathbf{a}', \mathbf{b}'$ on the model.

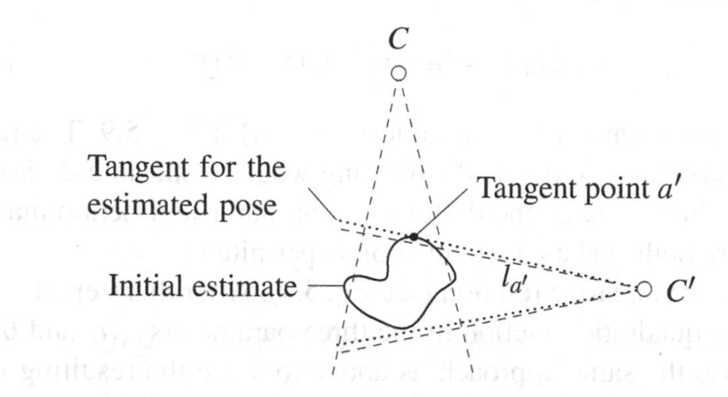

Fig. 5.8: Estimated bone position. We refine the estimate by minimizing the point-line distance between the original tangents (*dashed lines*) and the tangent points

As in the case of point-based registration, $\mathbf{R}$ is a rotation matrix with parameter θ and $\mathbf{t}$ is the translation vector with entries t_x and t_y.
The minimization problem is a slight variation of the function in Eq. 5.3:

$$f(\theta, t_x, t_y) = d(\mathbf{Ra} + \mathbf{t}, l_a)^2 + \cdots + d(\mathbf{Rb}' + \mathbf{t}, l_{b'})^2 \tag{5.6}$$

$d(\mathbf{p}, l)$ is the distance of point $\mathbf{p}$ from line l. We can compute the distance of the point $\mathbf{a}$ from the line l_a via:

$$d(\mathbf{a}, l_a)^2 = (\mathbf{a} - \mathbf{u} - \lambda_0(\mathbf{v} - \mathbf{u}))^2, \tag{5.7}$$

for appropriate λ_0, and $l_a = \mathbf{u} + \lambda(\mathbf{v} - \mathbf{u})$.
We minimize this expression by taking the derivative with respect to λ, and setting to zero:

$$(\mathbf{a} - \mathbf{u} - \lambda(\mathbf{v} - \mathbf{u}))(\mathbf{v} - \mathbf{u}) = 0. \tag{5.8}$$

The point on the line l_a which is closest to the point $\mathbf{a}$ thus has the λ-value

$$\lambda_0 = \frac{(\mathbf{a} - \mathbf{u})(\mathbf{v} - \mathbf{u})}{(\mathbf{v} - \mathbf{u})^2}. \tag{5.9}$$

Thus, for $\lambda = \lambda_0$ we obtain a closed formula for the quadratic distance $d(\mathbf{a}, l_a)^2$. We insert the values for λ_0 into the above function f. This way, we can resolve the distance expressions:

$$d(\mathbf{a}, l_a)^2 = (\mathbf{a} - \mathbf{u} - \lambda_0(\mathbf{v} - \mathbf{u}))^2. \tag{5.10}$$

Notice that we cannot cancel the term $(\mathbf{v} - \mathbf{u})$ in Eq. 5.9. The reason is: $\mathbf{a}, \mathbf{v}$ and $\mathbf{u}$ are vectors, and canceling would result in a division of vectors, which is undefined! But the nominator and denominator in Eq. 5.9 are both scalars, thus division is permitted.
As above, we linearize rotation (see Eq. 5.4). After this step, the function f is a quadratic function in the three parameters t_x, t_y and θ, and we can use the same approach as above to solve the resulting linear system of equations.
A minor problem remains. Tangent points may move by a large amount after a small rotation (see Fig. 5.9). To address this problem, we do not take just one initial position and solve the system of equations for this particular position. We take several initial positions, each with a slightly modified orientation.

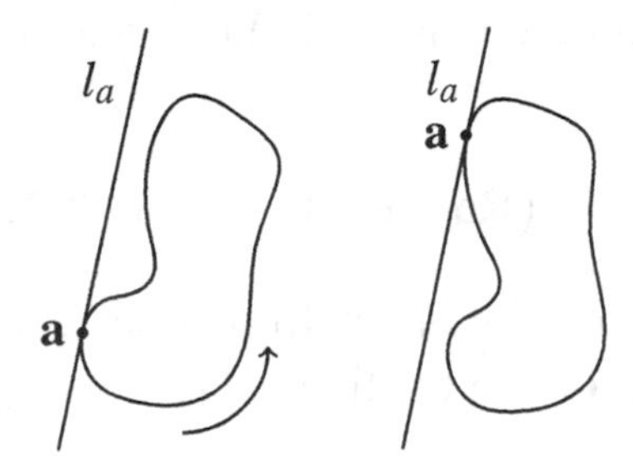

Fig. 5.9: Small rotations may move tangent points by large amounts

5.3.1 Three-Dimensional Case

In the three-dimensional case, the contours of the projections become curves in two dimensions. Now the contour does not consist of two points, but rather of a curve, or a set of image points. As in the 2D case, tangents are drawn connecting each contour point with the camera origin, and the tangent points are determined. These points lie on the surface model.

As above, our target function f has six parameters $t_x, t_y, t_z, \alpha, \beta, \gamma$, and we use the linear version of the rotation matrix given above to obtain a linear system of equations.

Example 5.2

In MR images, the surface of a bone is often not well visible. This is due to the fact that the tissue on the bone surface, or close to the bone surface gives the same MR-signal as the cortical bone. However, the *inner* contour of the bone (contour between cortical bone and spongy bone) is typically very clear in MR images (see also Fig. 1.6). This inner contour is also visible in X-ray images. This observation allows for a contour-based X-ray to MR registration.

(End of Example 5.2)

5.4 Intensity-Based Registration

For contour-based registration, it is necessary to find the contours first. To avoid this, another class of registration algorithms has been developed: intensity-based registration algorithms. No contours are needed and we only use the gray levels of the image pixels. The idea is shown in Fig. 5.10.

Obviously, for the example in Fig. 5.10, we obtain the registration position for the MR image by rotating in clockwise direction (90°).

However, images from two different sources might not assign the same gray levels to a given structure. As an example, look at the images from Fig. 1.6, showing two images of the same structure (femur bone) imaged with CT (left) and MR (right).

Since CT is X-ray-based, the bone appears white in the image, whereas it is black in the MR image. Then it would seem hard to match the structures, based on the pixel gray levels.

CT

1	1	3	3
1	1	3	3
2	2	3	3
2	2	3	3

MR

3	3	3	3
3	3	3	3
1	1	2	2
1	1	2	2

Fig. 5.10: Abstract example images. 16 pixels, only three potential gray values

CT

1	1	3	3
1	1	3	3
2	2	3	3
2	2	3	3

MR

2	2	2	2
2	2	2	2
3	3	1	1
3	3	1	1

Fig. 5.11: Abstract example images. An appropriate matching of gray levels must be computed by the registration algorithm

Look at the example in Fig. 5.11. Which should be the correct registration position of the images from Fig. 5.11? The answer is that the MR image should again be rotated clockwise by 90°. But now, we must additionally map the pixel intensities according to the following table:

CT	MR
1	$\rightarrow 3$
2	$\rightarrow 1$
3	$\rightarrow 2$

The mutual information algorithm (MI algorithm) solves both problems in an elegant way (computing the registration position and the table for the intensity mapping).
The mapping does not have to be one-to-one. Notice that all this can be achieved only by looking at the intensity values of the pixels, no

contour is needed! Thus MI registration is an ideal method for registering 3D CT images to 3D MR images.
One important application of MI registration is radiation therapy. CT images contain information on the Hounsfield units, i.e. the tissue density with respect to radiation. Therefore, CT is the standard image modality for radiation therapy planning. However, MR images often show a better contrast for soft tissues. Thus, a better delineation of tumors is possible.

5.4.1 Basic Definitions for MI-Registration

Assume an image is generated by a random process. We move through the pixels of the image line by line, from left to right. At each pixel we stop, and a random generator decides what color to give this pixel. More formally, $p_A(a)$ is the probability that the random experiment A gives result a. Then $p_A(a)$ is the probability that the current pixel obtains gray value a.
For two random variables A, B, the joint probability $p_{A,B}(a,b)$ is the probability that A gives outcome *a and* B gives outcome b. We will write (a,b) as an abbreviation for (a and b).
For two images, we have two random variables A and B. For simplicity, we also call the images A and B.
Now assume image A shows a landscape, and image B shows a dog. Thus the two images are completely different. Assume also we have not yet seen the images, we have only heard about them. Then knowing something about one pixel in image A will not tell us much about the corresponding pixel in image B. With other words, image A *does not contain much information* about image B.
Next, consider the opposite case: assume the two images are exactly the same, i.e. $A = B$. Again, we have not seen either of the two images. But here, knowing the value of one pixel in image A informs us about image B as well. We know that the gray level of this pixel must be the same.
In terms of the random variables producing the images, we have the following situation. In the first case (landscape and dog), the two random variables are independent.

In the second case ($A = B$), the random variables are maximally dependent.
We return to the problem of registration. We do the following experiment. Images A and B are still the same. But now, B is slightly moved to the left, i.e. the images are slightly out of registration. Now what will happen to the random variables? The random variables will no longer be maximally dependent. But since we only moved image B by a very small amount, they will be close to maximally dependent. Thus we could simply measure the degree of dependency of the two random variables, to find the registration position.

5.4.2 Mutual Information $I(A,B)$

Mutual information $I(A,B)$ is a measure related to the concept of independence. $I(A,B)$ is defined by

$$I(A,B) = \sum_{a,b} p_{A,B}(a,b) \log \frac{p_{A,B}(a,b)}{p_A(a)p_B(b)}. \tag{5.11}$$

The sum in this definition ranges over all outcomes a,b of the two random variables A,B. It can be shown that $I(A,B) \geq 0$ [7].
The connection between mutual information and independence becomes visible, if we observe the following: If A,B are independent, then

$$p_{A,B}(a,b) = p_A(a)p_B(b) \tag{5.12}$$

and

$$\log \frac{p_{A,B}(a,b)}{p_A(a)p_B(b)} = \log 1 = 0. \tag{5.13}$$

The next example illustrates mutual information for image pairs.

Example 5.3

Consider the two images A and B with only four "pixels" each (Fig. 5.12). They have only two gray levels: 0, or black, and 1, or white.

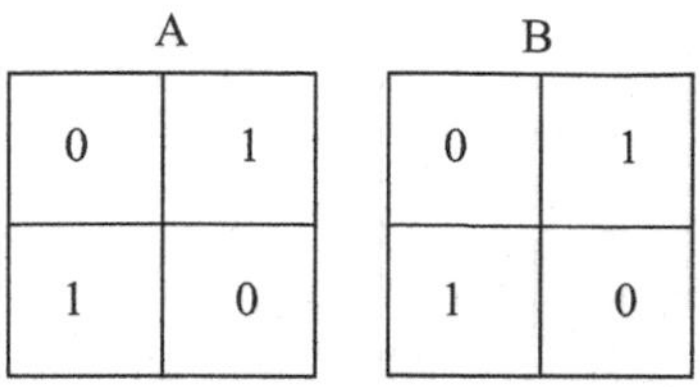

A	
0	1
1	0

B	
0	1
1	0

Fig. 5.12: Abstract example images. Four pixels, two gray values (0 and 1)

Obviously, both images are the same, so there is maximal dependency in the image information.
The distributions for A and B are

$$p_A(0) = 0.5 \quad p_A(1) = 0.5,$$

$$p_B(0) = 0.5 \quad p_B(1) = 0.5.$$

The joint distribution is calculated as follows:
$p_{A,B}(0,0)$ is the probability that a pixel in image A is black, while the same pixel is also black in image B, here

$$p_{A,B}(0,0) = 0.5. \tag{5.14}$$

Likewise,

$$p_{A,B}(1,1) = 0.5, \tag{5.15}$$

and of course

$$p_{A,B}(0,1) = 0, \tag{5.16}$$

$$p_{A,B}(1,0) = 0. \tag{5.17}$$

Thus, we can calculate the mutual information between the two images as

$$I(A,B) = 0.5\log\left(0.5/(0.5)^2\right) + 0.5\log\left(0.5/(0.5)^2\right) = 1. \tag{5.18}$$

The next example shows that the two images do not have to use the same colors (Fig. 5.13).

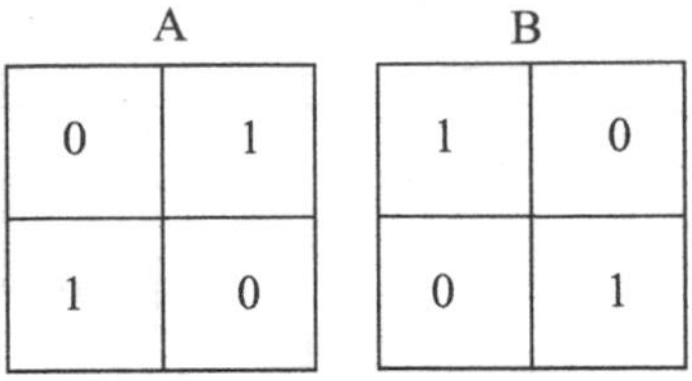

A

0	1
1	0

B

1	0
0	1

Fig. 5.13: Gray level 0 is mapped to gray level 1 and vice versa. Here the mutual information $I(A,B)$ also equals one!

Example 5.4

Before we look at the actual method of image registration with mutual information, we briefly return to the definition in Eq. 5.11. The entropy $H(A)$ is a measure for the degree of 'disorder' in a random variable A. It is defined as

$$H(A) = -\sum_{a} p_A(a) \log p_A(a). \tag{5.19}$$

Notice that the sum ranges over the possible outcomes of A. An example is a random variable with only two outcomes (namely 0 and 1). Then $H(A)$ is maximal if both outcomes have equal probability, i.e.

$$p_A(0) = 0.5 \quad p_A(1) = 0.5.$$

Now, by contrast, assume one outcome has probability 1 and the other 0, i.e.

$$p_A(0) = 1 \quad p_A(1) = 0.$$

Then the degree of 'disorder' is minimal, i.e. the entropy is 0 (apply the convention $0 \log 0 = 0$ in the above formula). Finally, if one outcome has the probability 0.25 and the other one 0.75, the entropy $H(A)$ is 0.811.

(End of Example 5.4)

From the definition, mutual information is closely related to entropy. The exercises at the end of this chapter discuss the connection between entropy and mutual information from a more theoretical point of view. We consider two more examples to further illustrate mutual information in the context of images.

Example 5.5

Figure 5.14 shows a case in which the mutual information of two images is zero.

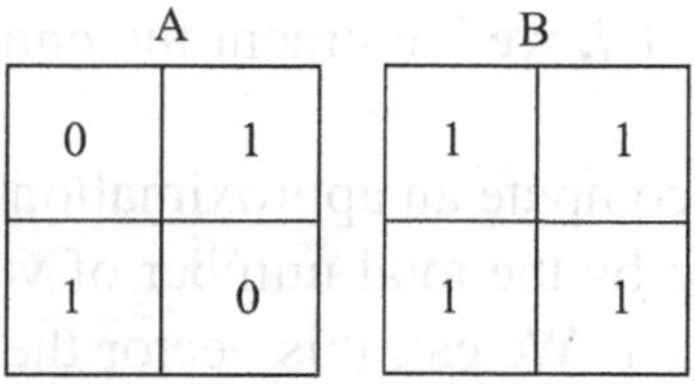

A

0	1
1	0

B

1	1
1	1

Fig. 5.14: Image A gives no information on the content of image B. In this case the mutual information $I(A,B) = 0$

This can be verified in the same way as in Example 5.3.

(End of Example 5.5)

Example 5.6

One final example is shown in Fig. 5.15. Three pixels are the same, but not the fourth.

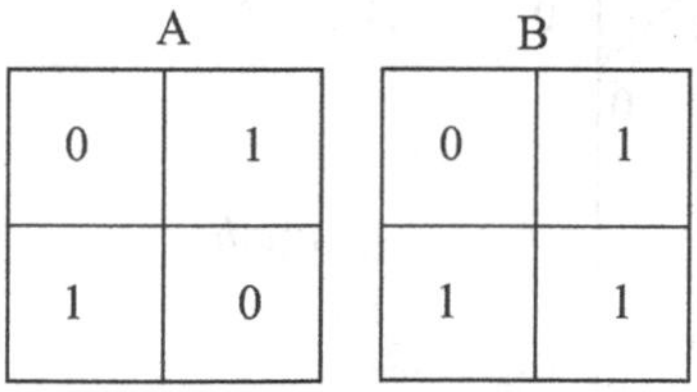

A

0	1
1	0

B

0	1
1	1

Fig. 5.15: In this example $I(A,B) = 0.32$

(End of Example 5.6)

5.4.3 Registration Method Based on Mutual Information

Assume there are 256 gray levels in both images A and B, $(0,\dots,255)$. The first step is to estimate the distribution p_A. Set up a vector with 256 entries, one entry for each possible gray level. We count the number of voxels (in 2D: pixels) for each gray level value. This means: we step through the image voxel by voxel. Whenever we meet a voxel with gray level j, we increment the entry with index j in the vector by 1.
From this vector, we compute an approximation for p_A: we normalize the vector by dividing by the total number of voxels, so that the sum of all entries becomes 1. We call this vector the gray level histogram for p_A. In the same way, we compute the histogram for p_B.
After calculating the two histograms, the only thing missing is the joint distribution of the two random variables. Therefore, consider a table with 256×256 entries as a joint histogram with all entries initialized to 0. First, bring the two images into an approximate matching position (i.e. by superimposing the images). For each voxel pair with gray levels (a,b) increment the table entry with index (a,b) by 1. Compute the estimate of the joint distribution by normalizing the table entries (divide by number of voxel pairs), so that the sum of all table entries becomes 1. The computation is illustrated in Fig. 5.16.

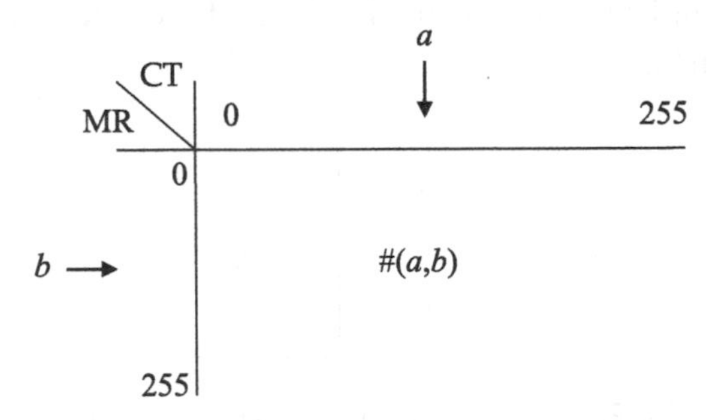

Fig. 5.16: Table for computing the joint distribution $p_{A,B}$. Place the number of voxels having gray level a in A and gray level b in B at the table position with index a,b

Notice that the joint distribution $p_{A,B}$ is position-dependent! This means $p_{A,B}$ depends on the relative position of image B with respect to image A. Notice also that p_A, p_B are independent of the relative position.
Having computed the three histograms for p_A, p_B and $p_{A,B}$, we have all the tools for evaluating the defining equation for mutual information (Eq. 5.11).

5.4.3.1 Registration Criterion

Let image A be the fixed image, image B be the floating image, i.e. B moves over image A (rotation and translation), until the final registration position is reached.
We move the floating image under six transformation parameters: three angles α, β and γ and three translations t_x, t_y and t_z.
Criterion: *For each position of B, evaluate the mutual information via Eq. 5.11. The images match optimally for the position where the mutual information is maximal.*

5.4.3.2 Interpolation in the Floating Image

One problem that arises is that the pixel (voxel) center in the floating image may not always be exactly above the pixel (voxel) center of the fixed image (Fig. 5.17). Thus, in Fig. 5.17, we have assumed that in one box-section of our CT image (fixed image) we have four voxels with gray levels of 97, 98, 102 and 103, respectively. And we assume a voxel of the MR, inside this box has gray level 13.
To compute the histogram-table for the joint distribution, we need to state which of the four gray levels in the bounding box we will update. There are three types of interpolation:

- nearest neighbour interpolation (NN)
- trilinear interpolation (TI)
- trilinear partial volume interpolation (TPV)

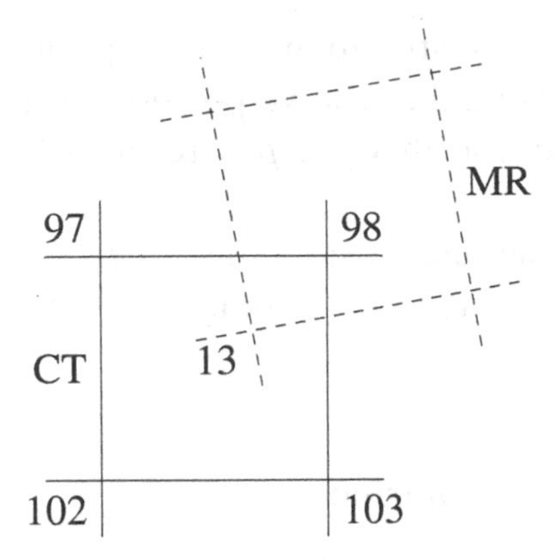

Fig. 5.17: Interpolation of the voxel position

Nearest Neighbor Interpolation

For the example of Fig. 5.17, the CT-voxel with gray level 98 is the nearest neighbour of the MR-voxel with grey level 13. We thus increment the table entry for the index pair $(98, 13)$ in the joint distribution.

Trilinear Interpolation

Trilinear interpolation takes the weighted mean of the neighboring gray levels. Notice that gray levels not actually occurring in the original image can be generated in this way. In the example of Fig. 5.17, we compute the distances d_1 to d_4, between the MR-voxel inside the box and the four corners of the box. Trilinear interpolation increments the table entry with index $(x, 13)$. Here, x is the weighted average of the neighboring gray levels. The weight is determined by the distance from the MR-voxel. The term trilinear stems from the fact that the interpolation is three-dimensional.

Trilinear Partial Volume Interpolation

Trilinear partial volume interpolation avoids generating new gray levels which do not occur in the image. We do not increment by 1, but by the weight obtained from the interpolation. All neighbors obtain increments corresponding to their distance.

Search for the Registration Position

The search for the registration position starts with the initialization, i.e. images are overlaid so that centers and axes match. The optimization is then decomposed into a separate search along several axes. Thus, we compute the mutual information $I(A,B)$ for the current position (start position) according to Eq. 5.11. We then move the floating image by a small amount along one of the six axes (three translational and three revolute axes). For this new position, we recompute the mutual information $I(A,B)$. This process is repeated to maximize the mutual information. Notice that the mutual information depends on the position of the floating image relative to the fixed image. As a consequence, we must recompute the joint distribution for each new position in this process. However, the distributions p_A and p_B remain unchanged when moving the floating image. The maximization process can, for example, be guided by Levenberg-Marquardt optimization [18].
Trilinear partial volume interpolation yields the smoothest optimization function. It is thus the preferable interpolation method.

Binning

The histograms described above provide an estimate for the distribution. The quality of this estimate depends on the number of observations. To obtain a better estimate, observations can be grouped together into so-called bins. For example, we return to the histogram describing p_A with 256 gray level values. Then we form 64 bins each representing four gray levels. We count the number of entries in each bin, rather than counting the number of entries for each gray level. In this example the width of the bins (four) has been chosen rather arbitrarily. Histograms depend on a good choice of the bin size, and even bins of different width can be useful. In practice it turns out that a reasonable approach is the following: take several bin sizes and average over the resulting histograms to obtain the final histogram.

Notice that intensity based registration (with mutual information) can be applied for two-dimensional and three-dimensional images as well.

So far, we saw several basic methods for registration. In each case, our registration was rigid. This means, potential deformations of any structures (in images) were taken not into account. In the next section, we will discuss image deformations.

5.5 Image Deformation

We will need methods for image deformation in two applications. In the first application, we must correct for distortions. Thus, the physical process of image acquisition can cause distortions of the image. The second application is elastic registration.
Both applications mentioned (distortion correction and elastic registration) share a common root, and we will start with a simple example illustrating this. In this case, we have two grids of points. We will call these grids G and G'. Let G be a grid of equidistant points. We assume G' is a (slightly) deformed version of G, and we know the point-to-point correspondences (see Fig. 5.18).

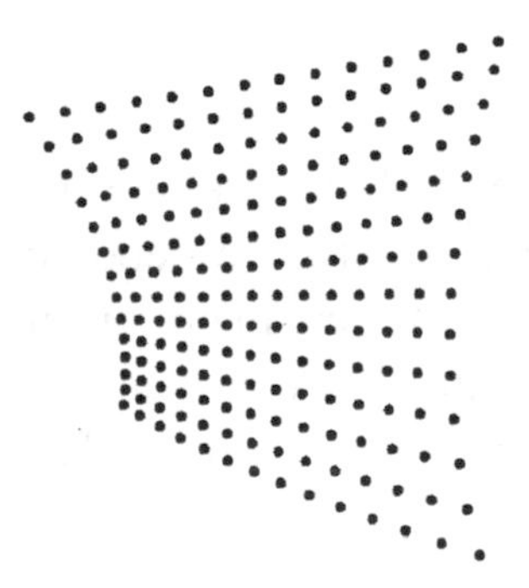

Fig. 5.18: Deformation of a grid of equidistant points

5.5.1 Bilinear Interpolation

Suppose the grid points in G and G' are landmarks in two images. Our goal is to deform the image underlying G', while moving each landmark point in G' to its target position in G. We find an initial

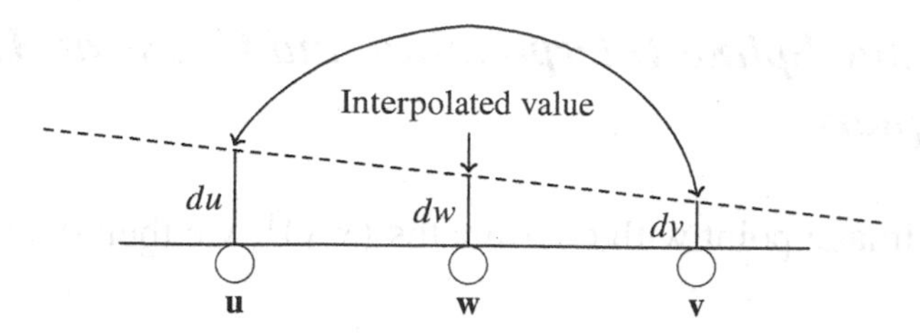

Fig. 5.19: Distortion correction with bilinear interpolation

registration position with landmark-based registration, as described above. After this step, the positions of the landmarks in G and G' may not match exactly, and we deform G' appropriately, to bring the points into a matching position. To this end, suppose we have two neighboring landmarks $\mathbf{u}$, and $\mathbf{v}$, both in G'. We treat shifts in x-and y-directions separately. Given the point-to-point correspondence, we know that the point $\mathbf{u}$ must be shifted by an amount du in x-direction, and $\mathbf{v}$ must be shifted by dv. We then shift each image point $\mathbf{w}$ in between $\mathbf{u}$ and $\mathbf{v}$ by an amount corresponding to the linear interpolation of its position (see Fig. 5.19). The figure shows the interpolation function, from which we read the shift for $\mathbf{w}$.

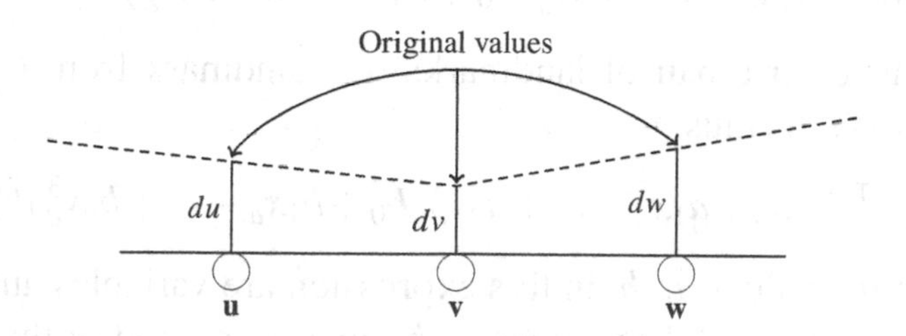

Fig. 5.20: Interpolation function

Interpolation is now applied in both the x-direction and the y-direction of the image, hence the name bilinear interpolation. The advantage of bilinear interpolation is its simplicity. The disadvantage is that our interpolation function is not smooth (Fig. 5.20). We will discuss a better method next.

5.5.2 Cubic Spline Interpolation and Gaussian Least Squares

Given an image point with coordinates $(x, y)^{\mathrm{T}}$, we then define a polynomial

$$a_0 + a_1x + a_2y + a_3xy + a_4x^2 + a_5y^2 + a_6x^2y + a_7xy^2 + a_8x^3 + a_9y^3. \tag{5.20}$$

This polynomial (in the two variables x and y) describes the shift of this image point in x-direction. Likewise,

$$b_0 + b_1x + b_2y + b_3xy + b_4x^2 + b_5y^2 + b_6x^2y + b_7xy^2 + b_8x^3 + b_9y^3 \tag{5.21}$$

describes the shift in y-direction.
The parameters a_i and b_i in this polynomial must be adjusted in such a way that the distances between the model points $(x_m, y_m)^{\mathrm{T}}$ (i.e. grid points in G) and the corresponding landmarks in G' are minimized. The coordinates of the landmarks in G' are given by $(x_d, y_d)^{\mathrm{T}}$. Shifting under the correction polynomials will give points

$$(a_0 + a_1x_d + \ldots + a_9y_d^3, b_0 + b_1x_d + \ldots + b_9y_d^3)^{\mathrm{T}}. \tag{5.22}$$

The distance for a pair of landmarks, i.e. landmark from G to landmark from G', is thus

$$\|(x_m, y_m)^{\mathrm{T}} - (a_0 + a_1x_d + \ldots + a_9y_d^3, b_0 + b_1x_d + \ldots + b_9y_d^3)^{\mathrm{T}}\|. \tag{5.23}$$

Note that the values a_i, b_i in this expression are variables and x_m, y_m, x_d, y_d are constants! The values a_i, b_i appear squared in the distance term. Now consider the sum of the squared distances for all such landmark pairs. The overall sum is still quadratic in the values a_i, b_i and the derivative of this term with respect to all 20 parameters a_i, b_i yields 20 linear equations in 20 unknowns. The solution of the linear equation system gives the optimal values for the parameters a_i, b_i. Transforming the entire image under the function

$$(x, y)^{\mathrm{T}} \rightarrow (a_0 + a_1x + \ldots + a_9y^3, b_0 + b_1x + \ldots + b_9y^3)^{\mathrm{T}} \tag{5.24}$$

gives the undistorted image. This method is called Gaussian Least Squares.

5.5.3 Thin-Plate Splines

The Gaussian least squares method in the last section provides a smooth deformation of the image. However, this method is purely mathematical, and does not necessarily represent the physical conditions that led to the deformation. The thin-plate spline method (which we will look at in this section) was designed to reflect physical characteristics of typical deformations.

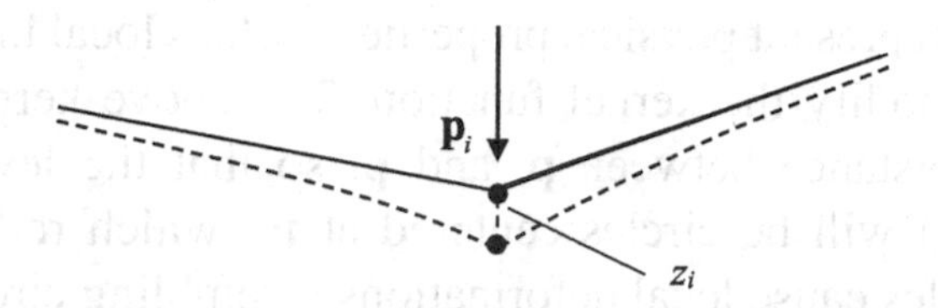

Fig. 5.21: Deforming a thin metal plate. The plate is deformed by a force pushing downwards at point $\mathbf{p}_i$. The magnitude of the displacement at $\mathbf{p}_i$ is z_i

Assume we have forces acting on a piece of sheet metal. For simplicity, the forces are assumed to be needles pushing in vertical direction onto the metal plate. Assume the metal sheet is completely flat initially. To be specific, we further assume the sheet is rectangular, and three of the four corner points are mechanically fixed. Now deform this plate by pushing a needle in downward direction. The amount of displacement at the needle tip $\mathbf{p}$ is given by a value z. The situation is illustrated in Fig. 5.21.

More generally, assume we have N needles, again pushing in vertical direction onto a metal sheet, where the position of the points $\mathbf{p}_i = (x_i, y_i)^T$ on the sheet is arbitrary. We are looking for a function $f(\mathbf{p})$ where $\mathbf{p} = (x, y)^T$ is a point on the sheet. f should assume the value z_i at point $\mathbf{p}_i$, i.e. it is used to model the displacement. The values z_i are real numbers.

Now set

$$f(\mathbf{p}) = \sum_{i=1}^{N} w_i F(\| \mathbf{p} - \mathbf{p}_i \|). \tag{5.25}$$

In this function, the values w_i are the parameters, i.e. the values w_i take the role of the values a_i, b_i in the previous section.

The function F is called a kernel function. For now, we set $F(r) = r^2$. Thus, for a point $\mathbf{p} = (x,y)^T$ the value of $F(\|\mathbf{p}-\mathbf{p}_i\|)$ increases with the squared distance of $\mathbf{p}$ from $\mathbf{p}_i$. But notice that the influence of the corresponding weight value decreases with the distance from the control point. Thus, we can simply insert our control points $\mathbf{p}_i = (x_i, y_i)^T$ into this function, and the desired output values z_i of f are known. In this way we obtain a linear equation system with N variables (the weights w_i) and N equations.
The flexibility of this method stems from the fact that we have a kernel function. To represent physical properties such as local inhomogeneities we can modify the kernel function. The above kernel F simply returns the distance between $\mathbf{p}_i$ and $\mathbf{p}$, so that the level curves of $F(\| \mathbf{p}-\mathbf{p}_i \|)$ will be circles centered at $\mathbf{p}_i$, which reflects the fact that the needles cause local deformations resembling circular basins.
To allow for translational displacement, the function f can be modified to

$$f(\mathbf{p}) = \sum_{i=1}^{N} w_i F(\| \mathbf{p}-\mathbf{p}_i \|) + a_0 + a_1 x + a_2 y. \tag{5.26}$$

We now have three new variables a_0, a_1, a_2. The resulting linear system is under-determined. To obtain a unique solution, we restrict the solution set appropriately. As an example, we can set

$$\sum_{i=1}^{N} w_i = 0, \quad \sum_{i=1}^{N} w_i x_i = 0, \quad \sum_{i=1}^{N} w_i y_i = 0. \tag{5.27}$$

The above version of the thin-plate-splines method only works for scalar-valued functions. To make it work for image deformation or warping, we need functions mapping from 2D to 2D, i.e. a control point (2D) in the image must be moved to a model point (also 2D).
Such a vector-valued function f can be generated by using two thin-plate-splines, one for the x-coordinate and one for the y-coordinate. In the same way this method can be extended to the 3D case.
Thin-plate-splines are rather expensive computationally. For every interpolation, the distance to all control points must be calculated and the kernel function must be evaluated.
One way to improve this is to use TPS only on the grid points of a coarse grid (e.g. ten pixel grid width). Within the grid, fast bilinear interpolation can be applied.

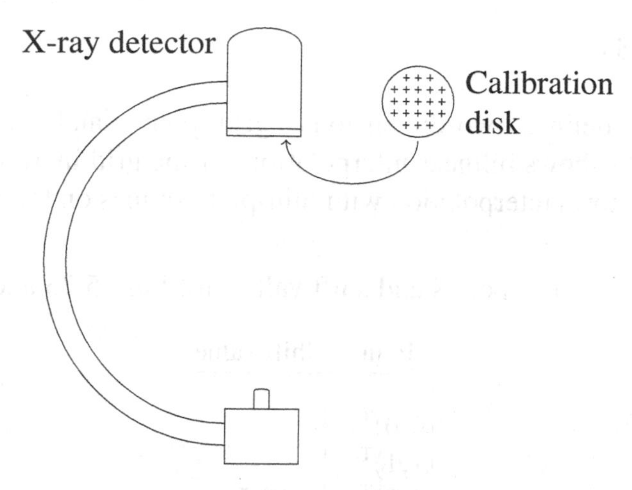

Fig. 5.22: Calibration disk

Example 5.7

The physical acquisition process for most image modalities causes small deformations of the image. The deformation may resemble the pattern shown in Fig. 5.18. Images produced by C-arms are deformed by the earth's magnetic field. Small deformations are tolerable as long as the images are only used for diagnosis. However, for navigation, deformations must be corrected. An example is shown in Fig. 5.22 A calibration disk is mounted in front of the detector of the C-arm. Small metal crosses form a regular grid of radio-opaque markers on the radio-translucent background of the disk. The markers are thus visible in the images. Notice that the distortion of images is position-dependent. Thus, if we move the C-arm (i.e. we vary the imaging direction), then the distortion pattern will change!

(End of Example 5.7)

The following example illustrates the difference between bilinear interpolation and thin-plate splines.

Example 5.8

Table 5.1 defines two-dimensional grid points and shift values. Figure 5.23 shows bilinear interpolation for the grid in Table 5.1 and Fig. 5.24 shows interpolation with thin-plate splines on the same grid.

Table 5.1: Grid points and shift values for Figs. 5.23 and 5.24

Point	Shift value
$(0,0)^{\mathrm{T}}$	1
$(1,1)^{\mathrm{T}}$	1
$(1,0)^{\mathrm{T}}$	0.5
$(0,1)^{\mathrm{T}}$	0
$(2,1)^{\mathrm{T}}$	0
$(0,2)^{\mathrm{T}}$	1

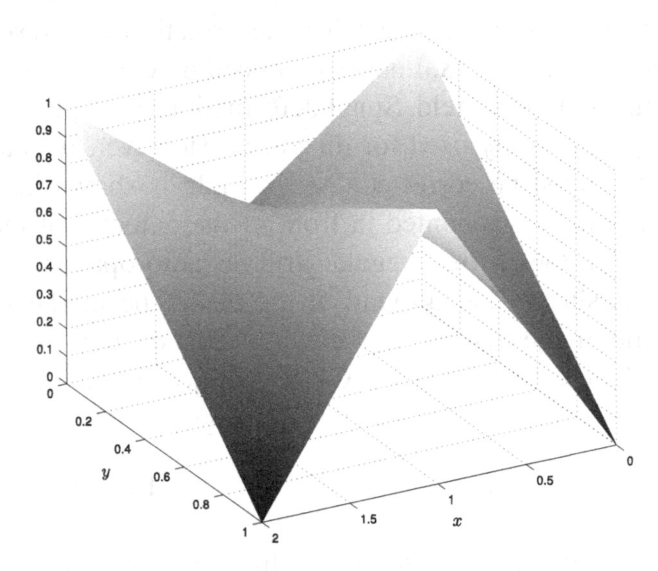

Fig. 5.23: Bilinear interpolation

(End of Example 5.8)

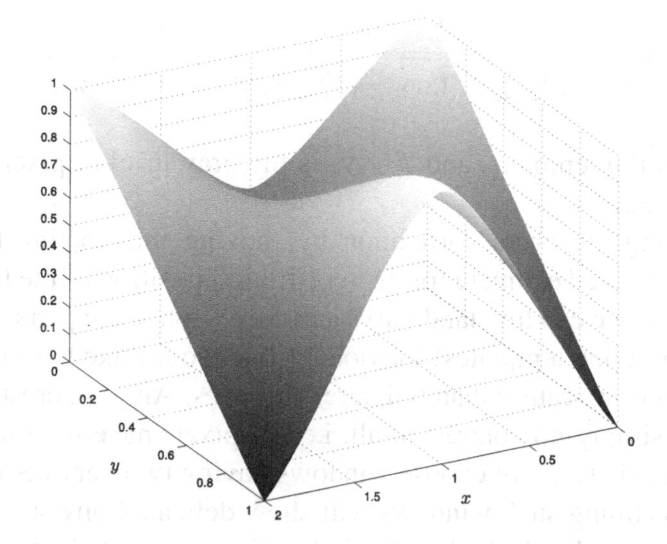

Fig. 5.24: Interpolation with Thin-Plate Splines

5.5.4 Elastic Registration

In elastic registration, we again have two images A and B, where A is the fixed image, and B is the floating image. Here, we allow the floating image B to deform during registration. Thus, assume we have two images of a lung, for the same patient, but taken at different points in time. The lung deforms as the patient breathes. To quantify the magnitude of the deformation, or to locate targets within the lung, we will need to deform images.

Cross Correlation Thin-plate splines need landmarks and correspondence pairs. Landmarks are not always available. A simple strategy to find landmarks automatically is template matching.
Consider a small window of image B. For example, this window can be a square region of 9×9 pixels.
The window will be called the template. Having a coarse alignment, we move the template (from image B) over the corresponding region in A, and find the best matching position. The motion of the template is purely translational. We compute the following value for each position, denoting translational displacements by (u, v):

$$C(u,v) = \frac{\sum_x \sum_y T(x,y)A(x+u,y+v)}{\sqrt{\sum_x \sum_y [T(x,y)]^2} \sqrt{\sum_x \sum_y [A(x+u,y+v)]^2}} \tag{5.28}$$

Here T is the template, and $T(x,y)$ is the gray level at pixel (x,y) in the template.

Maximizing the cross correlation by moving the floating template gives the desired estimate for the registration position of the template. In this way, we can find landmarks and correspondence pairs. But how do we find good templates? Obviously, one would like to select interesting windows rather than uninteresting ones. An uninteresting window has simply no contrast at all, i.e. all pixels have the same color or gray level. Thus we choose windows having two very distinct gray levels, assuming such windows will show delicate bony structures or salient landmarks. To find such windows, we compute histograms for each window in the floating image. A histogram simply plots the number of pixels having a given gray value over the x-axis with the gray levels. The histogram is called bimodal, if we can distinguish two distinct peaks.

This matching process described here can also be extended to mutual information matching.

Elastic registration in real-time is difficult and error-prone. In later chapters we will describe tracking methods based on motion correlation which allow for motion tracking in real-time.

5.6 Hand-Eye Calibration

Accurate navigation requires a further component, which we have not yet discussed. In practice, it is often necessary to register the robot effector to a camera image. This process is called hand-eye calibration. In a typical navigation scenario, for example an orthopedic drilling task, a robot program may look like this:

1. Point to the target position with the pointer of a tracking system
2. Compute the robot joint angles, given this target point
3. Move the robot to the target point/direction
4. Drill

In step one, we simply touch the target with the pointer of the tracking system. The tracking system then computes the position and orientation of the pointer with respect to its own internal coordinate system. The position and orientation data will then be returned to the host computer.
However, you may argue that we now have the position of the pointer with respect to the internal system of the camera. How does the robot know where the internal system of the camera is? This type of problem is a calibration problem, and this is what we will address in this section.
To illustrate hand-eye calibration in a more specific case, assume an LED marker is attached to a robot gripper. The tracking system reads the 3D position of the marker. We have attached the marker on the robot in a rather arbitrary position, and we have placed the tracking system on a floor stand in front of the robot. The situation is illustrated in Fig. 5.25.

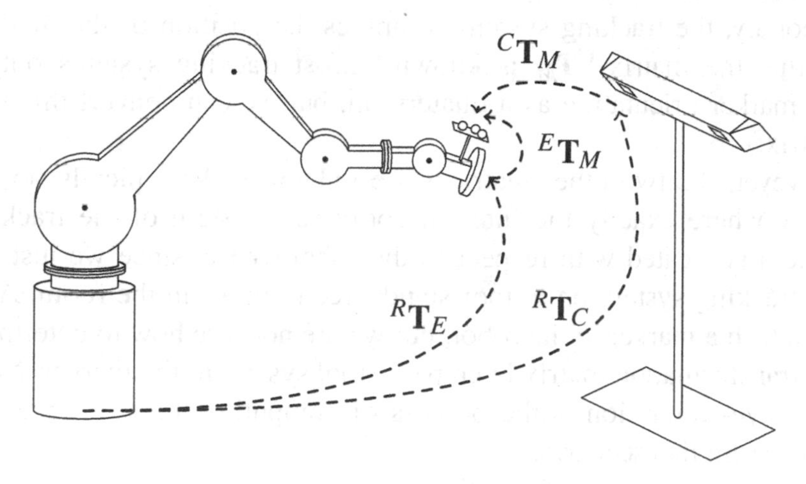

Fig. 5.25: Hand-eye-calibration

Now four transformations describe the spatial relationships. The first is the transformation from the robot's base coordinate system to the robot's effector. Call this transformation matrix $^R\mathbf{T}_E$. Then there is the transformation from robot effector coordinate system to the attached marker $^E\mathbf{T}_M$. The tracking system has an internal coordinate system. If the robot's base coordinate system is the fixed world coordinate

system, then the transformation from robot base to the coordinate system of the tracking system is needed. Call this transformation ${}^{R}\mathbf{T}_{C}$. (Here C refers to the tracking camera.) Finally, our tracking system reports the position of the marker. This position is the transformation between the amera coordinate system to the marker. Call this last transformation ${}^{C}\mathbf{T}_{M}$.
Hence, we have the following four matrices:

${}^{R}\mathbf{T}_{E}$ Robot base to tool flange/effector
${}^{E}\mathbf{T}_{M}$ Effector to marker
${}^{R}\mathbf{T}_{C}$ Robot base to tracking camera
${}^{C}\mathbf{T}_{M}$ Tracking camera to marker

Two of the four matrices are known. Firstly, the position of the tool flange/gripper coordinate system with respect to the robot base is known. The robot is a kinematic chain, and matrices describe the position of the gripper or tool flange with respect to the robot's base coordinate system. Thus ${}^{R}\mathbf{T}_{E}$ is known.
Secondly, the tracking system computes the position of the marker, so that the matrix ${}^{C}\mathbf{T}_{M}$ is known. (Most tracking systems output the marker orientation as a quaternion, but we can convert this to a matrix.)
However, the two other matrices are unknown. We typically do not know where exactly the internal coordinate system of the tracking system is located with respect to the robot's base, since we just put the tracking system on a floor stand, free to move in the room. Also we attach a marker to the robot, but we are not sure how to determine the transformation matrix from robot tool system to the marker. Now, hand-eye-calibration is the process of computing the two unknown matrices in this scenario.
We note that the transformation from robot base to marker via the robot gripper must give the same result as the transformation from robot base to marker via the tracking system. This observation can be expressed in an equation:

$$ {}^{R}\mathbf{T}_{E}\ {}^{E}\mathbf{T}_{M} = {}^{R}\mathbf{T}_{C}\ {}^{C}\mathbf{T}_{M} \tag{5.29} $$

Now recall that two of the four matrices are known, namely ${}^{R}\mathbf{T}_{E}$ and ${}^{C}\mathbf{T}_{M}$. Thus only two matrices will have to be computed from this equation.

We rename the above matrices to obtain a simpler notation.

$$\mathbf{AX} = \mathbf{YB} \tag{5.30}$$

So the last two equations are the same, only we have changed the names of the matrices. Now **A** and **B** are known, and **X** and **Y** are unknown.

But notice that we can move the robot. After moving to a second position, we obtain a second equation.

So assuming the first position gives

$$\mathbf{A}_1 \cdot \mathbf{X} = \mathbf{Y} \cdot \mathbf{B}_1. \tag{5.31}$$

The second position will give the equation

$$\mathbf{A}_2 \cdot \mathbf{X} = \mathbf{Y} \cdot \mathbf{B}_2. \tag{5.32}$$

We rearrange the two equations to have

$$\mathbf{A}_1 \cdot \mathbf{X} \cdot \mathbf{B}_1^{-1} = \mathbf{A}_2 \cdot \mathbf{X} \cdot \mathbf{B}_2^{-1}, \tag{5.33}$$

or

$$\mathbf{A'}\,\mathbf{X} = \mathbf{X}\,\mathbf{B'}, \tag{5.34}$$

where

$$\mathbf{A'} = \mathbf{A}_2^{-1}\mathbf{A}_1, \tag{5.35}$$

$$\mathbf{B'} = \mathbf{B}_2^{-1}\mathbf{B}_1. \tag{5.36}$$

Hence, it remains to solve for **X** alone. Daniilidis [8] presents a method for solving Eq. 5.36 using dual quaternions. Hence, Daniilidis starts from Eq. 5.36. We will not use the method by Daniilidis. Instead, we will start from a series of n equations of the form in Eq. 5.31. If we move the robot through a series of positions, then each position will give rise to an equation of the form Eq. 5.31. Thus, we will start from a series of equations of the type

$$\mathbf{A}_i\mathbf{X} = \mathbf{Y}\,\mathbf{B}_i, \quad i = 1, \ldots, n. \tag{5.37}$$

Setting $\mathbf{C}_i = \mathbf{B}_i^{-1}$, we have

$$\mathbf{A}_i \mathbf{X} \mathbf{C}_i = \mathbf{Y}. \tag{5.38}$$

The matrix $\mathbf{X}$ is a homogeneous 4×4-matrix, and hence there are 12 non-trivial entries in this matrix. Likewise, $\mathbf{Y}$ has 12 non-trivial entries. Thus Eq. 5.38 gives rise to a linear system of equations with $12 \cdot n$ equations and 24 variables.
Since we assume $n > 2$, the resulting system has more equations than variables. We have already encountered a method for solving such over-determined systems in the context of image reconstruction. The ART algorithm is a suitable method for this problem (see Exercise 1.2). After solving the linear system we obtain the values for the variables $x_{11}, \ldots, x_{34}$ and $y_{11}, \ldots, y_{34}$. This gives matrices describing the transformations needed for the calibration.

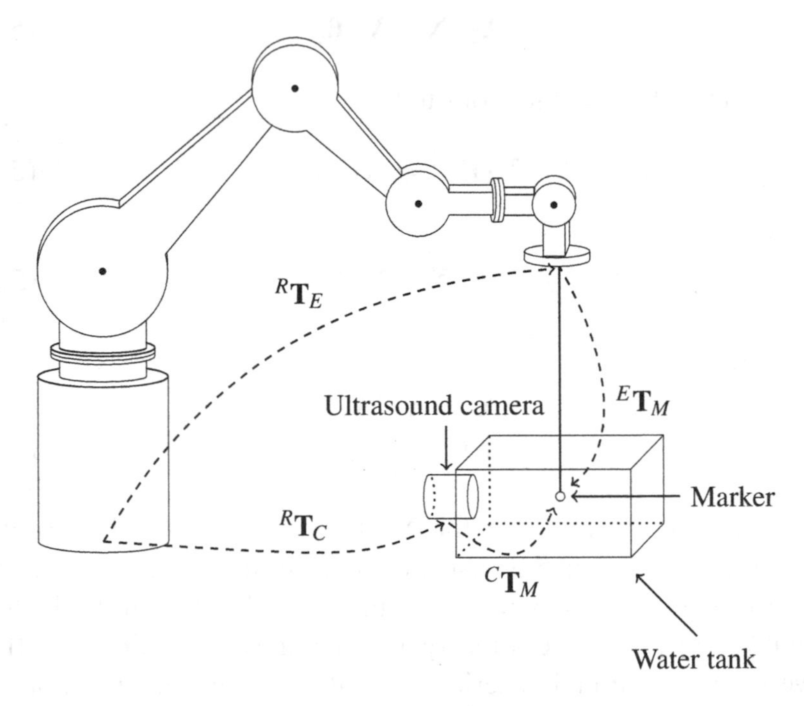

Fig. 5.26: Hand-Eye-Calibration for an ultrasound camera. A small lead ball acts as a marker. The marker is attached to the robot. The marker is in a water tank. The lead ball is detected in the ultrasound image

A further example for hand-eye calibration is shown in Fig. 5.26. The same methods apply.
Note that this method will not result in full 6D data for ${}^{E}\mathbf{T}_M$, since ${}^{C}\mathbf{T}_M$ is only 3D (position only). We can, however, fully determine ${}^{R}\mathbf{T}_E$ and the translational part of ${}^{E}\mathbf{T}_M$.

Exercises

Exercise 5.1

Verify the values $I(A,B)$ for the examples in Figs. 5.13, 5.14 and 5.15.

Exercise 5.2

Show that $I(A,B) = H(A)$ if the two images A, B are the same, i.e. $A = B$. Discuss this in the light of Example 5.3 above. Find the value for $H(A)$ in case the image A has an even distribution of gray levels, i.e. there are 256 gray levels, and all gray levels occur equally often in the image.

Exercise 5.3

Show that

$$\sum_{a,b} p_{A,B}(a,b) \log p_A(a) = \sum_{a} p_A(a) \log p_A(a). \tag{5.39}$$

Exercise 5.4

The joint entropy $H(A,B)$ is defined as

$$H(A,B) = -\sum_{a,b} p_{A,B}(a,b) \log p_{A,B}(a,b). \tag{5.40}$$

Let A, B be binary images, (i.e. p_A and p_B have only two outcomes 0 and 1). Based on the result in Eq. 5.39, show that

$$I(A,B) = H(A) + H(B) - H(A,B). \tag{5.41}$$

Exercise 5.5

Prove Eq. 5.41 for arbitrary, not necessarily binary images.

Exercise 5.6

Show that $H(A) \geq 0$ for a random variable A.

Exercise 5.7

The χ^2-function tests the hypothesis that two random variables are independent. It can also measure the degree of dependency between A and B. (Pronounce χ^2 as 'ki-squared', as in 'kite'). Thus, we measure the 'distance' between the observed joint distribution $p_{A,B}(a,b)$ and the hypothetic distribution which would be observed if A and B were independent:

$$\chi^2(A,B) = \sum_{a,b} \frac{(p_{A,B}(a,b) - p_A(a)p_B(b))^2}{p_A(a)p_B(b)} \tag{5.42}$$

This expression is zero (minimal) if A and B are independent.
Evaluate the two criteria in Eqs. 5.11 and 5.42 in experiments with simple synthetic images. Find the local maxima and the global optimum for both functions. Based on the two criteria (running in parallel), can we develop an ad hoc test for deciding which maximum is a global one?

Exercise 5.8

Set

$$\begin{aligned}
\mathbf{p}_1 &= 0 \qquad & f(\mathbf{p}_1) &= 0 \\
\mathbf{p}_2 &= 1 \qquad & f(\mathbf{p}_2) &= 1 \\
\mathbf{p}_3 &= 2 \qquad & f(\mathbf{p}_3) &= 0,
\end{aligned} \tag{5.43}$$

Evaluate the weights w_1, w_2, w_3, following the definition of the weights for thin-plate splines. Visualize the effect of thin-plate spline deformation for the constraints thus defined with a small program.

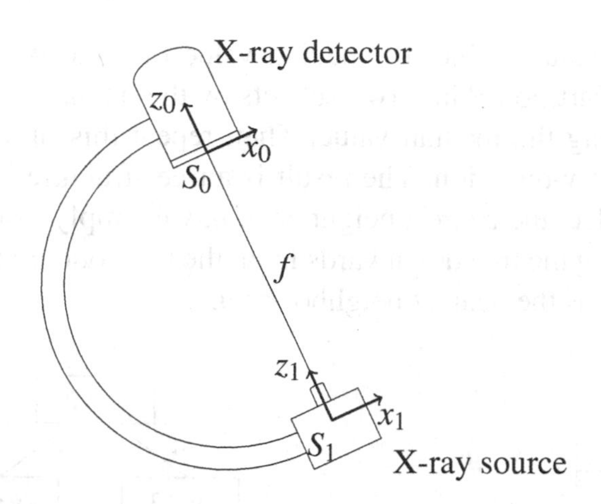

Fig. 5.27: Projection geometry of a C-arm. The focal length f is the distance between the source and the detector

Exercise 5.9

Place two coordinate systems S_0 and S_1 (the detector coordinate system and the source coordinate system of a C-arm) according to Fig. 5.27.
A marker is attached to the C-arm, and we assume this marker is already calibrated with respect to the detector coordinate system. A second marker is used as a calibration phantom. It consists of four (radiopaque) spheres, which mark the origin and the tips of the x-, y- and z-vectors in the marker coordinate system. The spheres can be distinguished in X-ray images.
We assume the pixel size of the detector is known. We also assume the source is a point, the origin of S_1. The focal length f of a C-arm is the distance between the center of the detector (origin of S_0), and the source. Derive a procedure for calibrating the focal length of a C-arm, with this calibration phantom.

Exercise 5.10

Let a be a point, and B be a cloud of points. The k-d-tree algorithm computes the nearest neighbor of a in the point cloud B. A simplified version works as follows. We sort the points in B according to ascending x-values. Find the median value of all x-axis values in B (Fig. 5.28). Partition B into two subsets by the median line, i.e. a vertical line along the median value. Then repeat this process for both subsets in the y-direction. The result is a tree structure, shown in the figure. To select the nearest neighbor of a, we simply insert a into the tree, following the tree downwards from the top node. In the example, we obtain b_3 as the nearest neighbor of a.

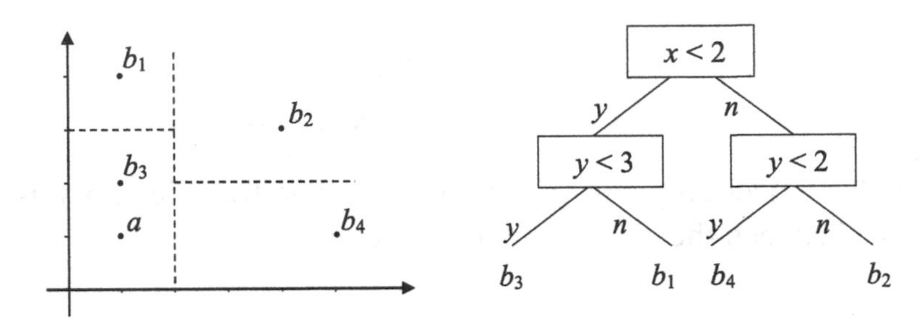

Fig. 5.28: k-d-tree

a) Find an example where this simplified version does not report the correct nearest neighbor.
b) Describe and implement a way to the repair the problem from part a).

Exercise 5.11

The matrices **X** and **Y** derived following Eq. 5.38 are estimates, and were obtained by solving an over-determined system. The rotational part of a 4×4-matrix describing a valid transformation should be an orthogonal 3×3-matrix (see also exercises for Chap. 2). The result of the estimation process contains inaccuracies. We must apply a procedure that computes an orthogonal matrix from an approximation matrix. This can be done by Gram-Schmidt orthonormalization. However, Gram-Schmidt orthonormalization is general, and not specifically designed for finding a valid three-dimensional orientation. A more dedicated way is obtained as follows. We extract Euler angles (α, β, γ) according to the convention (z, x, z) for standard Euler angles from the given 3×3 rotational input matrix. Likewise, we can extract such angles according to other conventions for Euler angles (i.e. (z,y,z)). There are 12 such conventions for Euler angles. In each case, we reassemble the resulting matrices from the extracted angles according to the conventions used. The resulting 12 matrices are orthogonal. But typically the 12 matrices will be different. We then extract Euler angles from each of the 12 matrices according to the same convention, e.g. (z,x,z). This will give 12 triples of Euler angles, typically all different. By averaging over the 12 sets (e.g. with a median selector) we obtain an estimate for the angles, and reassemble the matrix corresponding to this average. In an implementation, compare this strategy to the Gram-Schmidt orthonormalization.

Summary

Registration brings structures into alignment. Typically, two structures are given, and we compute the transformation for achieving the best match. Many navigation methods require a registration step. Digitally reconstructed radiographs (DRRs) provide a basic method for automatic registration during interventions. DRRs are synthetic X-ray images, computed from a CT data set, via projection from different angles. Other typical registration methods are: landmark-based registration, point-based registration, contour-based registration and intensity-based registration. For landmark-based registration, a small number of points with known correspondences is marked in both data sets. The registration problem then reduces to matching the two point sets, given information on which point should match which. We obtain a quadratic minimization function after introducing approximations of rotation matrices. A least-squares method is used to solve the minimization problem. Point-based registration finds the correspondences by itself. Iterative closest point matching (ICP) is a standard technique for this case. It is heuristic, and exact methods for large sets are not known. ICP alternates between a move step (as in landmark-based registration) and a match step. The match step computes the correspondences by a search for the nearest neighbor of each point. Contour-based registration is a direct extension of ICP. We replace the point-to-point distance in ICP by a point-to-line distance. MI registration allows for multi-modal image registration, by automatically finding correspondences between pixel intensities (or voxel intensities). We start by placing image B on top of image A. Then move B, and compute the value $I(A,B)$ for each position. The position giving the maximum is the registration position. The movement of B is guided by Levenberg-Marquardt optimization. To compute $I(A,B)$, we need the histograms for p_A, p_B, and $p_{A,B}$. Each histogram is a table. The table entries correspond to the image intensities. For each table entry, we count the number of pixels having the corresponding intensity. Normalizing gives an approximation for p_A, p_B, and $p_{A,B}$. Intensity-based registration is rarely used in navigation, due to limitations in speed and robustness. One typical application of MI-registration is CT-MRI fusion. In radiation therapy, tumors must be delineated in the CT. If the tumor boundary is not well visible, then the MRI can help improve the delineation.

To apply medical imaging in navigation, distortions must be corrected, and we must determine parameters describing the projection geometry. For X-ray camera calibration, calibration objects with grid patterns are placed into the beam path. The geometry of the grid pattern is known from measurements. Based on this, we deform the image such that the markers match the geometry of the grid. Thin-plate splines and cubic splines reduce the deformation problem to a linear equation system.

Hand-eye calibration aligns internal coordinate systems of cameras and robots. The problem of hand-eye calibration leads to a matrix equation of the form $\mathbf{AX} = \mathbf{YB}$, where $\mathbf{A}$ and $\mathbf{B}$ are known, and $\mathbf{X}$ and $\mathbf{Y}$ are unknown. We can set up a number of such equations, by moving the robot through a series of n different positions, giving n equations $\mathbf{A}_i\mathbf{X} = \mathbf{YB}_i$, where $i = 1, ..., n$. The resulting system is overdetermined for larger n. The ART algorithm provides a fast and practical solution method.

A simple scheme for elastic registration can be set up with thin-plate splines. But here landmarks must be known. We move small templates over the image, and evaluate cross-correlation, in order to find landmarks. Here, cross-correlation can be replaced by mutual information.

Notes

L. Brown [6] gives a summary of early methods for image registration. Introductions to the problem of medical image registration are contained in [20] and in the text book [21].
Frameless radiosurgery based on DRR registration has been in routine clinical use since the year 2000 [1]. X-ray images of the patient's skull are registered to DRRs taken before treatment.
Linear approximations for rotation matrices are a standard tool in robot kinematics. Point cloud registration can also be solved without an approximated rotation matrix [2, 14]. ICP methods were first described in [3]. S. Rusinkiewicz and M. Levoy [25] gives a survey of variants for ICP. Mutual information and joint entropy occur in many applications. $I(A,B)$ can be expressed as a direct function of joint entropy [7], see also the exercises for this chapter. Multi-modal image registration with mutual information was first described in 1996 by F. Maes et. al. and P. Viola and W. Wells [19, 34]. It is now a field of its own [23]. Phase-correlation based on Fourier transformation finds a translational displacement for aligning images [17]. More recent methods, including cross-correlation ratio, are described in [10, 24]. The thin-plate spline method is widely used for elastic registration [4]. A different method is the demon's algorithm [28].
The mechanical flex of a C-arm causes inaccuracies, since the source-detector distance is subject to small changes, depending on the position of the C-arm. Furthermore, the relative orientation of coordinate systems in the source and the detector is subject to mechanical instability. C-arm distortion correction and flex calibration is described in [5] and [13]. R. Tsai and R. Lenz [29, 30] investigate hand-eye calibration in the scenario given by Eq. 5.34. K. Daniilidis [8] extends this approach by representing rotational parameters with quaternions. Ernst et al. [9] considers hand-eye calibration for typical medical robotics scenarios.
It is useful to distinguish between 2D/3D registration and 3D/2D registration. An example for the first case is the following: we are given a 2D slice image. The goal is to find the matching placement of this (floating) slice in a fixed CT data set. By contrast, 3D/2D registration

does the opposite: we are given fixed 2D images taken from known positions. The goal is to register a 3D data set (see also [31]).
Soft tissue moves under respiration and pulsation. Beyond 2D-3D registration, so-called 2D-4D registration allows for navigation in soft tissue (see e.g. [26]). We will address the problem of tissue motion in Chap. 7.
Multi-modal image fusion is one of the main applications of MI-based registration. We have looked at CT-MRI fusion in this chapter. Beyond this, many other pairs of modalities require registration. Dedicated methods have been developed in [11, 15, 33]. Beyond cross-correlation and mutual information, many other similarity measures can be applied to intensity-based registration [22]. Diffusion-tensor imaging adds an extra data component to 3D image data. In this case, registration must include the additional information [35]. Methods for finding a good bin width for mutual information have been described in the literature, such as Scott's rule [16, 27].
Automatic registration typically does not make use of the surgeon's experience in recognizing anatomical structures. However, such experience can help. A method to include prior information on target shapes into the registration process via machine learning is given in [12].
A problem related to registration is image stitching. For example, C-arm images are arranged in a mosaic pattern to obtain a full image of a long bone or a chest [32].

References

[1] J. R. Adler, Jr., S. D. Chang, M. J. Murphy, J. Doty, P. Geis, and S. L. Hancock. The CyberKnife: A frameless robotic system for radiosurgery. *Stereotactic and Functional Neurosurgery*, **69**: 124–128, 1997. DOI 10.1159/000099863.
[2] K. S. Arun, T. S. Huang, and S. D. Blostein. Least-squares fitting of two 3-d point sets. *IEEE Transactions on Pattern Analysis and Machine Intelligence*, **9**(5):698–700, 1987.
[3] P. J. Besl and H. D. McKay. A method for registration of 3-D shapes. *IEEE Transactions on Pattern Analysis and Machine Intelligence*, **14**(2):239–256, 1992. DOI 10.1109/34.121791.

[4] F. L. Bookstein. Principal warps: thin-plate splines and the decomposition of deformations. *IEEE Transactions on Pattern Analysis and Machine Intelligence*, **11**(6):567–585, 1989. DOI 10.1109/34.24792.

[5] C. Brack, H. Götte, F. Gossé, J. Moctezuma, M. Roth, and A. Schweikard. Towards accurate X-ray camera calibration in computer assisted robotic surgery. In *Proceedings of the International Symposium on Computer Assisted Radiology (CAR)*, Paris, France, 1996. pages 721–728.

[6] L. G. Brown. A survey of image registration techniques. *ACM Computing Surveys*, **24**(4):325–376, 1992. DOI 10.1145/146370.146374.

[7] T. Cover and J. A. Thomas. *Elements of Information Theory*. Wiley Series in Telecommunications and Signal Processing. John Wiley & Sons, 2nd edition, 2008.

[8] K. Daniilidis. Hand-eye calibration using dual quaternions. *International Journal of Robotics Research*, **18**(3):286–298, 1999. DOI 10.1177/02783649922066213.

[9] F. Ernst, L. Richter, L. Matthäus, V. Martens, R. Bruder, A. Schlaefer, and A. Schweikard. Non-orthogonal tool/flange and robot/world calibration for realistic tracking scenarios. *International Journal of Medical Robotics and Computer Assisted Surgery*, **8**(4):407–420, 2012. DOI 10.1002/rcs.1427.

[10] B. Fischer and J. Modersitzki. Curvature based image registration. *Journal of Mathematical Imaging and Vision*, **18**(1):81–85, 2003. DOI 10.1023/a%3a1021897212261.

[11] C. Grova, A. Biraben, J.-M. Scarabin, P. Jannin, I. Buvat, H. Benali, and B. Gibaud. A methodology to validate MRI/SPECT registration methods using realistic simulated SPECT data. In W. J. Niessen and M. A. Viergever, editors, *Medical Image Computing and Computer-Assisted Intervention - MICCAI 2001*, volume 2208 of *Lecture Notes in Computer Science*, pages 275–282. Springer Berlin Heidelberg, 2001. DOI 10.1007/3-540-45468-3_33.

[12] C. Guetter, C. Xu, F. Sauer, and J. Hornegger. Learning based non-rigid multi-modal image registration using Kullback-Leibler divergence. In J. S. Duncan and G. Gerig, editors,

Medical Image Computing and Computer-Assisted Intervention - MICCAI 2005, volume 3750 of *Lecture Notes in Computer Science*, pages 255–262. Springer Berlin Heidelberg, 2005. DOI 10.1007/11566489_32.

[13] A. Gueziec, P. Kazanzides, B. Williamson, and R. H. Taylor. Anatomy-based registration of CT-scan and intraoperative X-ray images for guiding a surgical robot. *IEEE Transactions on Medical Imaging*, **17**(5):715–728, 1998. DOI 10.1109/42.736023.

[14] B. K. P. Horn. Closed-form solution of absolute orientation using unit quaternions. *Journal of the Optical Society of America A*, **4** (4):629–642, 1987. DOI 10.1364/JOSAA.4.000629.

[15] Y. Hu, H. U. Ahmed, C. Allen, D. Pendsé, M. Sahu, M. Emberton, D. J. Hawkes, and D. Barratt. MR to ultrasound image registration for guiding prostate biopsy and interventions. In G.-Z. Yang, D. J. Hawkes, D. Rueckert, A. Noble, and C. Taylor, editors, *Medical Image Computing and Computer-Assisted Intervention - MICCAI 2009*, volume 5761 of *Lecture Notes in Computer Science*, pages 787–794. Springer Berlin Heidelberg, 2009. DOI 10.1007/978-3-642-04268-3_97.

[16] A. Kraskov, H. Stögbauer, and P. Grassberger. Estimating mutual information. *Phys. Rev. E*, **69**(6):066138, 2004. DOI 10.1103/physreve.69.066138.

[17] C. D. Kuglin and D. C. Hines. The phase correlation image alignment method. In *Proceedings of the International Conference on Cybernetics and Society*, San Francisco, CA, USA, 1975. IEEE Systems, Man, and Cybernetics Society, pages 163–165.

[18] K. Levenberg. A method for the solution of certain problems in least squares. *Quarterly Applied Mathematics*, **2**:164–168, 1944.

[19] F. Maes, A. Collignon, D. Vandermeulen, G. Marchal, and P. Suetens. Multimodality image registration by maximization of mutual information. *IEEE Transactions on Medical Imaging*, **16**(2):187–198, 1997.

[20] J. B. Maintz and M. A. Viergever. A survey of medical image registration. *Medical Image Analysis*, **2**(1):1–36, 1998.

[21] J. Modersitzki. *Numerical Methods for Image Registration*. Numerical Mathematics and Scientific Computing. Oxford University Press, Oxford, UK, 2003.

[22] G. P. Penney, J. Weese, J. A. Little, P. Desmedt, D. L. G. Hill, and D. J. Hawkes. A comparison of similarity measures for use in 2-D-3-D medical image registration. *IEEE Transactions on Medical Imaging*, **17**(4):586–595, 1998. DOI 10.1109/42.730403.

[23] J. P. W. Pluim, A. Maintz, and M. A. Viergever. Mutual-information-based registration of medical images: A survey. *IEEE Transactions on Medical Imaging*, **22**(8):986–1004, 2003.

[24] A. Roche, G. Malandain, and N. Ayache. The correlation ratio as a new similarity measure for multimodal image registration. In *Proc. of First Int. Conf. on Medical Image Computing and Computer-Assisted Intervention (MICCAI'98)*, Cambridge, USA. Springer Verlag. Published in *Lecture Notes in Computer Science*, **1496**:1115–1124, 1998.

[25] S. Rusinkiewicz and M. Levoy. Efficient variants of the ICP algorithm. In *Third International Conference on 3D Digital Imaging and Modeling*, Los Alamitos, CA, USA, 2001. IEEE Computer Society, pages 145–152. DOI 10.1109/IM.2001.924423.

[26] A. Schweikard, H. Shiomi, J. Fisseler, M. Dötter, K. Berlinger, H. B. Gehl, and J. R. Adler, Jr. Fiducial-less respiration tracking in radiosurgery. In *Medical Image Computing and Computer-Assisted Intervention-MICCAI*. Springer. Published in *Lecture Notes in Computer Science*, **3217**:992–9, 2004.

[27] D. W. Scott. *Multivariate density estimation: theory, practice, and visualization*, volume 275 of *Wiley Series in Probability and Statistics*. John Wiley, New York, NY, 1992.

[28] J.-P. Thirion. Image matching as a diffusion process: an analogy with Maxwell's demons. *Medical Image Analysis*, **2**(3):243–260, 1998. DOI 10.1016/s1361-8415(98)80022-4.

[29] R. Y. Tsai and R. K. Lenz. A new technique for fully autonomous and efficient 3D robotics hand-eye calibration. In *Proceedings of the 4th international symposium on Robotics Research*, Cambridge, MA, USA, 1988. MIT Press, pages 287–297.

[30] R. Y. Tsai and R. K. Lenz. A new technique for fully autonomous and efficient 3D robotics hand/eye calibration. *IEEE Transactions on Robotics and Automation*, **5**(3):345–358, 1989. DOI 10.1109/70.34770.

[31] E. B. van de Kraats, G. P. Penney, D. Tomazevic, T. van Walsum, and W. J. Niessen. Standardized evaluation methodology for 2-D-3-D registration. *IEEE Transactions on Medical Imaging*, **24**(9):1177–1189, 2005. DOI 10.1109/tmi.2005.853240.

[32] L. Wang, J. Traub, S. Weidert, S. M. Heining, E. Euler, and N. Navab. Parallax-free long bone x-ray image stitching. In G.-Z. Yang, D. J. Hawkes, D. Rueckert, A. Noble, and C. Taylor, editors, *Medical Image Computing and Computer-Assisted Intervention - MICCAI 2009*, volume 5761 of *Lecture Notes in Computer Science*, pages 173–180. Springer Berlin Heidelberg, 2009. DOI 10.1007/978-3-642-04268-3_22.

[33] W. Wein, S. Brunke, A. Khamene, M. R. Callstrom, and N. Navab. Automatic CT-ultrasound registration for diagnostic imaging and image-guided intervention. *Medical Image Analysis*, **12**:577–585, 2008. DOI 10.1016/j.media.2008.06.006.

[34] W. M. Wells, III, P. A. Viola, H. Atsumi, S. Nakajima, and R. Kikinis. Multi-modal volume registration by maximization of mutual information. *Medical Image Analysis*, **1**(1):35–51, 1996.

[35] B. T. T. Yeo, T. Vercauteren, P. Fillard, X. Pennec, P. Golland, N. Ayache, and O. Clatz. DTI registration with exact finite-strain differential. In *5th IEEE International Symposium on Biomedical Imaging: From Nano to Macro (ISBI '08)*, 2008, pages 700–703. DOI 10.1109/isbi.2008.4541092.

Chapter 6
Treatment Planning

Most surgical interventions rely on a planning step. For example, in orthopedic surgery, angles or cutting planes must be defined before the intervention. This step requires image data. Given the image data, we could plan the intervention with paper and pencil. However, it seems reasonable to combine planning with navigation, since we must retrieve the geometric results of the planning steps during the intervention.
In radiosurgery, an optimal set of directions from which to irradiate the tumor must be defined. This gives rise to complex patterns of intersections between beam directions. For each beam direction, we must assign a dose weight. Then a motion path for the beam source must be computed with mathematical methods. This path must be collision free and dose constraints must be satisfied.

6.1 Planning for Orthopedic Surgery

In intertrochanteric osteotomy, a small bone wedge is removed to improve the posture of the femur head. Figure 6.1 shows the two cutting planes for removing the wedge. A metal implant (Fig. 6.1, left) joins the two bone fragments (femur head/femur shaft).
During the procedure, the surgeon drills a channel through the femur neck from the lateral direction Fig. 6.2. The channel will later hold the top part of the implant. It is necessary to drill the channel *before*

A. Schweikard, F. Ernst, *Medical Robotics*,
DOI 10.1007/978-3-319-22891-4_6

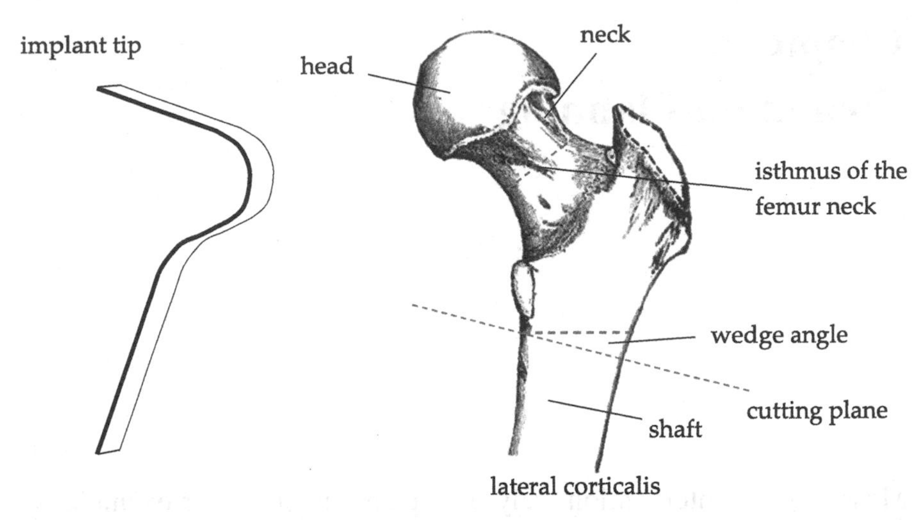

Fig. 6.1: Implant for intertrochanteric femur osteotomy. To adjust the position of the femur head, a small bone wedge is removed. The size, position and angle of the wedge are computed in the planning phase. During the intervention, a channel is drilled into the femur neck. The top part of the implant is then placed into this channel. The shaft of the implant is attached to the lateral femur shaft with screws

cutting the femur. Otherwise the femur head would be loose, making it hard to drill the channel. But now it is difficult to find the correct angle for the drill, since the implant shaft must touch the lateral femur shaft *after* removing the wedge.

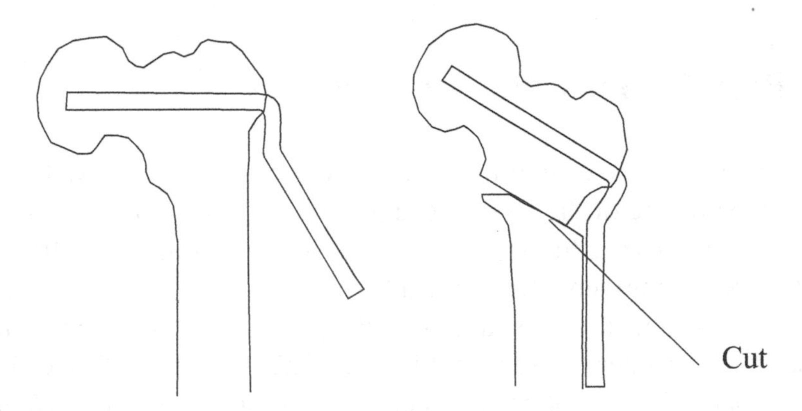

Fig. 6.2: The implant must be placed before the cut is made

To plan the intervention, a desired new position of the femur head with respect to the bone must be determined. Hence, three parameters are specified in the planning phase: channel direction, cutting plane and wedge plane.
The planning procedure consists of the following steps:

1. Take two X-ray images (anterior/posterior and axial)
2. Construct a simplified model of the femur bone before wedge removal
3. Determine the desired pose, based on this model
4. Plan the implant position

Images for step one are taken during the intervention. Planning is based on the X-ray images, hence no registration step is needed.
For step two, we extract the following five features from the X-ray images: femur shaft axis, center of the femoral neck isthmus (see also Fig. 6.1), femoral head center point, femoral shaft radius, and osteotomy plane. In the navigation set-up with an optical tracking system and the C-arm, we can obtain the spatial position of these features in the following way. In the simplest case, the feature is a point. The point is marked in both images on the computer screen. Cast a line in space from the X-ray source point to the marked image point on the detector. This is done for both images. The intersection point of the two lines gives the spatial position of the point. In a similar way, the spatial positions of the remaining features can be extracted.
The features thus extracted define a simplified bone model, and step three is done as follows: We define a coordinate system for the femur shaft. This coordinate system does not move with the shaft. All motions of the femur head and neck caused by repositioning are now described with respect to this coordinate system. The coordinate system is defined in the following way:

- The origin is the intersection point between the cutting plane and the shaft axis (defined in step 2).
- The z-axis is the extension of the shaft axis and points into the proximal direction (i.e. towards the patient's head).
- The y-axis is a vector in the AP-direction in the anatomy. Note that the AP-direction is defined implicitly by the user, when taking the

X-ray image in AP-direction under navigation. To obtain a valid coordinate system, we adjust this y-axis in such a way that it is orthogonal to the z-axis defined before.

- The x-axis completes the coordinate system such that we obtain a right-handed coordinate system.

In medical terminology, the three angles describing the orientation of the femur head are called:

- flexion/extension (tilting of the femur head into the anterior/posterior direction, this is the x-axis defined above)
- varus/valgus (tilting of the femur head downwards/upwards, this is a rotation about the y-axis of the above coordinate system, see also Fig. 6.3)
- rotation/derotation (rotating the femur head fragment about the femur shaft axis, which is our z-axis; the direction of rotation is clockwise when looking onto the x-y-plane from the proximal direction)

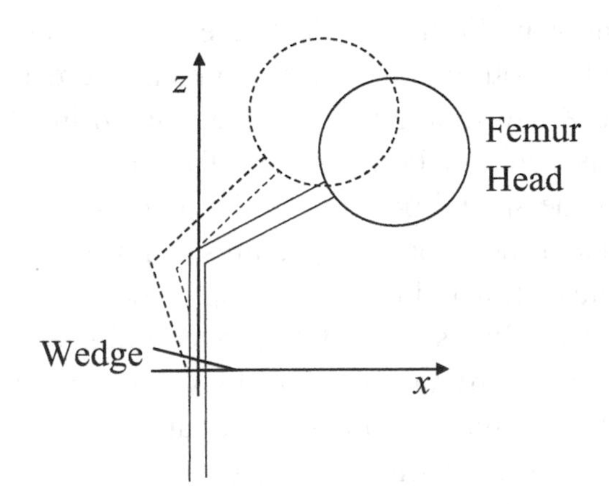

Fig. 6.3: Forward and inverse planning for intertrochanteric femur osteotomy. Frontal view onto the right femur. In this view, a valgus of 15° is specified. Original posture of the femur (*solid*) and new posture (*transparent*)

With the features defined above, a model of the femur can be visualized on the computer screen (Fig. 6.3).

Three rotational parameters and three translational parameters are set by the surgeon. In an inverse planning step, we compute the resulting wedge to be removed. Mathematically, this inverse step is very simple. We take the x-y-plane of the coordinate system defined above. The wedge (see Fig. 6.3) is between the original x-y-plane and the new x-y-plane. To obtain the new position of the x-y-plane, we rotate the coordinate system defined above by the three angles (x-rotation, followed by y-rotation, followed by z-rotation). The matrix operations involved are straightforward (see Chap. 2).

Finally, after planning the wedge, we plan the position of the implant (step 4). The implant tip must remain at a safe distance from the bone surface, and the shaft of the implant must be aligned with the femur shaft. To guide the positioning of the implant, we mark the lateral surface of the femur shaft in the images. We place and move the implant manually over the femur model (Fig. 6.3). To obtain correct alignment, the features extracted above are displayed in the same coordinate system. The position of the implant is now given in terms of the coordinate system specified for the femur. Thus all planning data refer to the same coordinate system. This coordinate system is defined directly on the images from the C-arm. Given the markers on the C-arm, we can locate all planning data in the anatomy.

6.2 Planning for Radiosurgery

In radiosurgery, tumors are irradiated from many different directions, to minimize dose in healthy tissue, and accumulate high dose in the tumor.

To plan a treatment in radiosurgery, the path of the radiation source must be computed. This path depends on the shape and size, and also on the anatomic position of the tumor. Specifically, we must avoid irradiating critical healthy organs close to the tumor. Such organs can be the lung, the spine, a blood vessel or a nerve. To avoid critical structures, the path of the robot must be computed given the individual anatomy. Images of the anatomy are available as CT or MR stacks.

First assume the tumor has spherical shape. To irradiate a spherical target, beams cross-fire from multiple directions at the target. This is

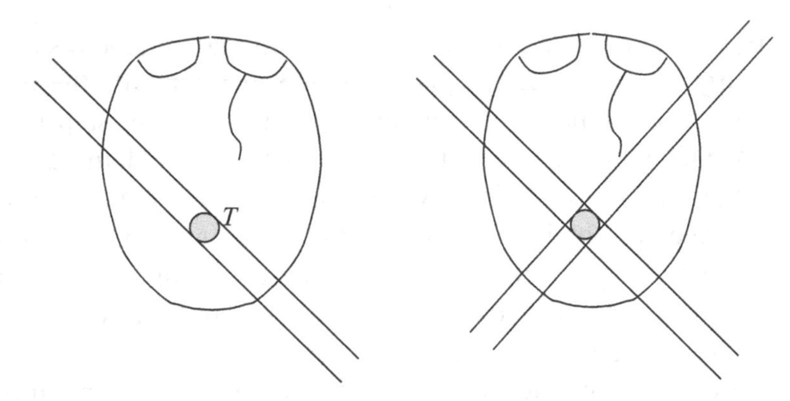

Fig. 6.4: Irradiating a spherical target from multiple directions. Dose is accumulated in the target region while healthy tissue is spared

shown in Fig. 6.4. The left part of the figure shows a treatment with one single beam direction. Such a treatment would be far from optimal, since the healthy tissue along the beam path will receive the same dose as the target. On the right side of the figure, two beams are used. Generally, the right plan is preferable over the left plan because we can ensure that the dose in most of the healthy tissue remains below a given threshold.
If we increase the number of beams in Fig. 6.4, we obtain a so-called isocentric treatment (Fig. 6.5). All beams intersect, so that the treated volume is a sphere.
In practice, the target region often is not spherical. Figure 6.6 shows an elongated tumor region T and a critical structure B.
During treatment, the beam is placed in a series of fixed positions (called treatment nodes). At each position the beam is activated for a certain amount of time. Thus, treatment planning consists of two phases:

Phase 1: Find irradiation directions (also called beam directions)
Phase 2: Find a weight for each beam direction (duration of activation of the beam at this irradiation direction)

For phase 1, we must choose the placement of the beams. The number of beams can be large (i.e. 1000 beams). For phase 2, the duration of

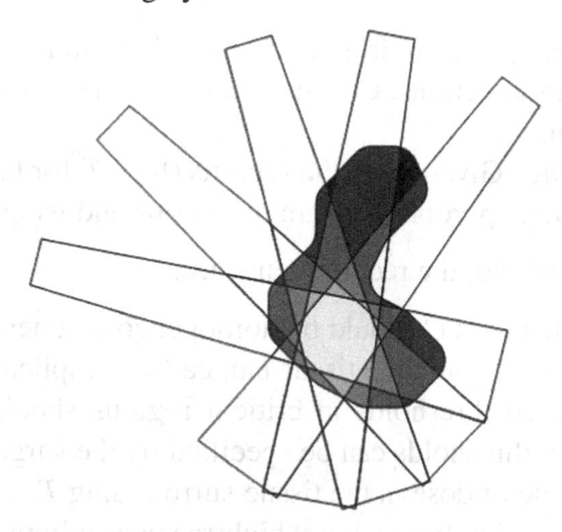

Fig. 6.5: Isocentric treatment. Beam axes cross in a single point, the treated volume is spherical

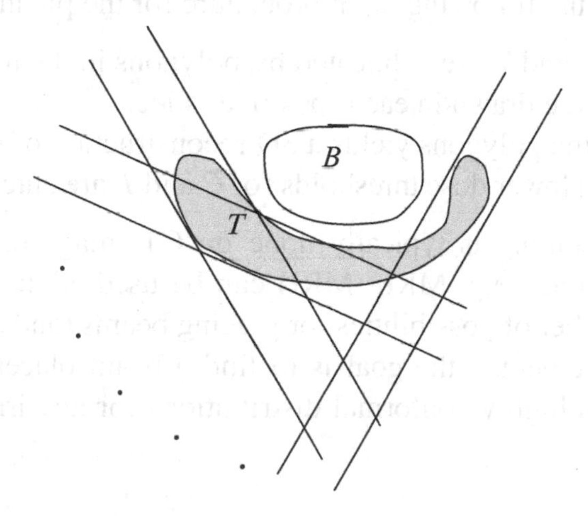

Fig. 6.6: Non-spherical target region T and critical region B

activation of each beam must be computed. This is an optimization problem. The computations for phase 1 and phase 2 interact. Thus it is useful to iterate over both phases.

After we have computed a treatment plan, we must simulate the effect of this plan in terms of dose delivered to the individual regions in the target area. Such a simulation must then be visualized. Thus we distinguish between forward and inverse planning:

Forward planning. Given: irradiation directions and the dose weights for all beam directions. Calculate and visualize the resulting dose distribution.

Inverse planning. Given: only the regions (here T for target and C for critical). Find appropriate beam directions and weights.

For inverse planning, the requirements are:

1. The dose in T and C should be homogeneous (uneven dose in the target and/or surrounding tissue can cause complications).
2. Maximal dose thresholds in critical regions should not be exceeded. Such thresholds can be specified by the surgeon.
3. Sharp decline of dose in the tissue surrounding T.
4. Conformality, i.e. the region which receives a high dose ('treated volume') should match T.

This leads to the following input procedure for the planning data:

1. Regions C and T are delineated by polygons in the tomography.
2. Polygons are drawn in each (positive) slice.
3. Stacking the polygons yields a 3D reconstruction of the regions.
4. Upper and lower dose thresholds for C and T are entered as inputs.

Treatment planning is typically done on CT image data, but other image modalities (e.g. MRI, fMRI) can be used additionally. Given the large number of possibilities for placing beams (and combinations of beam placements), the goal is to find a beam placement scheme which returns highly conformal distributions for any irregular target shape.

6.2.1 Beam Placement

When developing a scheme for beam placement, we will set up a hierarchy of shapes, from simple to more complex shapes. While it is impossible to find a global optimum for arbitrary target shapes, there is a straightforward method for special shapes: for a sphere, an isocentric beam placement is ideal (Fig. 6.5).

For non-spherical shapes, an isocentric treatment may not be optimal. To treat non-spherical volumes, one could pack several spheres together to cover the tumor (Fig. 6.7). However, this is also problematic. Overlap between spheres will often be unavoidable. (Fig. 6.7). Such overlap between the spheres must be minimized: overlap would result in hot spots, i.e. undesirable overdosage of subregions within the target.

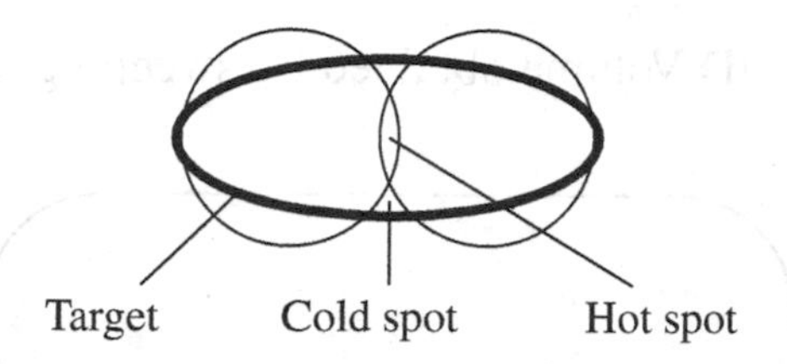

Fig. 6.7: Sphere packing for non-spherical target shape results in uneven coverage (hot spots)

Consider the target volume in the Fig. 6.8. This shape is obtained by sweeping a sphere. Now, instead of having a single isocenter, we sweep the isocenter along a line segment. This gives rise to a series of discretized isocenter points (Fig. 6.9b). Each of these new isocenter points is then treated as if it was the center of a spherical target volume. The result is an overlay of a series of spherical volumes. The main difference between this scheme and sphere packing is that now the spheres do overlap, while homogeneity is achieved by the sweeping process.
Now the question remains of how to place beams for arbitrarily shaped target volumes. A straight-forward extension of the above line-sweeping placement scheme is illustrated in Fig. 6.10. Thus, the outer boundary of the target volume is retracted, and a series of isocenter points are placed on the retracted surface. Sweeping is then applied to this retracted surface.

6.2.2 Beam Weights

In a second step, we compute the weights of the beams. We compute the beam weights with linear programming. Thus, linear programming

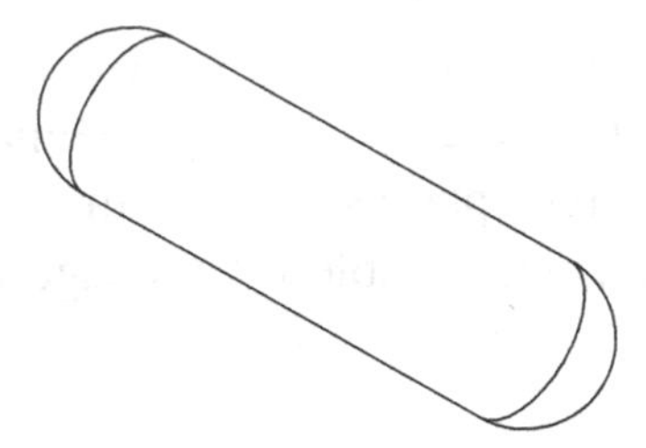

Fig. 6.8: 3D Volume obtained by sweeping a sphere

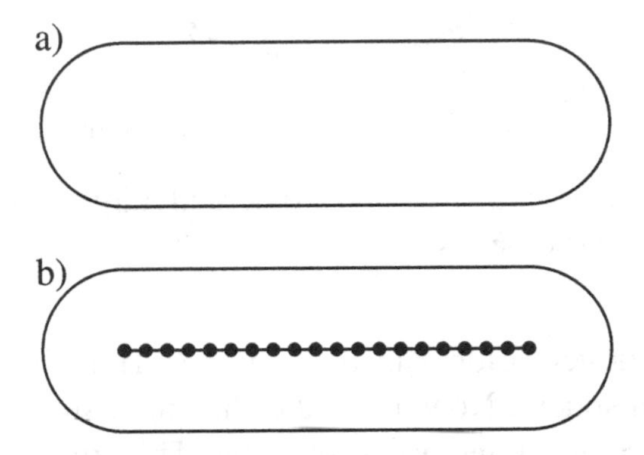

Fig. 6.9: Sweeping an isocenter point along a line segment

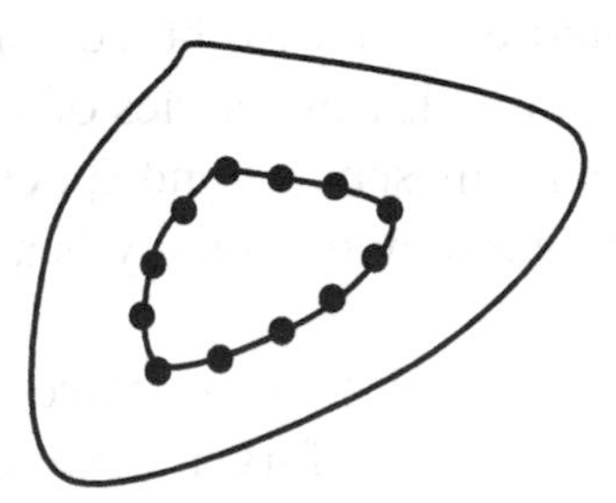

Fig. 6.10: Placement of isocenter points for irregular shapes

computes durations of activation for each beam by solving a large system of inequalities.

To set up the systems of inequalities, consider the situation in Fig. 6.11. The figure shows a target region (tumor T), a critical region C, and a polygon surrounding C and T. Furthermore, the figure shows three beams crossing the regions delineated. The polygons shown are bounded by line segments.

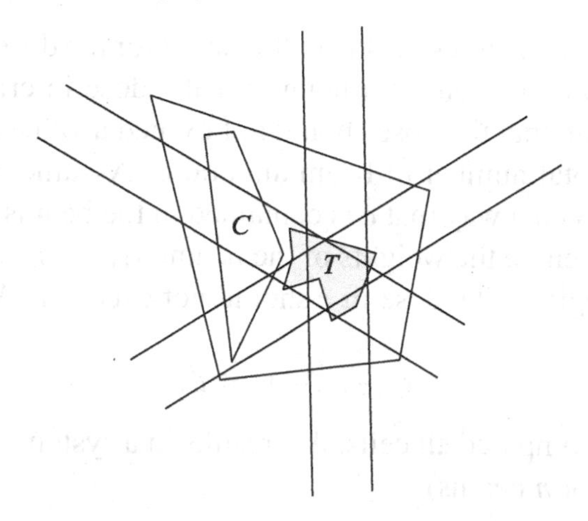

Fig. 6.11: Beam weighting and arrangements

We extend each line segment to a line. The lines partition the plane into so-called cells. Here, we define a cell as a maximally connected region containing no points on the given lines. (Thus, we consider geometric cells, not anatomic cells.) All cells thus defined are convex. Now we take a reference point in each cell. This is an arbitrary point inside the cell. For each such point we can compute a label. This label simply lists all regions which contain the cell. The label also includes the beams containing the cell. Our definition of geometric cells can be extended in two ways: first, the target is three-dimensional, and second, our beams are typically cylinders. For both extensions the necessary modifications are straightforward.

The partitioning of space which has been induced by the beams and the delineation gives rise to an equation system: We take the label of a single cell c. Assume c is contained in the target, and also in three of the beams, called s_1, s_2 and s_3. Then we wish to bound the dose in the target from below. Thus the dose should be above a given threshold value t.

Our goal is to compute the duration of activation of each beam. In our example (Fig. 6.11), we assign variables x_1, x_2, x_3 for these unknown durations of activation for the beams s_1, s_2 and s_3.

Overall we have an equation of the form

$$x_1 + x_2 + x_3 \geq t. \tag{6.1}$$

Here, the value t specifies the lower threshold for the dose in the target. In the same way we can set a bound for the dose in critical regions, i.e. we can state that the dose should not exceed a value t'.
Let n be the total number of beam directions. Assume the beams are numbered in such a way that c is contained in the beams $s_1, \ldots, s_k$. By $x_1, \ldots, x_k$ we denote the weights of the beams $s_1, \ldots, s_k$. Let c be a cell in a critical region. The dose in c should not exceed t'. We obtain the equation

$$x_1 + \ldots + x_k \leq t'. \tag{6.2}$$

After having computed all cells, this results in a system of inequalities of the form (for n beams)

$$\begin{aligned} a_{11}x_1 + \ldots + a_{1n}x_n &\leq t' \\ a_{21}x_1 + \ldots + a_{2n}x_n &\leq t' \\ &\vdots \\ a_{m1}x_1 + \ldots + a_{mn}x_n &\leq t', \end{aligned} \tag{6.3}$$

where the a_{ij} are 0 or 1.
If c is in T, then c corresponds to an inequality of the form

$$a_{11}x_1 + \ldots + a_{1n}x_1 \geq t, \tag{6.4}$$

where t is lower bound for the dose in T.
Exact methods for computing reference points for all cells are too slow for our application. For our purposes the following approximation suffices: choose a dense grid of the points in 3D, in an area containing the target. For each grid point **p**, test which beams contain **p**. Assume **p** is contained in the beams $s_1, \ldots, s_k$. From this, we can readily compute the label of **p**. The label of every grid point is a set. For each point we obtain one or more inequalities.

6.2.2.1 Linear Programming

In linear programming, we have a set of constraints given as linear inequalities, and our goal is to check whether this set of linear inequalities admits a solution. For example, consider the inequalities:

$$\begin{aligned} x_1 + x_2 &\leq 10 \\ x_1 &\geq 5 \\ x_2 &\geq 4 \end{aligned} \tag{6.5}$$

Obviously, these constraints are feasible, i.e. there are values for x_1 and x_2 satisfying these inequalities. The constraints are visualized in Fig. 6.12.

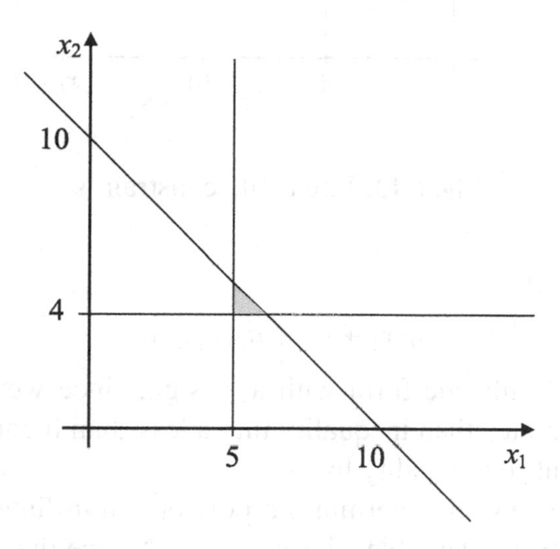

Fig. 6.12: Feasible region for the linear constraints in Eq. 6.5

On the other hand, the given inequalities will become *infeasible* if we apply the following small modification (see Fig. 6.13):

$$\begin{aligned} x_1 + x_2 &\leq 10 \\ x_1 &\geq 5 \\ x_2 &\geq 6 \end{aligned}$$

In general, we have an inequality system of the form

$$\begin{aligned} a_{11}x_1 + \cdots + a_{1n}x_n &\leq b_1 \\ a_{21}x_1 + \cdots + a_{2n}x_n &\leq b_2 \\ &\vdots \\ a_{m1}x_1 + \cdots + a_{mn}x_n &\leq b_m \end{aligned} \tag{6.6}$$

where m and n can be different. Notice that the $\leq$-sign used here is not a restriction. Inequalities in linear programming can also take the

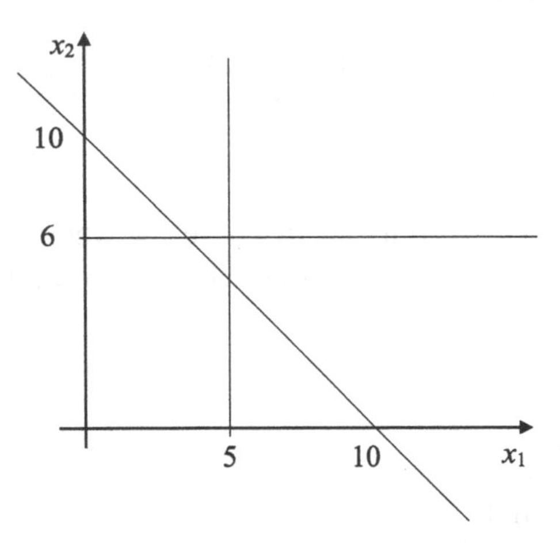

Fig. 6.13: Infeasible constraints

form

$$a_{i1}x_1 + \cdots + a_{in}x_n \geq b_i.$$

We have used only the form with a $\leq$-sign, since we could always transform a greater-than inequality into a less-than inequality by multiplying the entire inequality by -1.
The inequality system determines a polytope in n-dimensional space (n is the number of variables, i.e. $x_1, .., x_n$). Notice that n is not equal to two or three, although the system describes the constraints for the three-dimensional case. Rather, the dimension n is the number of variables in the system. A feasibility test (F) only checks whether this polytope is not empty, i.e. if there is a solution or not. Two problems are distinguished in linear programming:

(LP) 'search for a maximum under constraints'

and

(F) 'feasibility test'.

Notice that the above system of inequalities in Eq. 6.6 is not the standard form of linear programming in the literature. The standard linear programming (LP) is defined in the following way: Given constraints in Eq. 6.6, maximize the expression

$$c_1x_1 + \ldots + c_nx_n, \tag{6.7}$$

where all $x_i \geq 0$. The expression in Eq. 6.7 is called the objective function . Figure 6.14 shows the situation. Here the objective function is $1x_1 + 0x_2$.

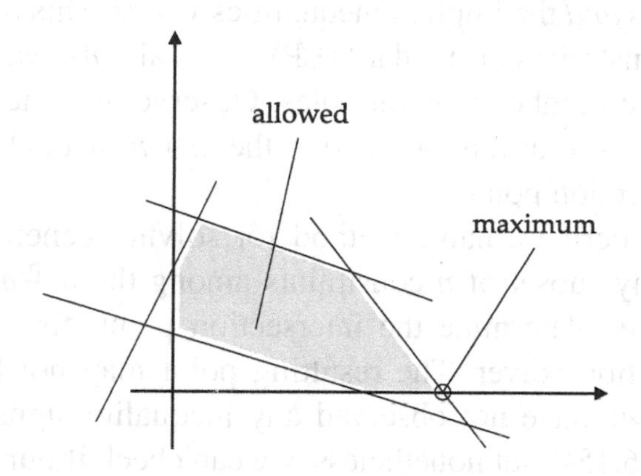

Fig. 6.14: Feasible region and objective function

The gray region is the feasible region. Notice that it does not extend into the negative quadrants, since we require all x_i to be positive. The values c_i determine a vector **c**. We maximize in direction of this vector **c**, while remaining within the feasible region.
Thus (LP) contains a maximization, which is more than (F) alone. However, in standard form, (LP) imposes the restriction that all x_i be positive. Convince yourself that this restriction can be removed: substitute each occurrence of the variable x_i in the given LP-problem by the expression $(y_i - y_i')$, where y_i and y_i' are new variables. After substitution, the new problem has the standard LP-form with all variables $y_i, y_i' \geq 0$.
The matrix form of the LP problem in Eqs. 6.6 and 6.7 is obtained by setting up a coefficient matrix **A** from the coefficients a_{ij}, and two vectors $\mathbf{b} = (b_1, \ldots, b_m)^{\mathrm{T}}$, $\mathbf{c} = (c_1, \ldots, c_n)^{\mathrm{T}}$. An LP problem can then be stated in the compact form

$$(\max \quad \mathbf{cx} \quad s.t. \quad \mathbf{Ax} \leq \mathbf{b}). \tag{6.8}$$

We have compared the two problem types (LP) and (F). We will now look at the connection between (LP) and the well-known linear equation systems. n equations (with n unknowns) determine (if independent) an intersection point in n-dimensional space. But notice that, in general, (LP) contains more than n inequalities, although we have not imposed any restrictions on the number m of constraints! The reason is that (LP) contains the actual inequalities with the a_{ij}- resp. b_i-coefficients *and* the implicit inequalities $x_i \geq 0$. This means that the number of constraints in standard (LP) is actually $n+m$. This value is larger than the number n of variables. Observe that each subset of n constraints, picked at random among the $m+n$ inequalities, determines an intersection point.

Now we can derive a naive method for solving general (LP) problems. Pick any subset of n constraints among the $n+m$ constraints. For this subset, determine the intersection point, for example with a linear equation solver. The resulting point may not be a feasible point, since we have not observed any inequality signs in our constraints (Fig. 6.15). But nonetheless, we can check if our point is feasible. Now repeat this for all n-element subsets of the $n+m$-element constraint set. Having checked all such points, we can either report infeasibility, or we can output the point which maximizes the objective function. But notice that this naive method will not help much in practice: the number of n-subsets of an $n+m$-set is exponential in general.

6.2.2.2 Finding Beam Weights with Linear Programming

As noted above, the planning process is interactive. The first step is to delineate the critical regions and the target. This is done in the CT data set. In each slice of the CT set, we delineate the relevant structures (both target and critical regions). After this, we need to find the beam directions. To this end, we specify the number of beams to be placed accordingto the heuristic method in the previous section. To each beam, we assign a variable x_i. We then place a dense grid of points over the region of interest and compute the labels of each grid point. Notice that many of the grid points will have the same label. We will return to this later.

When applying linear programming, we indeed solve the feasibility problem (F) discussed above for the constraint inequalities derived

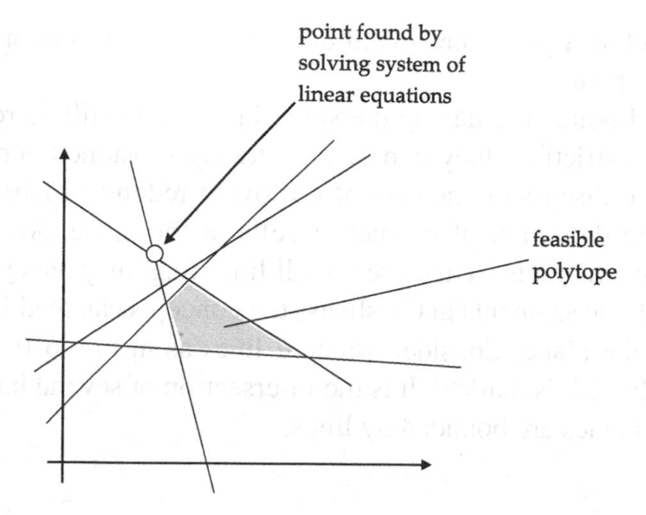

Fig. 6.15: Solving a system of linear equations does not necessarily yield a feasible point

from the labels of the grid points. We could include an objective function where $\mathbf{c} = (-1, \ldots, -1)^\mathrm{T}$. This objective function minimizes the total dose (sum of all variables x_i). In this form, we may simply obtain the answer that the given system is infeasible.
The problem that the given constraints may be infeasible can be solved by introducing so-called slack variables s_i, s'_i. The slack variables are treated in just the same way as the regular linear programming variables, i.e. we require s_i, s'_i be positive:

$$a_{11}x_1 + \ldots + a_{1n}x_n + s_1 - s'_1 \leq b_1 \tag{6.9}$$

$$\vdots$$

$$a_{m1}x_1 + \ldots + a_{mn}x_n + s_m - s'_m \leq b_m$$

After extending the input linear system in this way, the system will always be feasible. In the optimization step, we then minimize the sum of the slack variables, instead of the sum of the variables x_i.
As noted above, many of the grid points will have the same labels. Obviously, it is useful to have a small number of inequalities, since the computing time for solving the resulting system is often in the range of several hours. To this end, we remove grid points having the

same label as a grid point found earlier. This is straightforward, but we can do better.

Some grid points not having the same labels may still be redundant, since the restrictions they impose are already subsumed in other constraints. To discuss the process of removing redundant labels, we return to the definition of geometric cells in the plane. Although the geometric structures we use are not all lines (e.g. they are cylinders in space and line segments in CT slices) the concepts can readily be visualized in the plane. Consider oriented lines as in Fig. 6.16. One cell (shown shaded) is marked. It is the intersection of several half-planes. The half-planes are bounded by lines.

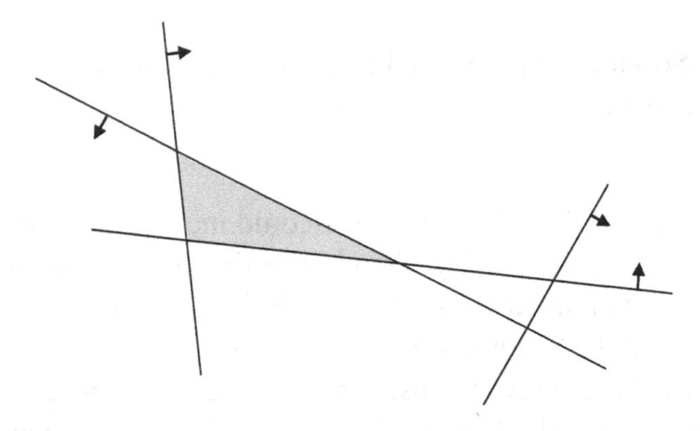

Fig. 6.16: Maximal cell. Lines are oriented, as indicated by *arrows*. The number of lines having the shaded cell in their interior half-space attains a local maximum

To define this orientation of lines, an arrow marks the 'upper' or 'inner' half-space for the line. The respective other half-space is the outer or lower half-space. Now we define a maximal cell: A cell c is maximal, if all lines directly bounding c have their inner half-space on the same side as c. Similarly, we can define minimal cells. To remove redundant constraints, we only retain constraints for maximal cells, if the dose is bounded from above. Likewise, only constraints for minimal cells are retained, in cases where the dose is bounded from below.

The interactive planning process for finding the dose weights now proceeds as follows:

After beam directions have been placed computationally, the threshold values for upper and lower dose limits in tumor and critical regions are set. These threshold values and region/beam boundaries determine a system of inequalities. Afterwards it is checked whether this system admits a solution, i.e. we perform a feasibility test (F).
Notice that the constants a_{ij} in the linear program can be set in such a way that depth in tissue is represented. A table listing dose attenuation with depth in tissue is the basis of this process. To adjust the values a_{ij}, we examine each of the points corresponding to our LP-constraints. The points correspond to the j-index in a_{ij}. Given the CT of the target region, we determine the depth in tissue of each point, depending on the beam direction.

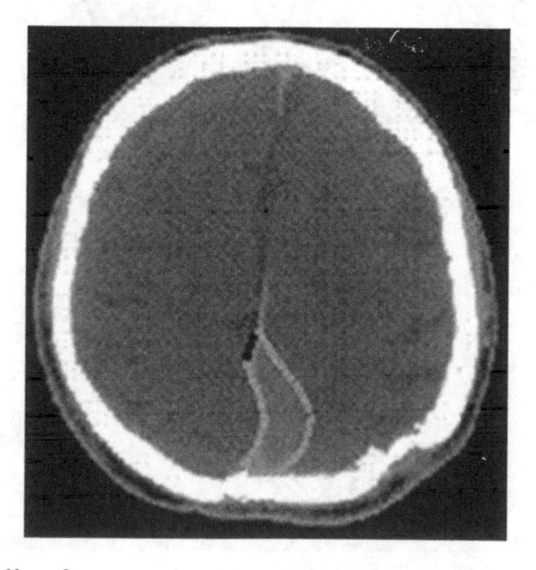

Fig. 6.17: CT slice for sample case with polygon delineating the target

Figure 6.17 shows a typical planning problem. The tumor is delineated by a polygon, shown in light gray in the back part of the head. In this case, there are no critical regions in direct vicinity of the target. The planning goal is to achieve high conformality and homogeneity. To specify constraints on the homogeneity of dose within the target, we require that the tumor dose stays between 2000 cGy and 2200 cGy (1 Gy = 1 Gray = 1 J/kg; 1 cGy is 0.01 Gy). An example result of inverse planning for this case is given in Fig. 6.18. When this plan is executed on a phantom, the dose actually delivered can be determined (see Fig. 6.19).

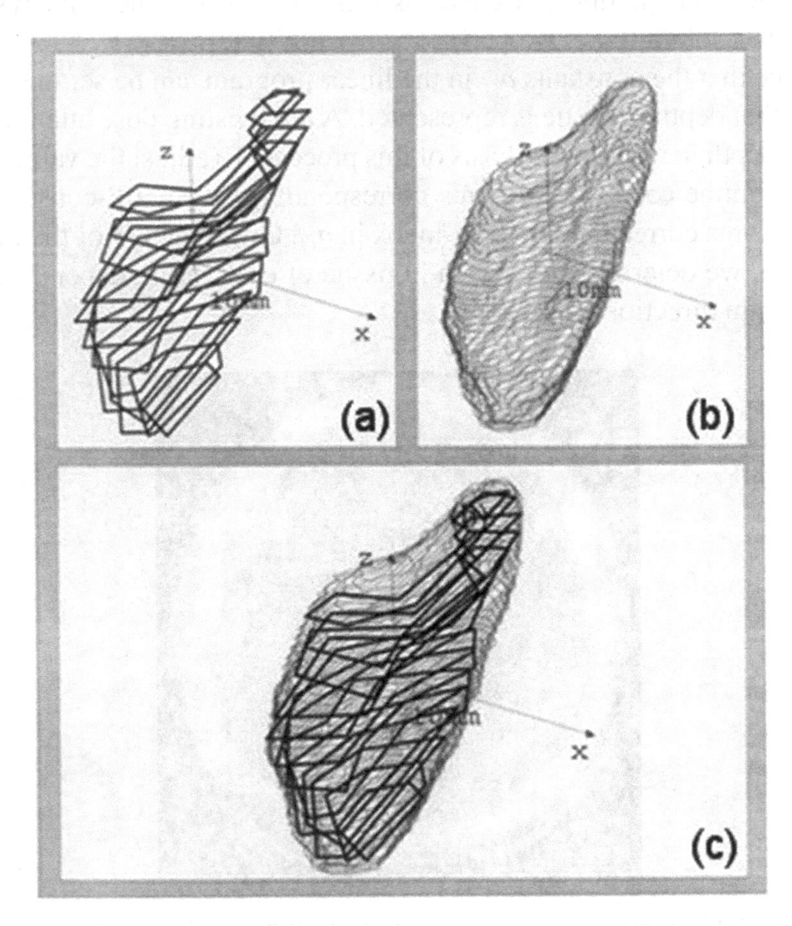

Fig. 6.18: Inverse planning input and output for sample case in Fig. 6.17. (**a**) Stack of tumor polygons in each positive slice. (**b**) 80 % isodose curve after computing the beam weights with linear programming. (**c**) Overlay of (**a**) and (**b**)

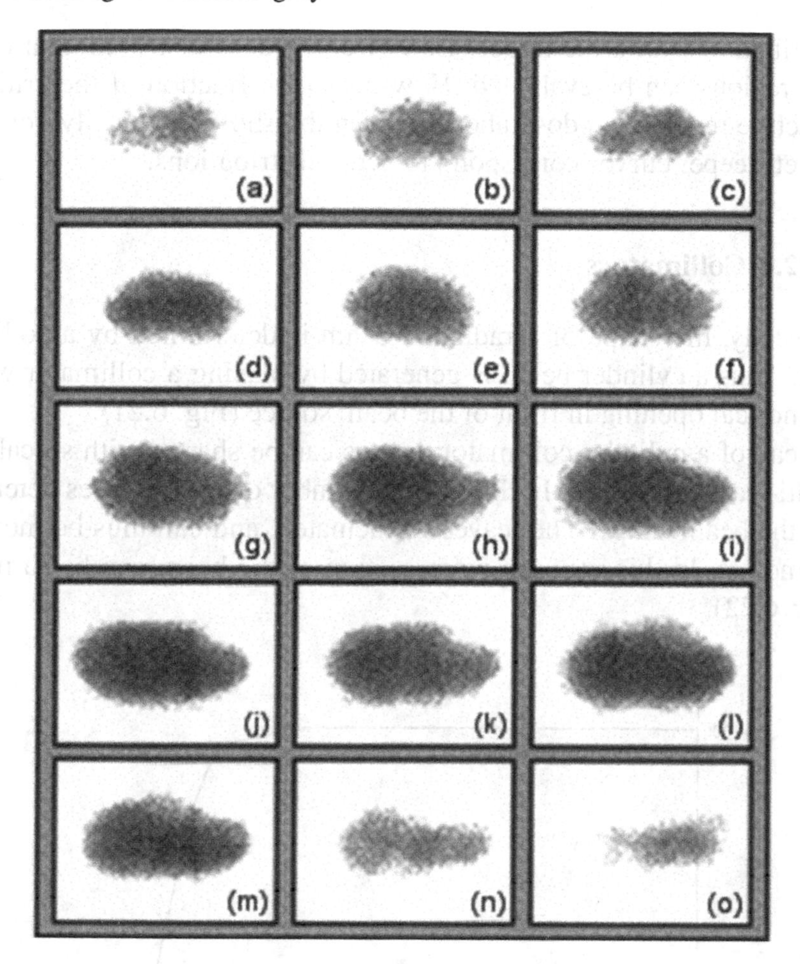

Fig. 6.19: Phantom: photographic film is exposed as the planned treatment for the case in Fig. 6.17 is executed (Notice treated region closely matches the input tumor shape.)

6.2.2.3 Dose Evaluation

We evaluate a dose distribution with a so-called dose volume histogram (Fig. 6.20). The x-axis lists dose values in cGy. The y-axis lists percentages of the total volume. Thus, the histogram gives percentages of volumes receiving specific amounts of dose. The histogram provides a way to evaluate a dose distribution at the target in several ways: how well is the target covered? How homogeneous is the distribution within the target? Likewise, the dose distribution at critical regions can be evaluated: How big is the fraction of the critical structure receiving a dose above a given threshold? Typically, for the target steeper curves correspond to better distributions.

6.2.2.4 Collimators

Typically, the shape of a radiation beam is determined by a collimator. Thus a cylinder beam is generated by placing a collimator with cylindrical opening in front of the beam source (Fig. 6.21).
Instead of a cylinder collimator, beams can be shaped with so-called multi-leaf collimators. In this case, a number of metal leaves determine the beam shape. The leaves are actuated, and can thus be moved be motors. In this way the cross-section of the beam can be formed (Fig. 6.22).

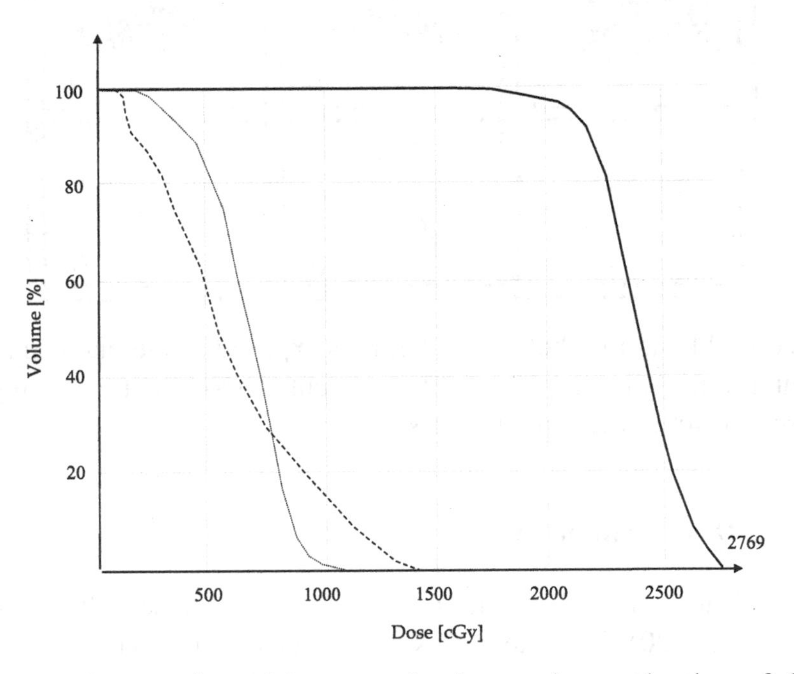

Fig. 6.20: Dose-volume histogram for interactive evaluation of dose distributions. Tumor volume (*bold curve*), esophagus (*thin dotted line*), spine (*dashed line*)

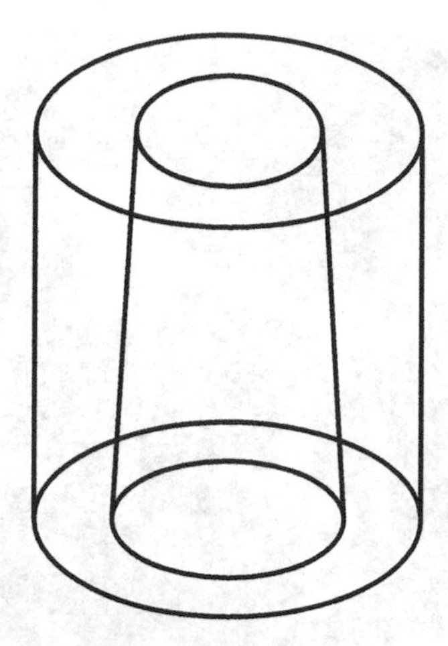

Fig. 6.21: Beam collimator. The beam is not cylindrical, but a cone. The radiation source is at the tip of the cone

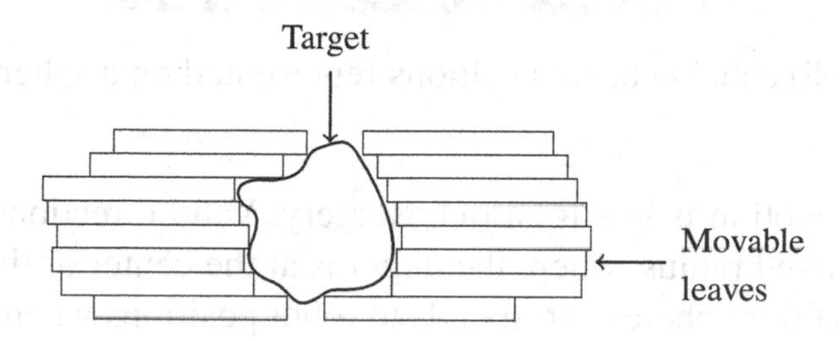

Fig. 6.22: Multi-leaf collimator

Reachable Robot Configurations and Treatment Planning

In robotic radiosurgery, we are given a set of beam directions, from which the target must be irradiated. Here it is necessary to find a valid robot path connecting these beam directions. The path must be collision-free with respect to the remaining work-space and the patient. The line-of-sight of imaging devices must not be blocked. To move along the path, any changes of robot configurations (elbow up/elbow down, robot left shoulder configuration/right shoulder configuration) should be avoided.

However, configuration changes become necessary whenever the robot reaches joint angle limits. Thus, it is useful to find a path with minimal number of configuration changes. Figure 6.23 shows an ex-

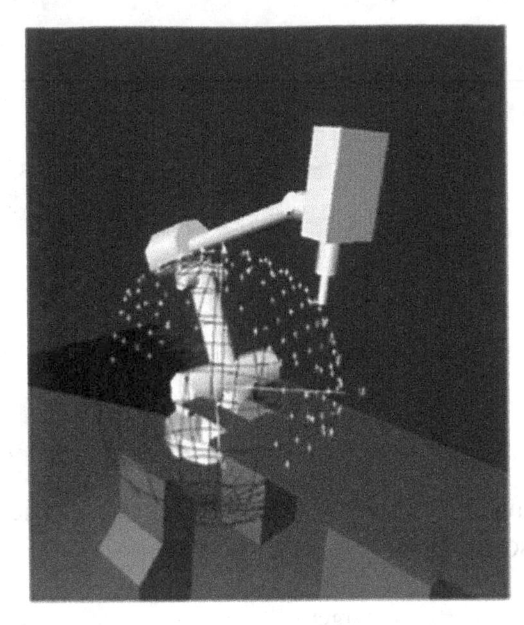

Fig. 6.23: Reachable beam positions represented on a spherical grid

ample for motion planning in radiosurgery. Valid directions are on a sphere of fixed radius, where the target is at the center of this sphere. A subset of this sphere corresponds to robot positions where no intersections between the robot arm and lines-of-sight of cameras will occur. This subset is marked by white points in the figure. The points in this set (node set) are connected by a series of standard paths, defined for individual anatomical locations.

6.3 Four-Dimensional Planning

Organs in soft tissue move during respiration. Critical regions close to the target may move at different velocities. For example, structures close to the spine may move less than organs further away. This is illustrated in Fig. 6.24.
We can address the problem of organ motion in the planning process. To this end, we must capture the motion of the organs with medical imaging. Four-dimensional CT is suitable for this purpose. Figure 6.25 illustrates four-dimensional CT. A four-dimensional CT

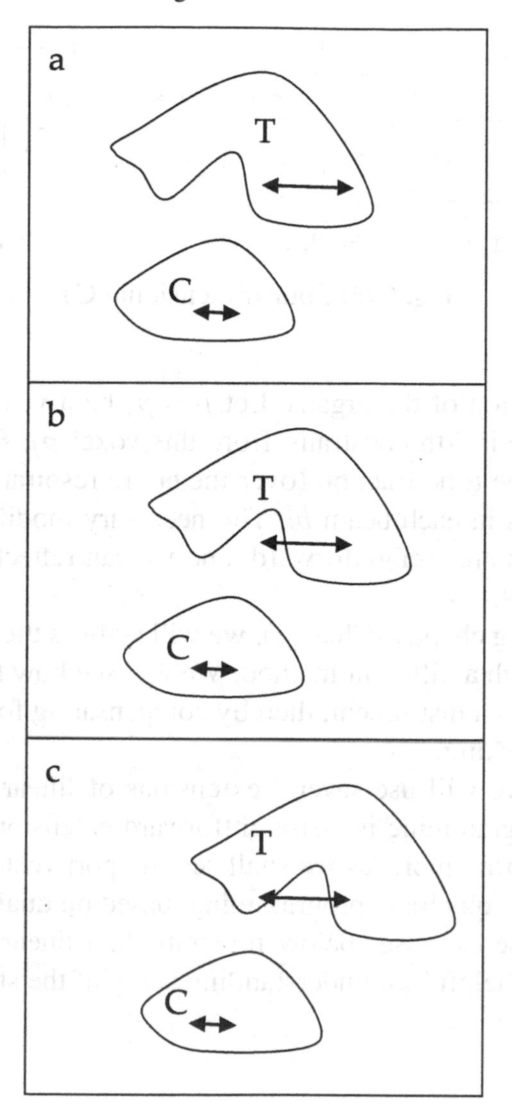

Fig. 6.24: Motion of organs in soft tissue. The target moves faster than a critical structure in the vicinity of the target

typically consists of 10 three-dimensional CT stacks, where each stack corresponds to one time point.
Having obtained a four-dimensional CT image set, we can incorporate organ motion into the planning process. Again we use linear programming. Recall that we computed values a_{ij} as coefficients of our linear program above. The computation of these values is now adapted to

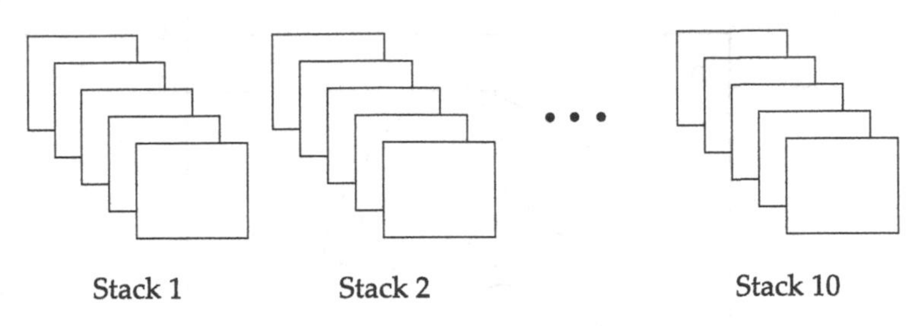

Fig. 6.25: Four-dimensional CT

reflect the motion of the organs. Let $p = p_j$ be a voxel. Assume we have derived our j-th constraint from this voxel p_j. For each beam, we compute the time fraction (over the entire respiratory cycle) during which p is in each beam b_i. The necessary modifications to our linear program are straightforward, and we can reflect the motion of organs in detail.
In the following chapter (Chap. 7), we will address the problem of organ motion with a different method. We will see how to track a moving target with an instrument, thereby compensating for organ motion with active tracking.
To this end, we will use several extensions of linear programming. Quadratic programming is a straightforward extension of linear programming. Furthermore, as we shall see, support vector regression is an extension of quadratic programming, based on dual quadratic programming. The exercises below illustrate dual linear programming, which will be helpful for understanding many of the steps involved.

Exercises

Exercise 6.1 *Graphical Solution of LP Problems*

Given the LP problem
Maximize

$$5x_1 + x_2$$

subject to

$$\begin{aligned} x_1 + x_2 &\leq 10 \\ x_1 &\geq 5 \\ x_2 &\geq 4. \end{aligned}$$

Determine a solution by computing all intersection points of bounding lines and inserting them into the objective function.

Exercise 6.2 *Dual of a Linear Program*

Suppose we are given a linear program in matrix form as in Eq. 6.10:

$$(\max \quad \mathbf{cx} \quad s.t. \quad \mathbf{Ax} \leq \mathbf{b}) \tag{6.10}$$

The so-called dual of an LP problem is also an LP problem. Here the roles of m and n, and the roles of the vectors $\mathbf{b}$ and $\mathbf{c}$ are exchanged. The dual LP is obtained by introducing new variables $(\alpha_1, \ldots, \alpha_m)^{\mathrm{T}}$:

$$(\min \quad \mathbf{b}\alpha \quad s.t. \quad \mathbf{A}^{\mathrm{T}}\alpha \geq \mathbf{c}) \tag{6.11}$$

Here, $\mathbf{A}^{\mathrm{T}}$ denotes the transpose of the matrix $\mathbf{A}$, and the vector α denotes the vector of the variables α_i, i.e. $\alpha = (\alpha_1, \ldots, \alpha_m)^{\mathrm{T}}$. The variables $(\alpha_1, \ldots, \alpha_m)^{\mathrm{T}}$ are called dual variables. To differentiate between the original version of the LP problem, i.e. as in Eq. 6.10, and the dual in Eq. 6.11, the original version is also called the primal linear program.

a) Set up the dual of the linear program in Exercise 6.1. Find a solution vector of the dual LP by evaluating the objective function at the intersection points defined by the (dual) constraints.
b) Let x_0 be a solution vector of a linear program. Then a solution vector y_0 of the dual linear program can also be found by the so-called equilibrium theorem of linear programming. This theorem relates inequalities of the primal problem to variables y_i of the dual problem. Notice that the number of inequalities of the primal is m, and the number of variables of the dual is also m. Specifically, from the above graphical solutions, you will find that

some of the inequalities are the carrier lines of the solution point. I.e. the solution point x_0 is the intersection point of two lines. These two lines will be called the carrier lines of the solution point. According to the equilibrium theorem, the carrier lines correspond exactly (in terms of their indexes) to the dual variables having non-zero values in the solution y_0. This theorem holds both ways. From this information alone, determine the solution of the dual for the LP problem in Exercise 6.1, given the solution x_0 for the primal problem.

Summary

Treatment planning relies on geometric constraints describing spatial relations of anatomical structures. Forward planning is the process of determining and visualizing the effects of a planned treatment. Inverse planning starts from a desired result, and parameters for achieving this result are computed.
In navigated femur osteotomy, anatomical features can be marked on X-ray image pairs, so that the spatial placement of these features can be found. With these features, the intervention can be planned interactively by a computer. Thus, for example, we assume the projection geometry of the C-arm is known. Then two circles delineating the femur head in a pair of X-ray images determine a pair of cones in space. The intersection of the cones gives the position of the femur head, and enables 3D navigation. In radiosurgery, the directions from which to irradiate a tumor must be computed. By using a very large number of beam directions, the dose distribution can often be improved. In this case, automatic inverse planning is needed. After finding the directions for irradiation, the activation duration (called weight) for each beam must be found. Linear programming provides an effective and fast way for computing such weights.
In linear programming, a set of linear constraints is checked with respect to feasibility. After computing a feasible point (i.e. a point satisfying the constraints), we can move this point in such a way that an objective function is maximized or minimized. This objective func-

tion is also a linear function. Assuming the dose from different beams add up to a total dose, we obtain a linear system of inequalities. In this system, the dose from each beam is represented as one variable, and points covering the target region give rise to linear constraints in these variables. We saw that linear programming directly extends methods for solving linear equation systems, which we have frequently applied in the previous chapters.
To reflect organ motion, we modify the linear program accordingly. Based on four-dimensional imaging, the organ motion can be quantified. We can thus protect critical structures which would receive too much dose if organ motion would bring this structure closer to the target during respiration or pulsation. In the exercises, at the end of this chapter, we look at duals of linear programs. Variables in the dual linear program correspond to inequalities in the primal and vice versa. In the next chapter, we will extend the mathematical tools used so far to address the problem of tracking soft tissue motion.

Notes

The use of linear programming in inverse radiation therapy planning was suggested in [1]. The inverse planning methods in [10, 11] have been clinical standard tools in robotic radiosurgery since 1997. Four-dimensional planning based on linear programming is described in [9].
In brachytherapy, small radioactive seeds are implanted into tumors. The position and weight for the seeds must be planned before treatment. Thus, as in radiation therapy and radiosurgery, dose constraints for critical regions and dose homogeneity constraints must be observed. The intervention can be guided by robots [3].
Further examples for inverse treatment planning in orthopedic surgery can be found in [4].
Treatment planning methods for vascular surgery based on simulation of vascular flow are described in [7, 13].
As an alternative to ionizing radiation, focused ultrasound can be used as an ablative surgical instrument [12]. As in radiosurgery and brachytherapy, the procedure is based on forward and inverse treatment

planning. Further applications are hyperthermia [6], thermo-ablation [8] and transcranial direct current stimulation [2].
Several authors have suggested to apply machine learning to treatment planning (see e.g. [5]). Thus, we can characterize recurring situations and geometric constraints to simplify and shorten the time-consuming interactive processes. For the case of radiosurgery, treatment planning can take several hours in each case. The quality of the plan depends to a large extent on the availability of resources and the expertise of the user.

References

[1] Y. Censor, M. D. Altschuler, and W. D. Powlis. On the use of Cimmino's simultaneous projections method for computing a solution of the inverse problem in radiation therapy treatment planning. *Inverse Problems*, **4**(3):607, 1988. DOI 10.1088/0266-5611/4/3/006.

[2] J. P. Dmochowski, A. Datta, M. Bikson, Y. Su, and L. C. Parra. Optimized multi-electrode stimulation increases focality and intensity at target. *Journal of Neural Engineering*, **8**(4):046011, 2011. DOI 10.1088/1741-2560/8/4/046011.

[3] G. Fichtinger, J. P. Fiene, C. W. Kennedy, G. Kronreif, I. Iordachita, D. Y. Song, E. C. Burdette, and P. Kazanzides. Robotic assistance for ultrasound-guided prostate brachytherapy. *Medical Image Analysis*, **12**(5):535–545, 2008. DOI 10.1016/j.media.2008.06.002.

[4] H. Gottschling, M. Roth, A. Schweikard, and R. Burgkart. Intraoperative, fluoroscopy-based planning for complex osteotomies of the proximal femur. *International Journal of Medical Robotics and Computer Assisted Surgery*, **1**(3):67–73, 2005. DOI 10.1002/rcs.29.

[5] M. Hauskrecht and H. Fraser. Planning treatment of ischemic heart disease with partially observable Markov decision processes. *Artificial Intelligence in Medicine*, **18**(3):221–244, 2000. DOI 10.1016/s0933-3657(99)00042-1.

[6] A. Jordan, R. Scholz, P. Wust, H. Fähling, and R. Felix. Magnetic fluid hyperthermia (MFH): Cancer treatment with AC magnetic field induced excitation of biocompatible superparamagnetic nanoparticles. *Journal of Magnetism and Magnetic Materials*, **201**(1-3):413–419, 1999. DOI 10.1016/s0304-8853(99)00088-8.

[7] S. Nakajima, H. Atsumi, A. H. Bhalerao, F. A. Jolesz, R. Kikinis, T. Yoshimine, T. M. Moriarty, and P. E. Stieg. Computer-assisted surgical planning for cerebrovascular neurosurgery. *Neurosurgery*, **2 41**:403–410, 1997.

[8] S. Rossi, M. Di Stasi, E. Buscarini, P. Quaretti, F. Garbagnati, L. Squassante, C. T. Paties, D. E. Silverman, and L. Buscarini. Percutaneous RF interstitial thermal ablation in the treatment of hepatic cancer. *American Journal of Roentgenology*, **167**(3): 759–768, 2014. DOI 10.2214/ajr.167.3.8751696.

[9] A. Schlaefer, J. Fisseler, S. Dieterich, H. Shiomi, K. Cleary, and A. Schweikard. Feasibility of four-dimensional conformal planning for robotic radiosurgery. *Medical Physics*, **32**(12):3786–3792, 2005. DOI 10.1118/1.2122607.

[10] A. Schweikard, M. Bodduluri, R. Tombropoulos, and J. R. Adler, Jr. Planning, calibration and collision-avoidance for image-guided radiosurgery. In *Proceedings of the IEEE/RSJ/GI International Conference on Intelligent Robots and Systems (IROS'94)*, 1994, pages 854–861. DOI 10.1109/iros.1994.407492.

[11] A. Schweikard, R. Tombropoulos, L. Kavraki, J. R. Adler, Jr., and J.-C. Latombe. Treatment planning for a radiosurgical system with general kinematics. In *IEEE International Conference on Robotics and Automation (ICRA 1994)*, 1994, pages 1720–1727. DOI 10.1109/robot.1994.351344.

[12] C. M. C. Tempany, E. A. Stewart, N. McDannold, B. J. Quade, F. A. Jolesz, and K. Hynynen. MR imaging-guided focused ultrasound surgery of uterine leiomyomas: A feasibility study. *Radiology*, **226**(3):897–905, 2003. DOI 10.1148/radiol.2271020395.

[13] N. Wilson, K. Wang, R. W. Dutton, and C. Taylor. A software framework for creating patient specific geometric models from medical imaging data for simulation based medical planning of vascular surgery. In W. J. Niessen and M. A. Viergever,

editors, *Medical Image Computing and Computer-Assisted Intervention - MICCAI 2001*, volume 2208 of *Lecture Notes in Computer Science*, pages 449–456. Springer Berlin Heidelberg, 2001. DOI 10.1007/3-540-45468-3_54.

Chapter 7
Motion Correlation and Tracking

To track the motion of an anatomic structure in real-time, we need very fast and robust imaging methods. However, this is often insufficient. A correlation-based approach can help here. Suppose we have an external structure (e.g. the patient's skin) which can be tracked easily, with optical methods. Then suppose we have an internal target, which is often very difficult to track.

Now we record the motion of the external structure (via highspeed imaging) and infer the position of the internal target via motion correlation. This can only work if the two motions (external and internal) are indeed correlated. Thus, we must establish that there is such a correlation, from physiological data. Clearly, such a correlation could be a complex mathematical dependency, subject to damping and hysteresis. Thus, it would seem likely that we can apply machine learning to the problem of finding the exact correlation pattern.

If we succeed in finding the correlation pattern, and if this pattern remains sufficiently stable throughout treatment, then we can track internal structures with high precision. The problem of learning such correlation patterns is one instance of motion learning. It seems reasonable to study the more general problem of motion learning in robotics, since many aspects of what we regard as dexterity rely on learning.

As discussed in Chap. 6, in external beam radiation therapy, tumors are irradiated with a moving beam of radiation. Tumors in the chest and abdomen move due to respiration. Our goal is to track this motion, see Fig. 7.1.

A. Schweikard, F. Ernst, *Medical Robotics*,
DOI 10.1007/978-3-319-22891-4_7

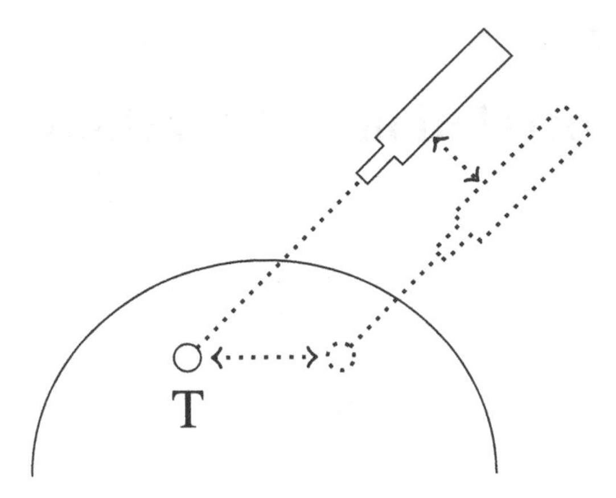

Fig. 7.1: Tracking a moving target in external beam radiation therapy

7.1 Motion Correlation

Respiratory motion is periodic. Furthermore, we observe that the motion of the target tumor and the motion of the patients's skin are correlated.

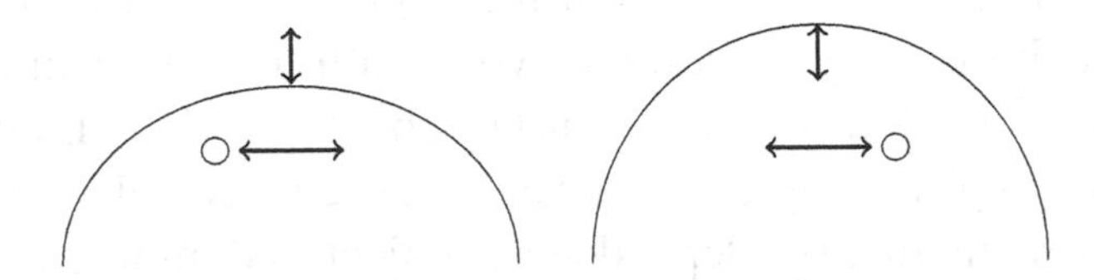

Fig. 7.2: Motion correlation

Figure 7.2 shows an example. In the figure, the motion of the skin surface is illustrated by the two vertical arrows. Thus, the skin surface (arc line in the figure) moves up and down during the respiratory cycle. The target (gray circle) moves in left-right direction. At full exhalation (left image), the target is on the left side. At full inhalation, the target is on the right side.
Our main observation is the following: tracking the skin surface is easier than tracking a tumor inside the body.
To track the skin surface, all we need is an optical or magnetic tracking marker placed on the skin. Optical tracking gives us exact position information in real-time, and no image analysis is needed.

Hence, we combine two sensors (X-ray and optical) in the following way: We take a stereo X-ray image pair and add a time-stamp to this image pair. We read the optical tracking system (or infrared tracking system) for the same point in time. This is done for several points in time. We then establish a correlation model between the motion of external markers visible with optical tracking and the internal motion of the target. The position of the internal target for images taken in the past is computed from X-ray images. From this correlation model, we infer the exact real-time position of the target tumor.
Intermediate positions of the target can now be computed by interpolation.
Figure 7.3 illustrates the process of correlation-based tracking.

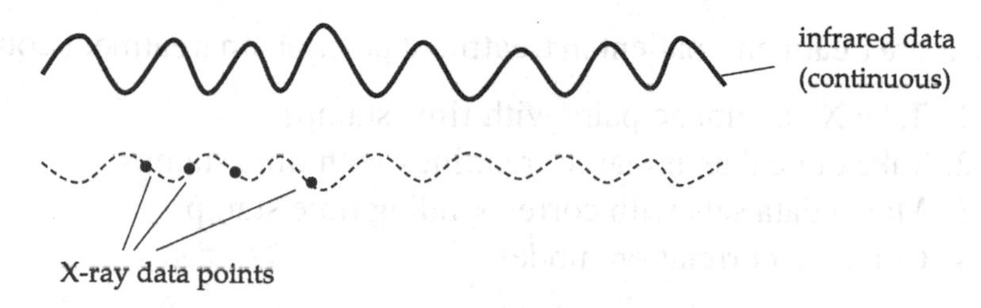

Fig. 7.3: Correlation-based tracking: the *bold curve* stems from the real-time sensor (here optical tracking). A series of points on the *dashed curve* are known (here: X-ray images), but these points are in the past, since we need segmentation time. The *bold curve* and the *dashed curve* (here: ground truth and target position) are in correlation. Our goal is to estimate the unknown dashed curve from this data

By taking more than two positions of the target, we can refine this correlation model. Thus curvilinear motion of the target can be approximated by a series of line segments, giving a model for this motion. The correlation model is continuously updated during treatment to reflect changes in breathing pattern.
As in the case of registration, we can replace specific image modalities but maintain the general method. In our description, optical tracking takes the role of a real-time sensor, and X-ray imaging computes ground truth intermittently. Motion correlation then determines the ground truth in real-time.

Example 7.1

Several scenarios for correlation-based tracking are possible. As discussed above, the first scenario links optical tracking and X-ray imaging. Tumors are not always visible in X-ray imaging. Then we can employ the following pseudo-stereotaxic scheme for tracking. Small gold landmarks are placed in the vicinity of the target before treatment. The relative position of the target with respect to the gold landmarks is known from a planning CT, also taken before the intervention.
During treatment, we take stereo X-ray images intermittently, and the position of the gold landmarks is determined in the images.
Thus, motion tracking consists of the following steps.

- Before treatment (patient in treatment position on treatment couch)
    1. Take X-ray image pairs with time stamps
    2. Take optical skin marker readings with time stamps
    3. Match data sets with corresponding time stamps
    4. Compute correlation model
- During treatment
    1. Take sensor reading
    2. Infer corresponding internal target position from optical data and correlation model
    3. Periodically (e.g. once every five seconds) take new X-ray image pair
    4. Compute an updated correlation model

(End of Example 7.1)

7.2 Regression and Normal Equations

To apply motion correlation, we must compute the correlation model. We are given data points with respiration data, taken before treatment. An exceedingly simple way to compute such a model is the following. We determine the coordinate axis with the largest excursion in the data points. This is done for both the X-ray image data and for the optical marker data. Both data consist of three-dimensional points. But we ignore the other two coordinate directions in favor of the one with largest excursion. Assume the coordinate with largest excursion is the z-coordinate for the optical data and the x-coordinate for the X-ray data. We take the two points with smallest and largest z-axis value (resp. x-axis value). Linear interpolation is then used to infer the internal target position from the external optical emitter position Fig. 7.4.

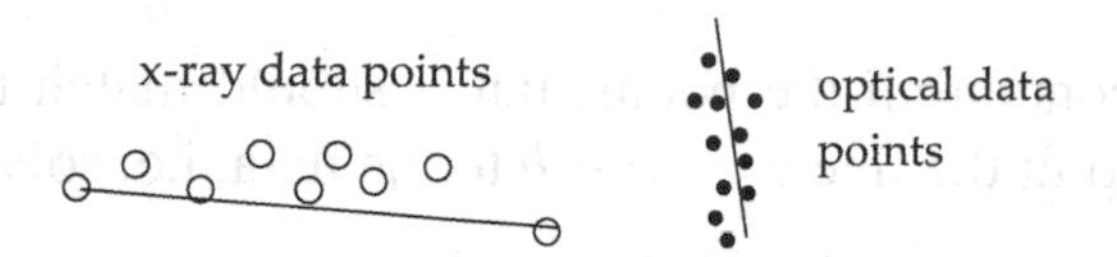

Fig. 7.4: Data points from optical tracking and X-ray imaging. Both types of sensor data points have time stamps. This allows for establishing the correspondences between the data points

Obviously this very simple technique has several drawbacks. It simply connects two data points by a line, and ignores all the other points. A more suitable method for fitting a line is described next. This technique takes all points into consideration, since they are valid data points. In Fig. 7.5 we select and visualize a single coordinate (here the x-coordinate) for both types of data. We do this for all three coordinates, and obtain a visualization for the correlation model.
Suppose now we are given data points as in the following table:

$(1, 9)$
$(2, 21)$
$(3, 33)$
$(4, 39)$
$(5, 50)$

If we take a closer look, we see that the data points are roughly on a line. We wish to find the line that best fits the data. This line does not

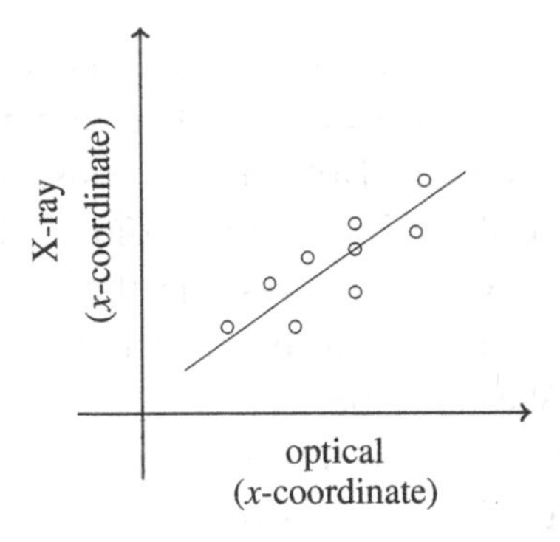

Fig. 7.5: Line regression

necessarily contain all the points, but it should match the data. Our goal is thus to fit the line $y = mx + b$ to the data, i.e. solve the system

$$\begin{aligned} b + 1m &= 9 \\ b + 2m &= 21 \\ b + 3m &= 33 \\ b + 4m &= 39 \\ b + 5m &= 50. \end{aligned} \tag{7.1}$$

The system is over-determined.
To find the solution for an overdetermined linear system, we could apply a method called the ART method. ART solves an overdetermined system by approximating the intersection of n planes chosen at random (n is the number of variables). This is based on the assumption that the intersection points are very close together. Simple examples show that this approach may not find very good regression lines. The ART method is discussed in detail in Exercise 1.2.
Instead, a better approach is to look for values $(b_0, m_0)^{\mathrm{T}}$ which minimize the expression:

$$(b + 1m - 9)^2 + \ldots + (b + 5m - 50)^2 \tag{7.2}$$

This is equivalent to finding a line that minimizes the sum of squared distances to the data points. We write the system in Eq. 7.1 in matrix form:

$$\mathbf{B} = \begin{pmatrix} 1 & 1 \\ 1 & 2 \\ 1 & 3 \\ 1 & 4 \\ 1 & 5 \end{pmatrix}, \mathbf{w} = \begin{pmatrix} b \\ m \end{pmatrix}, \mathbf{y} = \begin{pmatrix} 9 \\ 21 \\ 33 \\ 39 \\ 50 \end{pmatrix} \tag{7.3}$$

Then our system is:

$$\mathbf{Bw} = \mathbf{y} \tag{7.4}$$

Since $\mathbf{B}$ is a 5×2-matrix, $\mathbf{B}^{\mathrm{T}}$ will be a 2×5-matrix, and we can rewrite our system to:

$$\mathbf{B}^{\mathrm{T}}\mathbf{Bw} = \mathbf{B}^{\mathrm{T}}\mathbf{y} \tag{7.5}$$

This equation is called the normal equation for the system in Eq. 7.4. $\mathbf{B}^{\mathrm{T}}\mathbf{B}$ is a 2×2-matrix. Now this system can be solved by Gaussian elimination. Notice that the transition from $\mathbf{Bw} = \mathbf{y}$ to $\mathbf{B}^{\mathrm{T}}\mathbf{Bw} = \mathbf{B}^{\mathrm{T}}\mathbf{y}$ substantially reduces the matrix size. It can be shown that solutions of the least-squares problem (Eq. 7.2) are solutions of Eq. 7.5 and vice versa (see Exercise 7.1 at the end of this chapter).

7.3 Support Vectors

The method described in the last section has a remaining drawback. It does fit a line to a cloud of points, and does take into account all of the points equally. However, in practice it turns out that respiration data is subject to hysteresis. This means that the inhale curve of a point may be different from the exhale curve, as shown in Fig. 7.6.

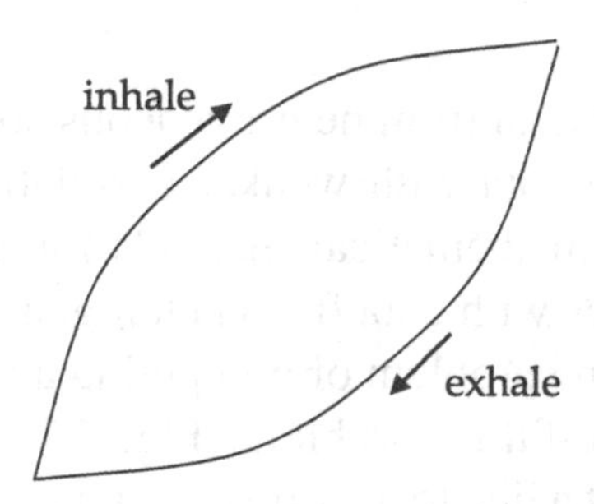

Fig. 7.6: Hysteresis: inhale path of target differs from exhale path

The difference can be quite large. A simple way to address this problem is to fit two lines to the data instead of just one. Here, we would use the optical tracking data to determine a gradient in the data, i.e. decide whether a given data point is an inhale or an exhale point. We would then map to one of the two regression lines. It turns out that respiratory traces are indeed curves and not just lines, so obviously we should attempt to fit curves to the data points. Polynomials of degree two or higher can be fit to the points by least squares methods. However, it is useful to include more sensor information. Beyond gradient information on the motion, speed and acceleration can be measured. A breath temperature sensor distinguishes between respiratory phases. A spirometer measures respiratory air flow. Similarly, data for pulsation can be acquired in a variety of ways.
Support vector methods collect heterogeneous data to set up training samples. Support vector regression computes a functional representation of correlations in the data. In the most simple form, the process resembles line regression. However, very complex correlations can be captured.

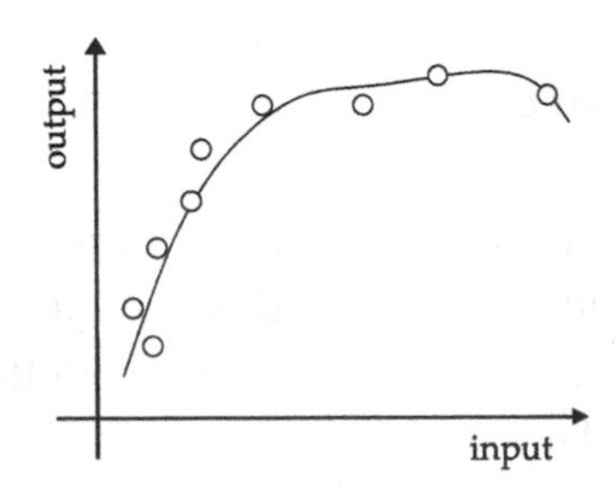

Fig. 7.7: Regression function for a cloud of points

Furthermore, having data from heterogeneous sources, it would seem necessary to remove data with weaker correlation to the target motion. Thus we need mathematical methods for analyzing correlation patterns in time series with data from heterogeneous sources.
Above we saw that the problem of computing a correlation model can be regarded as a line-fitting problem (Fig. 7.5). With support vector regression, we can fit a line to a cloud of points. Support vector regression can also fit a curve to such a cloud (Fig. 7.7). Of course there are

many mathematical methods to do just this: fit a curve to a point cloud. The advantage of support vector regression is the enormous flexibility. But more than that, support vector regression relies on a globally convergent optimization engine. This engine (called quadratic programming) performs the basic computation. You may not think much of this latter advantage. However, it is a big advantage in practice. No divergence will occur, and the optimization will not get stuck in local minima.

In the previous chapter, we saw applications of linear programming in treatment planning. Support vector methods emerged from linear programming and can be regarded as a direct extension.

To emphasize the fact that support vectors work in higher dimensions as well, we write the input values as vectors $\mathbf{x}_i$.

Hence, we have assumed a function with vector input $\mathbf{x}_i$ has a scalar function output y_i. Since we wish to work in high-dimensional space, we must think of our regression function to be a plane in space rather than a line in the plane. More generally, the regression function will be a hyperplane in a space of dimension n. Or even more generally, it will be a curved surface in high-dimensional space.

Before we look at regression with support vectors, we will look at the problem of separating two point clouds by a line. We will address this problem by support vector theory. It will turn out that the two problems (separating and regression) are related, but the basic concepts can be illustrated more easily if we look at the problem of separation first. Assume we have a planar example with only four points $\mathbf{x}_1, \mathbf{x}_2, \mathbf{x}_3$, and $\mathbf{x}_4$. We seek a line such that $\mathbf{x}_1$ and $\mathbf{x}_2$ are above and $\mathbf{x}_3$ and $\mathbf{x}_4$ are below this line. The situation is illustrated in Fig. 7.8.

7.3.1 Representation of Lines

Typically, lines are represented by equations of the form $y = mx + b$. For our application, we will not use this representation of lines. Instead, we will represent lines (in the plane) in the form

$$w_1 x_1 + w_2 x_2 + d = 0. \tag{7.6}$$

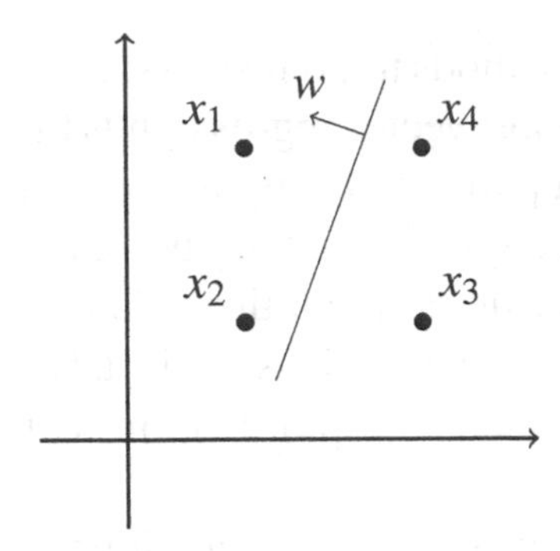

Fig. 7.8: Separating two clouds of points

To visualize this representation of lines, notice that $\mathbf{w} = (w_1, w_2)^T$ is the normal vector of the line. But furthermore, the direction of this normal vector $\mathbf{w}$ indicates an orientation of the line. Thus a point $\mathbf{p} = (p_1, p_2)^T$ is above the line (in the direction into which $\mathbf{w}$ is pointing), if

$$w_1 p_1 + w_2 p_2 + d > 0. \tag{7.7}$$

And $\mathbf{p}$ will be below the line if $w_1 p_1 + w_2 p_2 + d < 0$. The representation of lines discussed here also has a close relationship to distances. Namely, if $\mathbf{w}$ is a unit vector, then we know the distance of $\mathbf{p}$ from the line. It is simply the magnitude of the value $w_1 p_1 + w_2 p_2 + d$.
Notice also that this representation of lines is not unique. If $\mathbf{wx} + d = 0$ is a line, then $(\lambda \mathbf{wx}) + \lambda d = 0$ is the same line. Thus, we can scale our line equations. The scaling that turns the normal vector into a unit vector (i.e. $\lambda = 1/||\mathbf{w}||$) is often useful. One advantage of this representation of lines is that it works in any dimension. Hence,

$$w_1 x_1 + w_2 x_2 + w_3 x_3 + d = 0 \tag{7.8}$$

is a plane in space, with much the same distance properties we just discussed. And the same holds for higher dimensions.

7.3.2 Linear Programming for Separating Point Clouds

Assume as above we have a planar example with only four points $\mathbf{x}_1, \mathbf{x}_2, \mathbf{x}_3$, and $\mathbf{x}_4$. We seek a line such that $\mathbf{x}_1$ and $\mathbf{x}_2$ are above and $\mathbf{x}_3$ and $\mathbf{x}_4$ are below this line. This is the situation from Fig. 7.8.
Consider the linear program

$$\begin{aligned} x_{11}w_1 + x_{12}w_2 + d &\geq 0 \\ x_{21}w_1 + x_{22}w_2 + d &\geq 0 \\ x_{31}w_1 + x_{32}w_2 + d &\leq 0 \\ x_{41}w_1 + x_{42}w_2 + d &\leq 0. \end{aligned} \tag{7.9}$$

This is indeed a linear program, but here the objective function is empty, i.e. $(c_1, c_2)^{\mathrm{T}} = (0, 0)^{\mathrm{T}}$. Notice that the values w_i and d are the variables of this program! And the x_{ij} are the constant coefficients. A solution of this linear program will assign values to $\mathbf{w} = (w_1, w_2)^{\mathrm{T}}$ and d. Then the separating line is given by the normal vector $\mathbf{w}$ and the value d.
We will use values $y_i = \pm 1$ to indicate whether our data points x_i should be above the line or below. We rewrite the above linear program to include the values y_i:

$$\begin{aligned} y_1(\mathbf{w}\mathbf{x}_1 + d) &\geq 0 \\ y_2(\mathbf{w}\mathbf{x}_2 + d) &\geq 0 \\ y_3(\mathbf{w}\mathbf{x}_3 + d) &\geq 0 \\ y_4(\mathbf{w}\mathbf{x}_4 + d) &\geq 0 \end{aligned} \tag{7.10}$$

The system in Eq. 7.10 is the same as the system in Eq. 7.9. We have turned all inequalities into $\geq$-inequalities.
Now the linear program above will return a line such as the line shown in the next figure (Fig. 7.9). Notice that two of the points in Fig. 7.9 are actually on the separating line, hence not strictly below or above it. These are the points $\mathbf{x}_2$ and $\mathbf{x}_4$. Indeed linear programming will typically return this type of separating line. One can argue that this type of separating line does not represent the data points very well.

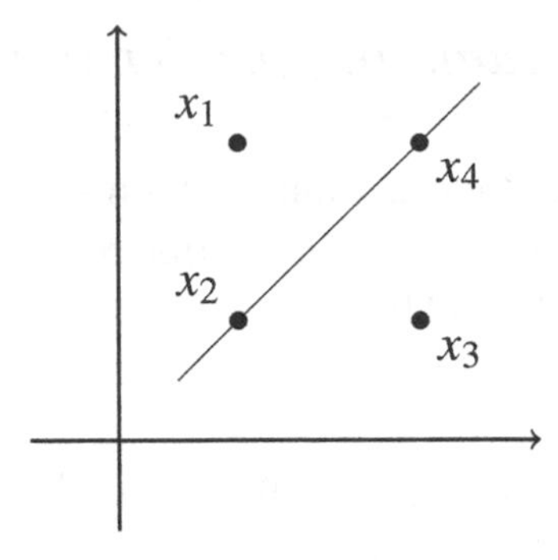

Fig. 7.9: Separator line for the classification problem in Eq. 7.10

Assume the points $\mathbf{x}_1, \mathbf{x}_2, \mathbf{x}_3$, and $\mathbf{x}_4$ are samples from a larger data set with more (unknown) sample points. We would again like to classify the data into two subsets. It would then seem more reasonable to use the dashed line in Fig. 7.10 as a separator line.

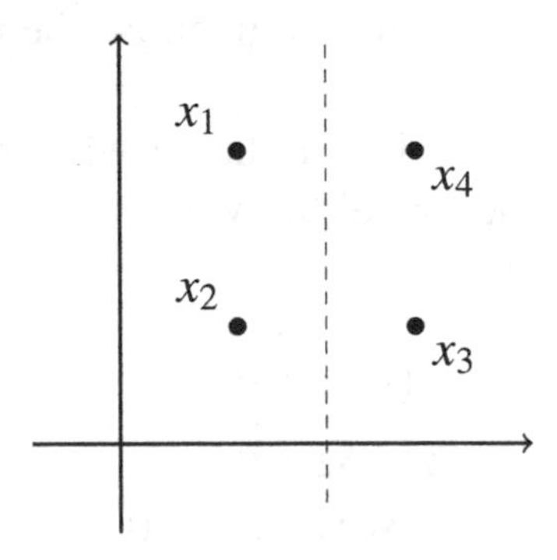

Fig. 7.10: Maximum margin separator line for the classification problem in Eq. 7.10

The advantage of this dashed line is that the margin between the separating line and the data points is maximal. In the picture, the data points can be thought of as repelling points which push the separating line away by the maximum amount. Likewise, we may say the data points 'support' the dashed separator line.
The basis of support vector theory is the observation that one can find such a maximum margin separator plane with quadratic programming.

Specifically, we replace the above linear program for finding the separator plane by the program:
Minimize

$$w_1^2 + w_2^2$$

subject to

$$y_1(\mathbf{wx}_1 + d) \geq 0$$
$$y_2(\mathbf{wx}_2 + d) \geq 0$$
$$y_3(\mathbf{wx}_3 + d) \geq 0$$
$$y_4(\mathbf{wx}_4 + d) \geq 0. \tag{7.11}$$

Recall that linear programs typically have an objective function as well. However, the program in Eq. 7.11 is not a linear program, since here the objective function is quadratic.
One would certainly want to know why the quadratic program in Eq. 7.11 does indeed compute a maximum margin line. For those who want to know, we give an example at the end of this chapter (see Exercise 7.2).

7.3.3 Regression

Having looked at maximum margin separator lines, we return to the problem of finding a regression line. We saw that quadratic programming does give a maximum margin separating line. Likewise it can be shown that quadratic programming can provide a regression line amidst a point cloud such that certain optimality criteria (resembling the optimal margin) are satisfied.
The regression line (or plane) can be found with quadratic programming:
Minimize

$$\mathbf{ww}^{\mathrm{T}} \tag{7.12}$$

subject to

$$y_i - (\mathbf{wx}_i + d) \leq \varepsilon$$
$$(\mathbf{wx}_i + d) - y_i \leq \varepsilon.$$

The constraints mean that the distance between the value $(\mathbf{w}\mathbf{x}_i + d)$ and the value y_i should not be bigger than ε. Recall that the values y_i in the case of regression are the function values at the points $\mathbf{x}_i$. Thus we no longer have $y_i = \pm 1$. Instead the values y_i are real numbers. Notice also that there are two constraints per sample point $\mathbf{x}_i$. The two constraints bound the distance from below and above. This means that the regression line must not have a distance more than ε from all samples $(\mathbf{x}_i, y_i)$. This may not always be feasible, i.e. if ε is too small. To allow for finding a regression line, even if the points are far apart, we introduce slack variables. Slack variables allow for a violation of the constraints. (We already saw a very simple application of slack variables in chapter Chap. 6.)
Thus, instead of requiring

$$y_i - (\mathbf{w}\mathbf{x}_i + d) \leq \varepsilon, \tag{7.13}$$

we ask for a little less, namely

$$y_i - (\mathbf{w}\mathbf{x}_i + d) \leq \varepsilon + \xi, \tag{7.14}$$

where ξ is a variable (ε is a constant)!
ξ is treated just like any other variable in quadratic programming (or linear programming), i.e. $\xi \geq 0$. You should take a minute to see why Eq. 7.14 is indeed a *weaker* constraint than Eq. 7.14.
We would like ξ to be as small as possible, since ξ is the amount by which the original constraint is violated.
Thus we include the minimization of the ξ-values into the above quadratic program:
Minimize

$$\mathbf{w}\mathbf{w} + \xi_1 + \xi_1' + \xi_2 + \xi_2' \ldots$$

subject to

$$\begin{aligned} y_1 - (\mathbf{w}\mathbf{x}_1 + d) &\leq \varepsilon + \xi_1 \\ (\mathbf{w}\mathbf{x}_1 + d) - y_1 &\leq \varepsilon + \xi_1' \\ y_2 - (\mathbf{w}\mathbf{x}_2 + d) &\leq \varepsilon + \xi_2 \\ (\mathbf{w}\mathbf{x}_2 + d) - y_2 &\leq \varepsilon + \xi_2' \\ &\ldots \\ \xi_i, \xi_i' &\geq 0. \end{aligned} \tag{7.15}$$

We introduce a constant C, which represents a trade-off between the weight of the quadratic part of the objective function ($\mathbf{ww}$) and the linear part. Thus, we modify the objective function in Eq. 7.15 to:
Minimize

$$\mathbf{ww} + C(\xi_1 + \xi_1' + \xi_2 + \xi_2' \ldots).$$

7.3.3.1 Dualization

Support vector machines do not employ quadratic programming in the form in Eq. 7.15. Rather, they rely on dualization. Dualization is a standard technique in linear programming (see also the exercises for Chap. 6 for a graphical visualization of this technique). Similar to linear programs, quadratic programs can be written in dual form.
As we shall see, the dual form has several advantages.
The dual QP for regression is:
Maximize

$$-\frac{1}{2}\sum_{i,j=1}^{m}(\alpha_i - \alpha_i')(\alpha_j - \alpha_j')\mathbf{x}_i\mathbf{x}_j - \varepsilon\sum_{i=1}^{m}(\alpha_i + \alpha_i') + \sum_{i=1}^{m} y_i(\alpha_i - \alpha_i')$$

subject to

$$\sum_{i=1}^{m}(\alpha_i - \alpha_i') = 0$$

and

$$\alpha_i, \alpha_i' \in [0, C]. \tag{7.16}$$

Unfortunately, the dual does not look much like the primal in Eq. 7.15 from which we started. However, we can recognize the constant C from the primal. Also, we still find ε.

Remark 7.1

The process of computing the dual from a given primal is based on Lagrange multipliers: We start from the so-called Lagrange function of the primal input system, take derivatives with respect to the (primal) variables $\mathbf{w}$, d, and ξ_i, ξ_i', set the resulting expressions to zero and substitute them back into the Lagrange function. Lagrange functions are

illustrated in the exercises below. Given a small amount of theory on Lagrange multipliers, the derivation of the dual quadratic program from the primal quadratic program is not difficult. One of the exercises at the end of this chapter shows that the dual in Eq. 7.16 is indeed a quadratic program in the first place (Exercise 7.3). As a further exercise (see end of this chapter), we show how to derive a very simple dual linear program from a primal linear program, all based on Lagrange theory.
The Exercise 7.3 at the end of this chapter not only illustrates the theory behind support vector machines in much more detail, but it also allows you to implement an exceedingly simple support vector machine. To be able to apply support vector machines in other contexts, this will turn out to be most helpful. Likewise, Exercises 7.4 and 7.5 will help to get a sense how the dual quadratic program in Eq. 7.16 is derived from the primal. Finally, you may again consider solving Exercise 7.2, since it further illustrates why we have set up the primal in Eq. 7.11 the way we did.

(End of Remark 7.1)

We mentioned the fact that the dual has several most surprising advantages over the primal. We will now set out to include kernel functions into the dual system in Eq. 7.16. This will allow us to find non-linear regression functions, which we need in our application.
But before we do that, one more thing remains:
Having solved the quadratic program in Eq. 7.16, e.g. with the Matlab routine *quadprog*, we get values for the variables α_i, α_i'. How can we get back to the values for $\mathbf{w}$ and d from the values for α_i, α_i'? The answer is: As part of the dualization process, we obtain equations (setting to zero derivatives with respect to dual variables). These equations state that

$$\mathbf{w} = \sum_{i=1}^{m} (\alpha_i - \alpha_i')\mathbf{x}_i = 0. \tag{7.17}$$

The value d can be computed in the following way:

$$d = y_j - \sum_{i=1}^{m} (\alpha_i - \alpha_i')\mathbf{x}_i\mathbf{x}_j - \varepsilon, \tag{7.18}$$

for a j with $\alpha_j \neq 0$, or

$$d = y_j - \sum_{i=1}^{m} (\alpha_i - \alpha_i')\mathbf{x}_i\mathbf{x}_j + \varepsilon, \tag{7.19}$$

for a j with $\alpha_j' \neq 0$.
Finally, we must evaluate the function value y for an unknown sample $\mathbf{x}$.
Here, of course, we have

$$f(\mathbf{x}) = \mathbf{w}\mathbf{x} + d, \tag{7.20}$$

but it is preferable to write

$$f(\mathbf{x}) = \sum_{i=1}^{m} (\alpha_i - \alpha_i')\mathbf{x}_i\mathbf{x} + d, \tag{7.21}$$

where we have simply inserted our formula for $\mathbf{w}$ derived above. The reason for this rewriting will become clear after we have discussed kernel functions. We will do this next.

7.3.4 Kernels

Consider the function F which maps points $\mathbf{x} = (x_1, x_2)^{\mathrm{T}}$ in two dimensions to

$$F : \begin{pmatrix} x_1 \\ x_2 \end{pmatrix} \rightarrow \begin{pmatrix} x_1 x_1 \\ x_1 x_2 \\ x_1 x_2 \\ x_2 x_2 \end{pmatrix}. \tag{7.22}$$

Hence, F maps from the input space (2D) to four-dimensional space. Here, 4-space is called the feature space of the mapping.
The reason why we would map samples from 2D space into 4D space is again best illustrated for the context of separation: In higher dimensions, it may be easier to separate the sample points by a plane. This is illustrated by the following example. Three points in 2D (two positive/one negative) can always be separated by a line. However, for four such points (two positive/two negative) this may not be the case.

(Try to find a 2D example for this case.) But in 3D, four points can always be separated by a plane. This generalizes to higher dimensions. In n-space, $n+1$ points can always be separated. Thus there is heuristic motivation to map the input sample points to a space of higher dimension, in order to simplify the separation. An example below will further illustrate this observation.
We again consider the above map F. Then for two points **x**, **y** we have

$$F(\mathbf{x})F(\mathbf{y}) = (\mathbf{xy})^2. \tag{7.23}$$

To see this, simply evaluate the left hand side:

$$F(\mathbf{x})F(\mathbf{y}) = \begin{pmatrix} x_1x_1 \\ x_1x_2 \\ x_2x_1 \\ x_2x_2 \end{pmatrix} \begin{pmatrix} y_1y_1 \\ y_1y_2 \\ y_2y_1 \\ y_2y_2 \end{pmatrix} = x_1^2y_1^2 + 2x_1x_2y_1y_2 + x_2^2y_2^2 \tag{7.24}$$

Likewise, the right hand side evaluates to:

$$(\mathbf{xy})^2 = x_1^2y_1^2 + 2x_1x_2y_1y_2 + x_2^2y_2^2 \tag{7.25}$$

The effect of the mapping is shown in Figs. 7.11 and 7.12. For the first figure, random data points uniformly distributed in the rectangular region $[-2, 2]$ by $[-2, 2]$ were generated. We mark all data points within the unit circle (i.e. points $(x_1, x_2)^{\mathrm{T}}$ in the plane with $x_1^2 + x_2^2 < 1$) as positive, and we mark the points outside the circle as negative.
In the second picture, the same points were mapped under F. Notice that the original (unmapped) points cannot be separated by a line. However, after the mapping under F, the points can be separated by a plane! Notice that the figure shows a 3D subspace of the 4D output space of F.
Hence, after mapping to higher dimensions under F, the data become linearly separable. This is in accordance with the above observation that separating points by hyperplanes is easier in higher dimensions.

Kernels and Quadratic Programming

We return to the problem of finding a regression plane. Instead of computing the regression plane in the original data space, we will compute

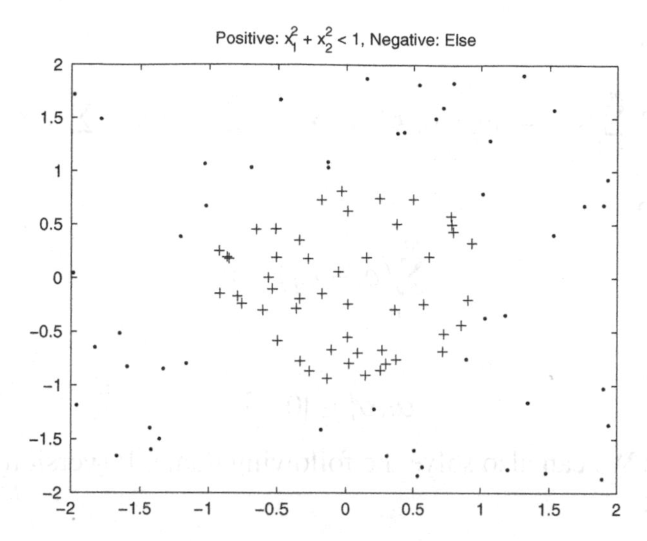

Fig. 7.11: Random sample points in interval [−2,2] by [−2,2]. Positive samples marked as *plus sign*, negative samples marked as *dots*

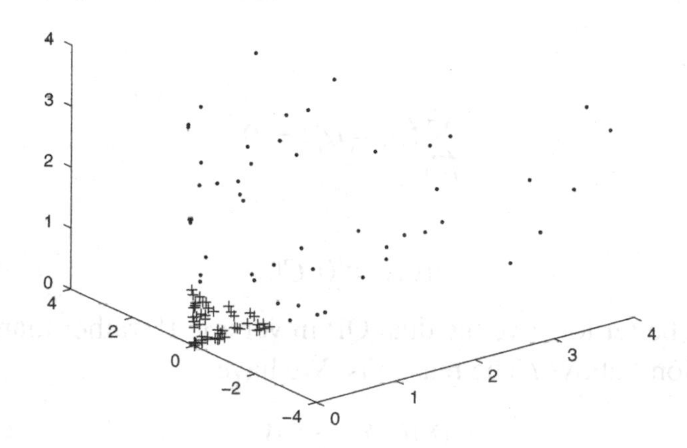

Fig. 7.12: Sample points from Fig. 7.11 mapped under $F : (x_1, x_2)^{\mathrm{T}} \rightarrow (\tilde{x}_1, \tilde{x}_2, \tilde{x}_3, \tilde{x}_4)^{\mathrm{T}} = (x_1x_1, x_1x_2, x_2x_1, x_2x_2)^{\mathrm{T}}$. Cross-sectional $(\tilde{x}_1, \tilde{x}_2, \tilde{x}_4)$-subspace

the regression plane in high-dimensional feature space. To this end, it suffices to map the input data points $\mathbf{x_i}$ under a mapping F. To find a regression plane, one could solve the following dual quadratic program (version I):

Maximize

$$-1/2\sum_{i,j=1}^{m}(\alpha_i-\alpha_i')(\alpha_j-\alpha_j')F(\mathbf{x}_i)F(\mathbf{x}_j)-\varepsilon\sum_{i=1}^{m}(\alpha_i+\alpha_i')+\sum_{i=1}^{m}y_i(\alpha_i-\alpha_i')$$

subject to

$$\sum_{i=1}^{m}(\alpha_i-\alpha_i')=0$$

and

$$\alpha_i,\alpha_i'\in[0,C]. \tag{7.26}$$

However: We can also solve the following dual QP (version II):
Maximize

$$-1/2\sum_{i,j=1}^{m}(\alpha_i-\alpha_i')(\alpha_j-\alpha_j')(\mathbf{x}_i\mathbf{x}_j)^2-\varepsilon\sum_{i=1}^{m}(\alpha_i+\alpha_i')+\sum_{i=1}^{m}y_i(\alpha_i-\alpha_i')$$

subject to

$$\sum_{i=1}^{m}(\alpha_i-\alpha_i')=0$$

and

$$\alpha_i,\alpha_i'\varepsilon[0,C]. \tag{7.27}$$

Why is it better to solve the dual QP in version II, rather than solving it in version I above? The reason is: We have

$$F(\mathbf{x})F(\mathbf{y})=(\mathbf{xy})^2. \tag{7.28}$$

Thus, the two programs are the same, and give the same solution. But it can be hard to compute $F(\mathbf{x})$ and $F(\mathbf{y})$ explicitly, while it is often much easier to compute $(\mathbf{xy})^2$. Specifically, the above function F is only one example for such a function. For other functions, $F(\mathbf{x})$ is much harder to compute.

Example 7.2

It can be shown that there is a function F, for which

$$F(\mathbf{x})F(\mathbf{y})=(1+\mathbf{xy})^k. \tag{7.29}$$

But computing $F(\mathbf{x})$ explicitly in this case would require evaluating an exponential number of terms (exponential in k), and this function F maps vectors to a space of dimension exponential in k.
The advantage of solving the dual QP in version II is that F is never computed explicitly. Instead, one only evaluates terms of the form $(1+\mathbf{xy})^k$.
This is much more efficient.

(End of Example 7.2)

Remark 7.2

An important point to note is that the last observation also holds for the step of computing $\mathbf{w}$ and d, from the values α_i and α_i'. You may wish to check this in the formulas defining the values for $\mathbf{w}$ and d (Eqs. 7.17 and 7.19). (End of Remark 7.2)

Hence, Eq. 7.27 gives the final method for finding a regression function with support vector machines. Notice that the use of kernels allows for finding non-linear regression functions as in Fig. 7.7. Equation 7.27 could be implemented in Matlab, e.g. by calling the Matlab-function *quadprog*. However, some minor rearrangement would be necessary to do this. Furthermore, the quadprog() module in Matlab does not give very good results in this case. Only very small data sets can be handled. A much better way to implement support vector methods is to use specialized algorithms for solving the optimization problem in Eq. 7.27. While this problem is indeed a quadratic program, more efficient algorithms for solving this special type of problem have been developed [16]. Such algorithms are provided in dedicated libraries for support vector methods [4].

(End of Remark 7.2)

The following example illustrates the difference between simple line regression and support vector regression.

Example 7.3

Support vector regression does not compute an explicit curve representing the correlation, such as a linear or polynomial curve, but rather a high-dimensional regression hyperplane which is then mapped back to the low-dimensional data space. The hyperplane is linear, but the mapping can be non-linear if we use a kernel function.
To illustrate the difference between explicit regression and support vector regression and evaluate practical benefits, we need respiratory data, ideally without relative latency between different image sources. Fluoroscopy is an X-ray image modality, and acquires images in real-time. Both LED skin markers and implanted gold markers are visible in fluoroscopic images. Hence, we do not need to calibrate relative acquisition latencies.
For explicit regression (i.e. line regression with normal equations, or polynomial curve fitting), we can visualize the dependency between motions of LED markers and fiducial markers as a line or a curve. Figure 7.13 shows the result of a measurement with two-plane fluoroscopy. Due to hysteresis, the point cloud is partitioned into two subregions. The figure also shows a regression line.
Figure 7.14 shows the results for support vector regression. We see that support vector methods can represent hysteresis directly.
Instead of fitting a single line to the data, we can also fit polynomials to the data points. Figure 7.15 shows two polynomial curves. The curves are blended at both ends to obtain a better match to the data and to avoid extrapolation errors.
Figure 7.16 compares polynomial fitting (degree less than 6) to support vector regression. The improvement obtained by support vector regression is clearly visible.
It is often difficult or undesired to record fluoroscopic data. Thus it is useful to look for other ways to validate and compare correlation methods. Ultrasound is non-invasive. Figure 7.17 shows a set-up for recording correlation data via ultrasound imaging.
A robotic arm holds the ultrasound camera. Optical markers (LEDs) are placed in a belt on the patient's chest. The ultrasound images do not show the positions of both types of markers. Thus, the latency of ultrasound image acquisition must be determined.

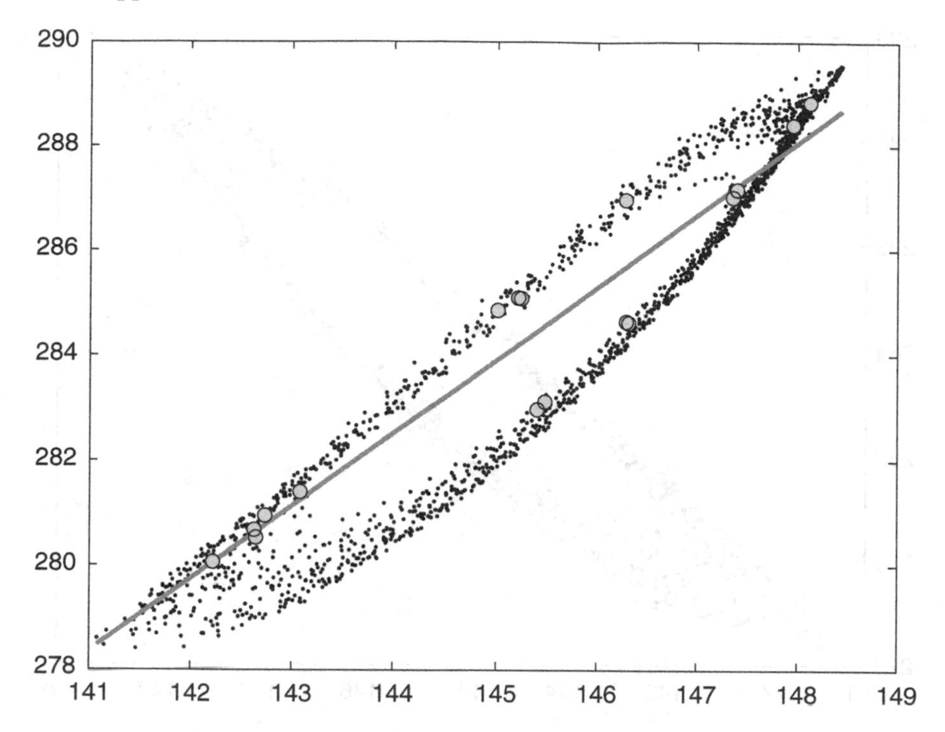

Fig. 7.13: Motion correlation measured with two-plane fluoroscopy. The x-axis shows the motion of an optical marker along a single coordinate in space. The y-axis shows the motion of an internal marker, again along a single coordinate. We fit a line to the training data points (*large dots*). The *small dots* represent the data points from fluoroscopy. The effect of hysteresis is clearly visible

In Fig. 7.18, a robot arm moves a phantom object in a water tank. The phantom is a small lead ball attached to a fixture, moved by the robot. The ultrasound camera tracks the motion of the phantom. This process generates two curves. The delay between the two curves represents the relative latency of ultrasound acquisition. Here, relative latency means the latency between ultrasound imaging and robot motion. By bringing the two curves into a matching position, we can calibrate the relative latency time.

However, now we only have the relative latency. To compute absolute latencies, we can proceed as follows. We first calibrate the latency of a fast optical tracking system: By means of an oscilloscope and

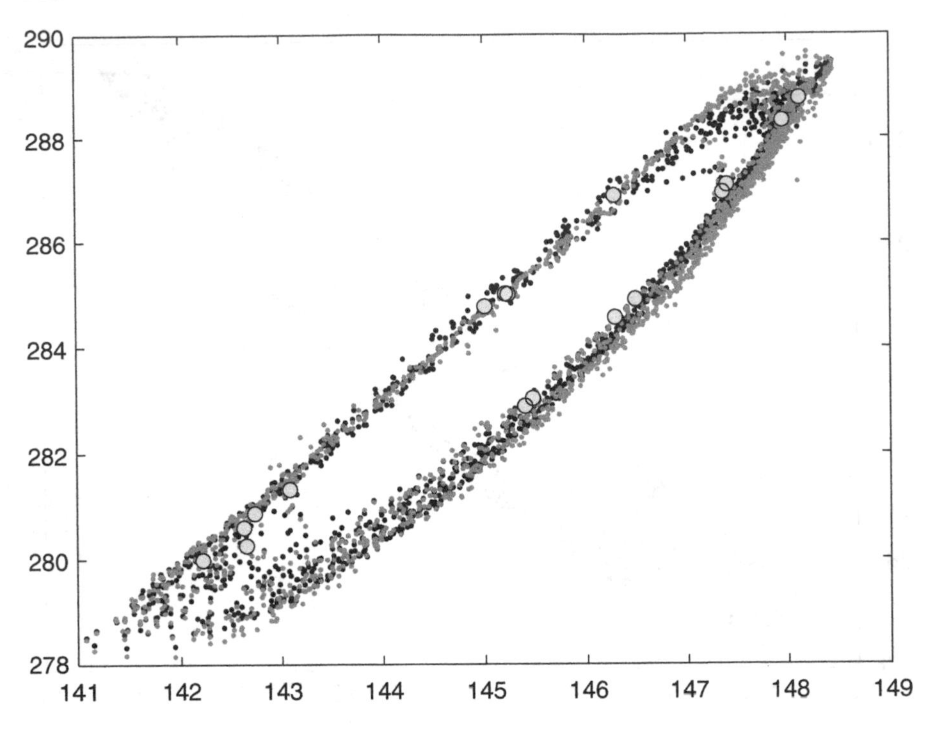

Fig. 7.14: Support vector regression for motion correlation. *Large gray dots*: training data. *Small black dots*: fluoroscopy data. *Small gray dots*: points computed by support vector regression. Same data as in Fig. 7.13

additional electronics, this can be done within an accuracy of below 0.5 ms. We then determine robot latency with a set-up of two robots of the same type. A motion command for the first robot is issued at time point t_0. This motion is detected by an optical marker attached to the first robot.

At this point in time, we trigger a motion command for a second robot. The second robot also carries an optical marker. The two markers are visible for the same tracking camera. We determine the graph for both marker motions, and compute the delay from the graph (Fig. 7.19).

(End of Example 7.3)

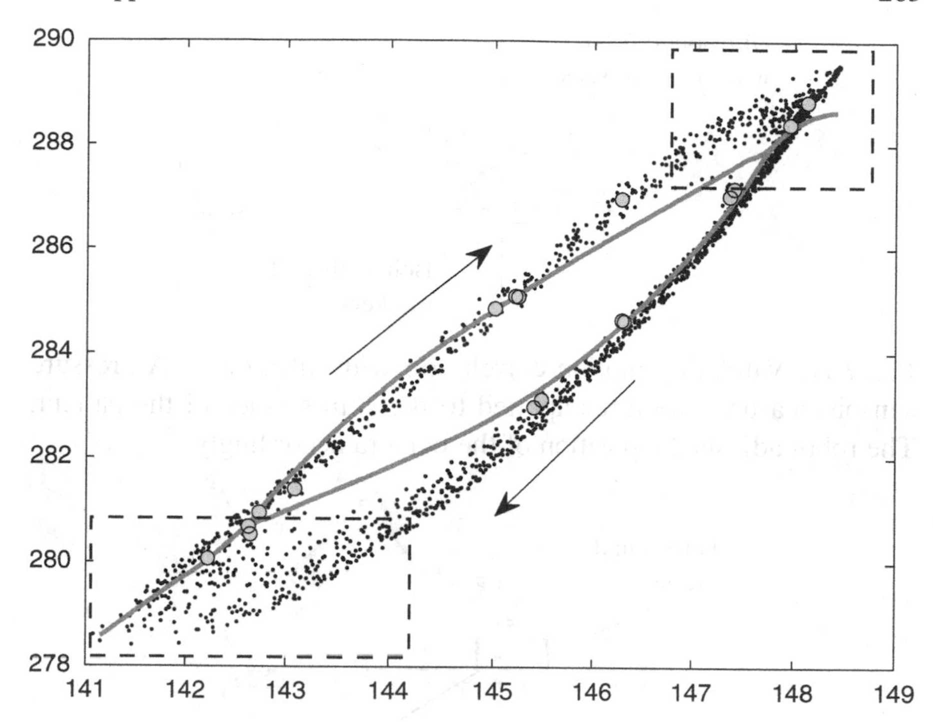

Fig. 7.15: Representing hysteresis by a correlation model consisting of two polynomial segments. Data as in Fig. 7.13

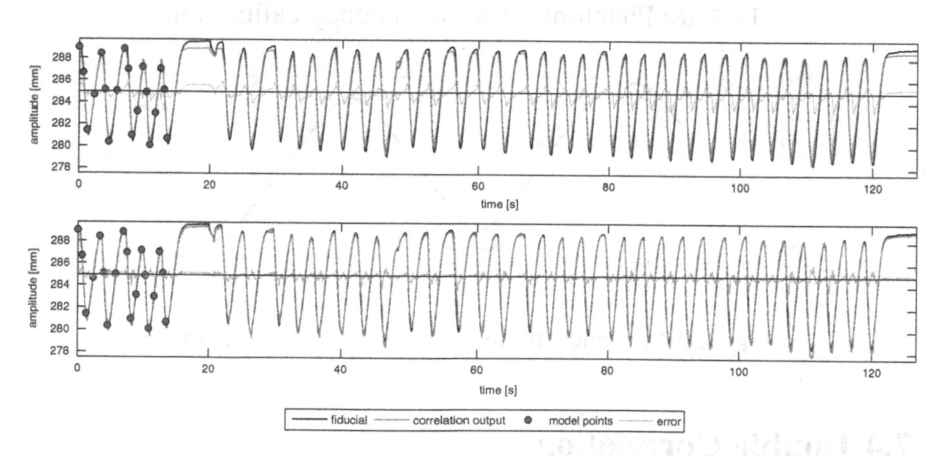

Fig. 7.16: Motion traces for the data in Fig. 7.13. *Top row*: polynomial fitting. *Bottom row*: support vector regression

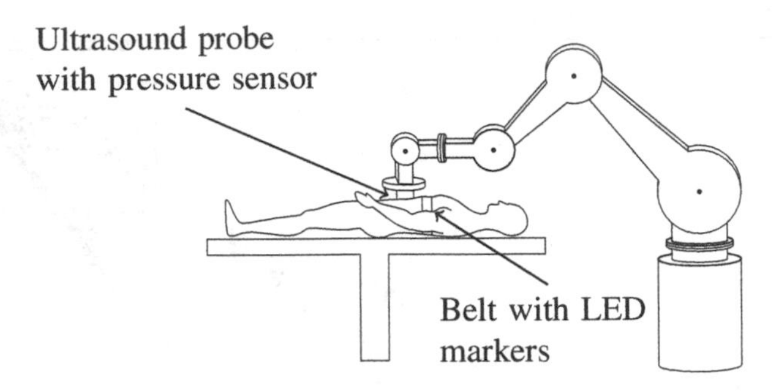

Fig. 7.17: Validating motion correlation with ultrasound. A pressure sensor measures the force applied to the skin surface of the patient. The robot adjusts the position of the camera accordingly

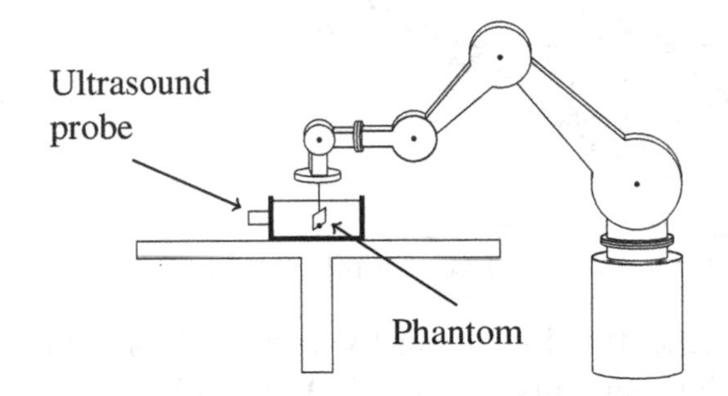

Fig. 7.18: Phantom set-up for latency calibration

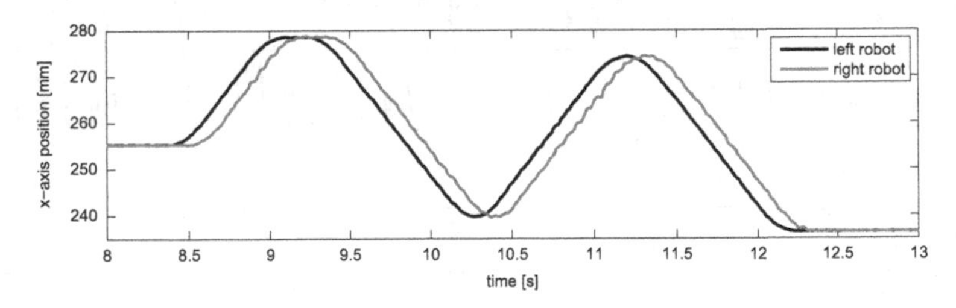

Fig. 7.19: Latency measurement with two robots

7.4 Double Correlation

Implanted markers have several disadvantages. Firstly, implanting is invasive, and requires an additional procedure before treatment. Secondly, the markers can move with respect to the target. This can cause inaccuracies. We see the rib cage in X-ray images, but the tumor is not always visible. The rib cage moves during respiration. To obviate the need for implanted markers, we can use two correlation models, both of which are established before treatment:

- model 1: external marker motion to rib cage motion
- model 2: rib cage motion to target motion

We combine the two correlation models in a chain to infer the target position in real-time (Fig. 7.20).

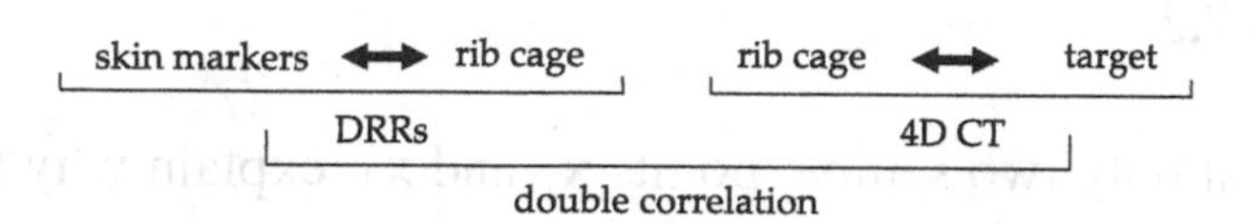

Fig. 7.20: Double correlation. The motion of the rib cage is detected by digitally reconstructed radiographs (DRRs). Before treatment the target is marked in a series of CT scans, showing distinct respiratory states (4D CT). DRRs are computed from a 4D CT data set. Live shots are matched to the DRRs to detect the current respiratory state, and compute ground truth location of the target.

To establish the correlation between external marker motion and bone motion, we need a substep, involving registration. We can use the DRR-technique from Chap. 5 (see also Fig. 5.3), but now we apply it to 4D CT images. As discussed in Chap. 5, a DRR (digitally reconstructed radiograph) is a projection image of a given CT image.
During treatment, we take stereo X-ray images, also called live images. When a new live image is taken, we compare it to each of the DRRs. (Recall that the DRRs now stem from 4D CT.) The comparison selects the best matching DRR. We identify the CT scan from which this DRR was generated. This allows for determining a time step in the 3D CT series. The given DRR also corresponds to a projection angle and a translational shift. Thus, after the matching step, we know the position, orientation and respiratory phase of the patient in the live image.

Exercises

Exercise 7.1

For the example in Eq. 7.1, show that the least squares solution obtained by direct differentiation of Eq. 7.2 with respect to b and m is the same as the solution obtained from the normal equation.

Exercise 7.2

Looking at only two sample points $\mathbf{x}_1$ and $\mathbf{x}_2$, explain why the quadratic program

Minimize

$$w_1^2 + w_2^2$$

subject to

$$\begin{aligned} y_1(\mathbf{w}\mathbf{x}_1 + d) &\geq 0 \\ y_2(\mathbf{w}\mathbf{x}_2 + d) &\geq 0, \end{aligned} \tag{7.30}$$

where $y_1 = 1$ and $y_2 = -1$, computes a maximum margin separator line.

Hints:
Represent the line by its parameters $(\mathbf{w}, d)$, where $\mathbf{w}$ is the normal vector of the line. Then this representation of a line can be multiplied by a factor λ, without changing the line. Thus $(\lambda\mathbf{w}, \lambda d)$ for non-zero λ is the same line as $(\mathbf{w}, d)$. First show that it suffices to consider only those lines having

$$\begin{aligned} y_1(\mathbf{w}\mathbf{x}_1 + d) &= 1, \\ y_2(\mathbf{w}\mathbf{x}_2 + d) &= 1. \end{aligned} \tag{7.31}$$

Now recall that for any line, we obtain the point-line distance by scaling the normal vector $\mathbf{w}$ to unit length, so that the margin is given by:

$$\frac{\mathbf{w}}{||\mathbf{w}||}\mathbf{x}_1 + \frac{d}{||\mathbf{w}||} \quad (7.32)$$

Hence the margin is simply $\frac{1}{||\mathbf{w}||}$. To maximize the margin, we must minimize the length of $\mathbf{w}$.

Exercise 7.3

The Matlab routine *quadprog* implements quadratic programming. Hence we can write our own support vector machine by calling the routine *quadprog* simply for the system in Eq. 7.11. This will actually work! (But do not be disappointed to see that this program will be very slow, and will not be able to handle more than 20 data points. There are other methods to implement support vector machines much more efficiently.) Similar to the Matlab routine for linear programming, the quadprog-routine expects input parameters in matrix and vector form. The parameters are: $\mathbf{H}$ is a symmetric matrix, $\mathbf{A}$ is a matrix, and $\mathbf{b}$ and $\mathbf{f}$ are vectors. Then $\mathbf{u} = quadprog(\mathbf{H}, \mathbf{f}, \mathbf{A}, \mathbf{b})$ minimizes $\frac{1}{2}\mathbf{u}^{\mathrm{T}}\mathbf{H}\mathbf{u} + \mathbf{f}^{\mathrm{T}}\mathbf{u}$ subject to $\mathbf{A}\mathbf{u} \leq \mathbf{b}$.

a) Write a program for the system in Eq. 7.11 with input points as in Fig. 7.5, and visualize the resulting regression line. This is an exceedingly simple support vector machine. Again, it will not be a very effective support vector machine, but will serve to illustrate the basics.
b) Show that the system in Eq. 7.16 is actually a quadratic program. Thus, show that input parameters in the form $\mathbf{H}, \mathbf{f}, \mathbf{A}, \mathbf{b}$ can be set up for the system in Eq. 7.16. One seemingly simple way to do this would be to set $\theta_i = \alpha_i - \alpha_i'$, and use the θ_i as variables, i.e. minimize $\frac{1}{2}\theta^{\mathrm{T}}\mathbf{H}\theta + \mathbf{f}^{\mathrm{T}}\theta$ subject to $\mathbf{A}\theta \leq \mathbf{b}$ However, this will fail, since we have the subexpression $\alpha_i + \alpha_i'$ in the objective function. Hint: Use the $2m$ variables $\theta_1, \ldots, \theta_{2m}$ by setting:
$\theta_i = \alpha_i - \alpha_i'$ for $i = 1, \ldots, m$
and
$\theta_{i+m} = \alpha_i'$ for $i = 1, \ldots, m$.
Then $\alpha_i = \theta_i + \alpha_i'$, and $\mathbf{H}$ is a $2m$ by $2m$ matrix.
Run this as a program for the same points as in part a), to compute and visualize the regression line with dual quadratic programming.

c) Run your program (now for more than just two points) with the kernel function in Eq. 7.22, and show that non-linear regression functions can be found.

Exercise 7.4 *Lagrange Multipliers*

Consider the optimization problem

Max $f(x,y)$

Subject to $g(x,y) = c$

Here, f and g are functions of two variables x and y. For example, f and g could be the functions

$$f(x,y) = -x^2 - y^2, \tag{7.33}$$

$$g(x,y) = x + 2y. \tag{7.34}$$

The function f can be visualized via its level curves (Fig. 7.21). The level curves are obtained as curves where $f(x,y) = c$ for various constants c. Likewise, we can visualize the constraint $g(x,y) = c$ as a curve. Looking again at the above optimization problem, two cases are possible: the curves $f(x,y) = c$ and $g(x,y) = c$ can cross, or they can meet tangentially. The key observation for Lagrange multipliers is the following: f can attain a maximum under the constraint $g(x,y) = c$ only if the level curves meet as tangents.
The gradient vector

$$\nabla f = \left(\frac{\partial f}{\partial x}, \frac{\partial f}{\partial y} \right)^{\mathrm{T}} \tag{7.35}$$

is orthogonal to the level curve. Thus, if f and g meet tangentially, their gradient vectors must be an α-multiple of each other for a non-zero α. Therefore, we have

$$\nabla f = \alpha \nabla g. \tag{7.36}$$

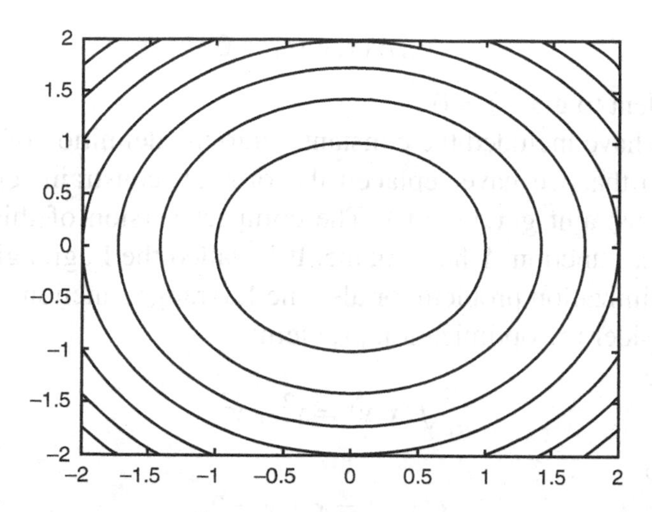

Fig. 7.21: Level curves of the function $f(x,y) = -x^2 - y^2$

α is called Lagrange-multiplier. To summarize, we can state the so-called Lagrange system for the above optimization problem in the following form:

$$\frac{\partial f}{\partial x} = \alpha \frac{\partial g}{\partial x}$$
$$\frac{\partial f}{\partial y} = \alpha \frac{\partial g}{\partial y}$$
$$g(x,y) = c$$

A more compact form is obtained in the following way. Here, the whole system (now with three equations) can be stated in a single equation.
Set

$$\Lambda(x,y,\alpha) = f(x,y) - \alpha(g(x,y) - c). \tag{7.37}$$

Then all three above equations are obtained by setting derivatives of Λ to 0. Specifically, the system

$$\nabla_{(x,y,\alpha)}\Lambda(x,y,\alpha) = 0 \tag{7.38}$$

condenses the three equations above into a single one. Note that differentiating Λ with respect to α, we obtain the original constraint $g(x,y) = 0$. Hence,

$$\nabla_\alpha \Lambda(x,y,\alpha) = 0 \tag{7.39}$$

is equivalent to $g(x,y) = 0$.
(Here we have included the constant c into the definition of the function g, so that we have replaced the original constraint $g(x,y) = c$ by the constraint $g(x,y) = 0$). The compact version of this system, namely the function Λ has a name. It is called the Lagrangian of the given optimization problem, or also the Lagrange function.
Now consider the optimization problem:
Minimize

$$f(x,y) = x^2 + y^2$$

subject to

$$g(x,y) = x + y = 2.$$

a) Find the Lagrange function for this system
b) Find the optimum with the help of the Lagrange function

Notice that the theory of Lagrange multipliers extends to the case of inequality constraints (see e.g. [9, 12]).

Exercise 7.5

The optimization problem

Max $c_1x + c_2y$

subject to

$$\begin{aligned} a_{11}x + a_{12}y &= b_1 \\ a_{21}x + a_{22}y &= b_2 \end{aligned} \tag{7.40}$$

is a linear program as defined in Eqs. 6.6 and 6.7, since each of the two equality constraints can be resolved to two inequality constraints. The Lagrange technique for solving optimization problems can be extended to the case of several constraint functions g_i in the following way.

Given m constraints, in a problem of the form:

Maximize

$$f(x_1,\ldots,x_n)$$

subject to

$$g_1(x_1,\ldots,x_n)=0$$
$$\vdots$$
$$g_m(x_1,\ldots,x_n)=0, \tag{7.41}$$

we must use m Lagrange multipliers $\alpha_1,\ldots,\alpha_m$.
Here, the tangent condition used above (gradient vectors of f and g aligned) is not as obvious. In fact, for multiple constraints, the tangent condition requires that the gradient vector of f is a linear combination of the gradient vectors of the g-functions.
Specifically, in this case, the Lagrange function is

$$\Lambda(x_1,\ldots,x_n,\alpha_1,\ldots,\alpha_m)=f(x_1,\ldots,x_n)-\sum_{k=1}^{m}\alpha_k g_k(x_1,\ldots,x_n). \tag{7.42}$$

At the optimum, the partial derivatives of the Lagrange function with respect to the variables x_i and α_i must vanish.

a) Set up the Lagrange function Λ for the optimization problem in Eq. 7.40. (You will need two Lagrange multipliers α_1,α_2, for the two constraints.) Take derivatives of Λ with respect to the Lagrange multipliers α_i and the primal variables x,y, and set the resulting expressions to zero. Inserting these equations back into Λ, show that $\Lambda=\mathbf{b}\alpha$, and $\mathbf{A}^{\mathrm{T}}\alpha=\mathbf{c}$. Compare to the dual of a linear program defined in Exercise 6.2.
b) Apply the strategy from part a) to the optimization problem:

Minimize

$$\mathbf{ww}+\xi_1+\xi_1'+\xi_2+\xi_2'\ldots$$

subject to

$$
\begin{aligned}
y_1 - (\mathbf{w}\mathbf{x}_1 + d) &= \varepsilon + \xi_1 \\
(\mathbf{w}\mathbf{x}_1 + d) - y_1 &= \varepsilon + \xi_1' \\
y_2 - (\mathbf{w}\mathbf{x}_2 + d) &= \varepsilon + \xi_2 \\
(\mathbf{w}\mathbf{x}_2 + d) - y_2 &= \varepsilon + \xi_2' \\
&\dots,
\end{aligned}
$$

taking derivatives with respect to the slack variables ξ_i, ξ_i' as well. This is a slight modification of the primal quadratic program for regression in Eq. 7.15. Compare your result to the dual quadratic program for regression in Eq. 7.16.

Exercise 7.6

Having acquired some background on mutual information and support vector machines, we can now combine the two techniques. Hence, for heterogeneous data streams (i.e. multiple infrared-markers, breath temperature sensors, strain gauges, acceleration sensors in the infrared markers), discuss the process of searching for tight correlations between heterogeneous data streams in the training phase, and then improving reliability and accuracy by merging several tightly coupled sensor data streams.

Summary

Targets in soft tissue move. Tracking such targets with registration alone is difficult. By contrast, the skin surface can be tracked with real-time imaging. Motion correlation can then provide an alternative to registration. Typically, the correlation between the motion of the skin surface and the motion of the target is computed prior to treatment. Here, so-called surrogates can take the role of the skin surface.
Hysteresis is a problem in this context. Inhale curves differ from exhale curves. Thus we have two curves in our correlation, and this situation cannot be represented by a single function. We saw that support vector methods can address this problem. Typically, support

vector regression does not compute an explicit regression function. Instead, a dual quadratic program is solved to obtain parameters specifying a plane in high-dimensional space. This plane determines a (not necessarily linear) mapping in low-dimensional space. Support vector methods are a direct extension of linear programming. The first step in this extension was the introduction of separating planes for classification. Such planes can also be found with linear programming alone. But support vector methods allow for finding separating planes with maximum margins. This leads to quadratic programming, and with the dual of a quadratic program we can include kernel functions to represent non-linear correlations.
The rib cage moves with respiration as well. Thus we can track without implanted markers using DRRs and four-dimensional CT scans.
We must validate the hypothesis that motions of organs are indeed correlated. Furthermore, we must measure the strength of the correlation. To this end, it would be ideal to have all structures visible in a single stream of images, so that we can ignore latencies in image acquisition. Two-plane fluoroscopy is a useful tool in this case, but typically too invasive for routine use. We can replace fluoroscopy by ultrasound, where the ultrasound is calibrated with respect to acquisition latency.

Notes

Motion correlation for tumor tracking was introduced in [19], and is now in routine clinical use in radiosurgery [5]. A variety of further applications for motion correlation has since been investigated. Surveys are given in [17] and [21], see also [1, 6, 8, 10, 11, 14, 22]. Validation methods for motion correlation, i.e. based on ultrasound imaging are given in [7].
Organs do not only move, but also deform during respiration. The methods in this chapter avoid direct image registration. However, several authors describe methods for addressing the problem of respiratory motion tracking with registration (see e.g. [15, 18]), or by combining motion correlation with direct registration.

A library for support vectors is available from [4], see also [3, 16, 20]. Additional background on normal equations and least squares problems is given in [13]. The text book by C. Bishop [2] discusses learning methods and regression.

References

[1] M. Baumhauer, M. Feuerstein, H.-P. Meinzer, and J. Rassweiler. Navigation in endoscopic soft tissue surgery: Perspectives and limitations. *Journal of Endourology*, **22**(4):751–766, 2008. DOI 10.1089/end.2007.9827.

[2] C. M. Bishop. *Pattern Recognition and Machine Learning*. Information Science and Statistics. Springer, New York, Berlin, Heidelberg, 2006.

[3] B. E. Boser, I. M. Guyon, and V. N. Vapnik. A training algorithm for optimal margin classifiers. In *Proceedings of the Fifth Annual Workshop on Computational Learning Theory*, New York, NY, USA. ACM. Published in *COLT '92*, pages 144–152, 1992. DOI 10.1145/130385.130401.

[4] C.-C. Chang and C.-J. Lin. *LIBSVM: a library for support vector machines*, 2001.

[5] È. Coste-Manière, D. Olender, W. Kilby, and R. A. Schulz. Robotic whole body stereotactic radiosurgery: clinical advantages of the Cyberknife® integrated system. *The International Journal of Medical Robotics and Computer Assisted Surgery*, **1** (2):28–39, 2005. DOI 10.1002/rcs.39.

[6] T. Depuydt, D. Verellen, O. C. L. Haas, T. Gevaert, N. Linthout, M. Duchateau, K. Tournel, T. Reynders, K. Leysen,M. Hoogeman, G. Storme, and M. de Ridder. Geometric accuracy of a novel gimbals based radiation therapy tumor tracking system. *Radiotherapy and Oncology*, **98**(3):365–372, 2011. DOI 10.1016/j.radonc.2011.01.015.

[7] F. Ernst, R. Bruder, A. Schlaefer, and A. Schweikard. Correlation between external and internal respiratory motion: a validation study. *International Journal of Computer*

Assisted Radiology and Surgery, **7**(3):483–492, 2012. DOI 10.1007/s11548-011-0653-6.

[8] R. Ginhoux, J. Gangloff, M. de Mathelin, L. Soler, M. M. A. Sanchez, and J. Marescaux. Active filtering of physiological motion in robotized surgery using predictive control. *IEEE Transactions on Robotics*, **21**(1):67–79, 2005. DOI 10.1109/tro.2004.833812.

[9] W. Karush. Minima of functions of several variables with inequalities as side conditions. Master's thesis, Department of Mathematics, University of Chicago, Chicago, IL, 1939.

[10] P. J. Keall, G. S. Mageras, J. M. Balter, R. S. Emery, K. M. Forster, S. B. Jiang, J. M. Kapatoes, D. A. Low, M. J. Murphy, B. R. Murray, C. R. Ramsey, M. B. V. Herk, S. S. Vedam, J. W. Wong, and E. Yorke. The management of respiratory motion in radiation oncology. Report of AAPM task group 76. *Medical Physics*, **33** (10):3874–3900, 2006. DOI 10.1118/1.2349696.

[11] A. Khamene, J. K. Warzelhan, S. Vogt, D. Elgort, C. Chefd'Hotel, J. L. Duerk, J. Lewin, F. K. Wacker, and F. Sauer. Characterization of internal organ motion using skin marker positions. In C. Barillot, D. R. Haynor, and P. Hellier, editors, *MICCAI 2004, Part II*, St. Malo, France. MICCAI, Springer. Published in *LNCS*, **3217**:526–533, 2004.

[12] H. W. Kuhn and A. W. Tucker. Nonlinear programming. In J. Neyman, editor, *Proceedings of the Second Berkeley Symposium on Mathematical Statistics and Probability*. University of California, University of California Press, 1951, pages 481–492.

[13] C. L. Lawson and R. J. Hanson. *Solving Least Squares Problems*, volume 15 of *Classics in Applied Mathematics*. Society for Industrial and Applied Mathematics, Englewood Cliffs, NJ, 1987.

[14] T. Neicu, H. Shirato, Y. Seppenwoolde, and S. B. Jiang. Synchronized moving aperture radiation therapy (SMART): average tumour trajectory for lung patients. *Physics in Medicine and Biology*, **48**(5):587–598, 2003. DOI 10.1088/0031-9155/48/5/303.

[15] G. P. Penney, J. M. Blackall, M. S. Hamady, T. Sabharwal, A. Adam, and D. J. Hawkes. Registration of freehand 3D ultrasound and magnetic resonance liver images. *Medical Image Analysis*, **8**(1):81–91, 2004. DOI 10.1016/j.media.2003.07.003.

[16] J. C. Platt. Fast training of support vector machines using sequential minimal optimization, pages 185–208 in B. Schölkopf, C. J. C. Burges, and A. J. Smola, editors, *Advances in kernel methods: Support Vector Learning*. MIT Press, Cambridge, MA, USA, 1999.

[17] C. N. Riviere, J. Gangloff, and M. de Mathelin. Robotic compensation of biological motion to enhance surgical accuracy. *Proceedings of the IEEE*, **94**(9):1705–1716, 2006. DOI 10.1109/jproc.2006.880722.

[18] T. Rohlfing, C. R. Maurer, W. G. O'Dell, and J. Zhong. Modeling liver motion and deformation during the respiratory cycle using intensity-based nonrigid registration of gated MR images. *Medical Physics*, **31**(3):427–432, 2004. DOI 10.1118/1.1644513.

[19] A. Schweikard, G. Glosser, M. Bodduluri, M. J. Murphy, and J. R. Adler, Jr. Robotic Motion Compensation for Respiratory Movement during Radiosurgery. *Journal of Computer-Aided Surgery*, **5**(4):263–277, 2000. DOI 10.3109/10929080009148894.

[20] A. J. Smola and B. Schölkopf. A tutorial on support vector regression. *Statistics and Computing*, **14**:199–222, 2004.

[21] D. Verellen, M. de Ridder, N. Linthout, K. Tournel, G. Soete, and G. Storme. Innovations in image-guided radiotherapy. *Nature Reviews Cancer*, **7**(12):949–960, 2007. DOI 10.1038/nrc2288.

[22] J. Wilbert, M. Guckenberger, B. Polat, O. Sauer, M. Vogele, M. Flentje, and R. A. Sweeney. Semi-robotic 6 degree of freedom positioning for intracranial high precision radiotherapy; first phantom and clinical results. *Radiation Oncology*, **5**:42, 2010. DOI 10.1186/1748-717x-5-42.

Chapter 8
Motion Prediction

In the previous chapter we discussed motion correlation. With motion correlation, we compute the current position of a moving target. Then we must move the robot so that it follows the target. The robot motion will thus always lag behind the moving target. This time lag is illustrated in Fig. 8.1. In the figure, the x-axis represents time, while the y-axis shows target position.

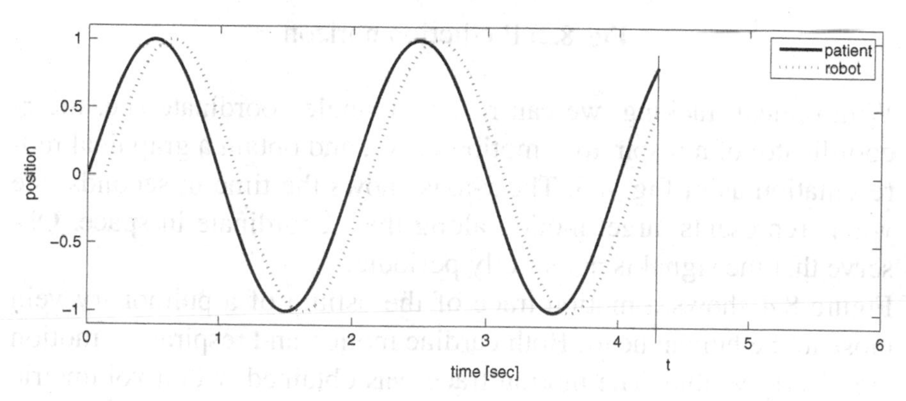

Fig. 8.1: Signal prediction

The figure shows an ideal situation, with a perfect sine wave. At time point t shown in the figure, the position of the target and the robot position are known. Time is discretized, i.e. at fixed time intervals (i.e. every 50 ms) we must send a motion command to the robot. By the time we have computed the target position and the robot has reached its new position, the target will have moved. This time lag (computing time, robot motion time, etc.) is typically constant (e.g. 100 ms).

A. Schweikard, F. Ernst, *Medical Robotics*,
DOI 10.1007/978-3-319-22891-4_8

The idea of motion prediction is the following. We send a motion command to the robot. The command tells the robot not to move to the current position of the target, but to the position where the target will be in 100 ms. Based on the past history of the motion curve, we can determine this future position. Thus it is our goal to extrapolate the patient's motion curve by a fixed amount δ_t. δ_t is called the prediction horizon (Fig. 8.2).

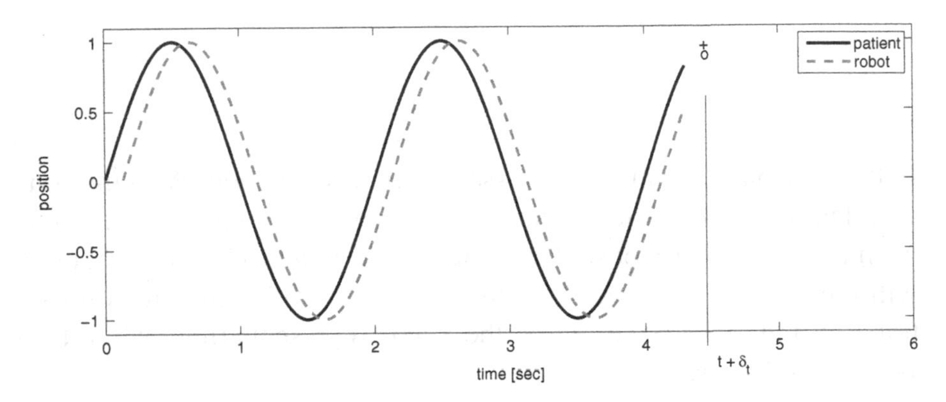

Fig. 8.2: Prediction horizon

With optical tracking, we can record a single coordinate (i.e. the z-coordinate) of a respiratory motion curve, and obtain a graphical representation as in Fig. 8.3. The x-axis shows the time in seconds, the y-axis represents target motion along the z-coordinate in space. Observe that the signal is not strictly periodic.

Figure 8.4 shows a motion trace of the ostium of a pulmonary vein close to the human heart. Both cardiac motion and respiratory motion are clearly visible. The motion trace was obtained with a volumetric ultrasound setup.

In principle, we could apply regression methods to the problem of prediction. Thus, for example support vector regression computes a value y for an unknown sample point $\mathbf{x}$, given training data pairs $(\mathbf{x}_1, y_1), \ldots, (\mathbf{x}_m, y_m)$. However, we will regard motion correlation and motion prediction as separate problems. There are several reasons for this: in prediction, we have time points with equidistant spacing, and we have a fixed prediction horizon. Furthermore, in prediction, the last known time point is more relevant for the computation than points

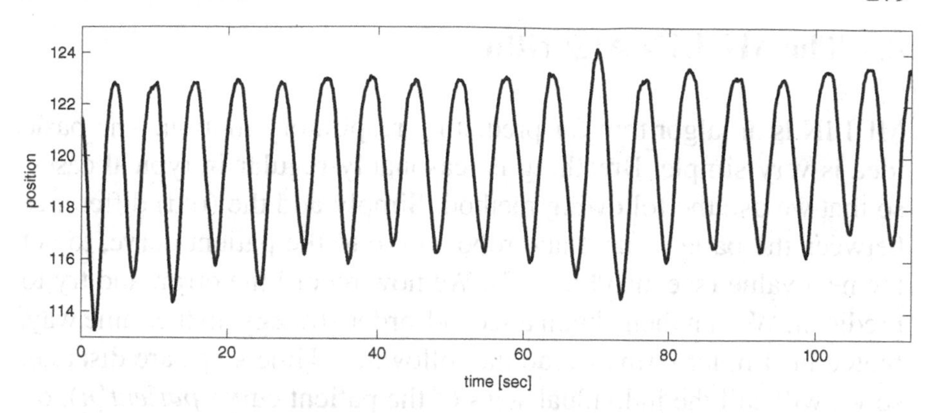

Fig. 8.3: Respiratory signal (measured with infrared tracking)

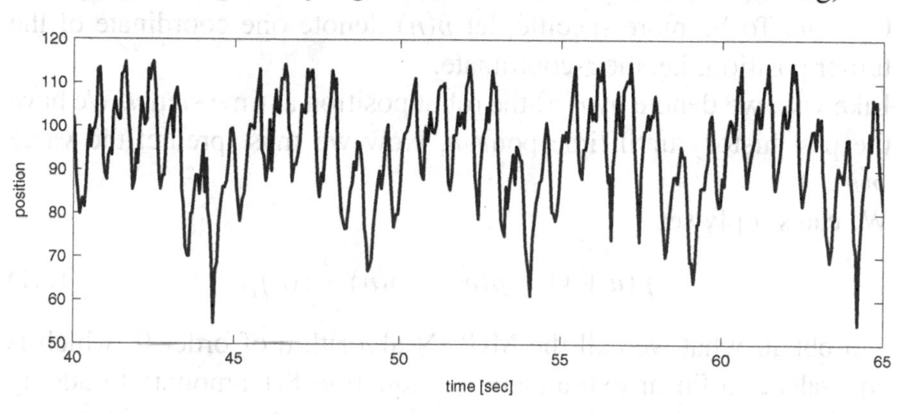

Fig. 8.4: Cardiac motion and respiratory motion, measured with ultrasound. Typically, the frequency of cardiac motion is four times larger than the frequency of the respiratory signal alone. The amplitude of respiratory motion is larger than the amplitude of cardiac motion at this target location

further in the past. Finally, we need a prediction result within a robot command cycle, thus within a few milliseconds. Standard methods for correlation often require substantial computing time. While support vectors provide a valid method for prediction, we will need so-called warm-start methods, capable of both learning and un-learning in real-time. We will find that other, more dedicated methods are more suitable.

8.1 The MULIN Algorithm

MULIN is an algorithm for predicting respiratory motion. The basic idea is very simple. Breathing is reasonably regular in typical cases, so that we use the following method. Simply add the (old) difference between the patient curve and robot curve to the patient curve, to get the next value (see also Fig. 8.2). We now record the error, and try to predict it. We can then obtain a second-order strategy, in the same way. Stated in simpler terms we do the following: Time steps are discrete, so we will call the individual steps of the patient curve $patient(n)$, or, for short $p(n)$ (see Fig. 8.2). Then p is a function of the time points $0,\ldots,m$. To be more specific, let $p(n)$ denote one coordinate of the tumor position, i.e. the z-coordinate.
Likewise, we denote by $r(n)$ the robot position at time step n. We have the past history until time point n. Now we must predict the value $p(n+1)$.
We can simply set

$$p(n+1) = p(n) + [p(n) - r(n)], \tag{8.1}$$

and obtain what we call the MULIN algorithm of order 0 (which is equivalent to linear extrapolation). Equation 8.1 amounts to adding the error made in the last step, just assuming the error will remain constant. But of course it will not. We now plot the error curve with the other curves. The dash-dotted curve shows the error, i.e. the difference between the patient curve and the robot curve (see Fig. 8.5).
Thus the error curve $e(n)$ (e for error) is given by

$$e(n) = p(n) - r(n). \tag{8.2}$$

The key to the MULIN algorithm is now the following: The error curve is also periodic, but has a smaller amplitude. So it should be easier to predict! Thus we delay the error curve by one time step, calculate the difference between the error curve and the delayed error curve, and add that to the last known value of the error curve. The result will change the above error term $[p(n) - r(n)]$. To delay the error curve, we simply use older values. I.e. if $e(n)$ is the value of the error curve at time point n, then $e(n-1)$ is the value of the delayed curve.

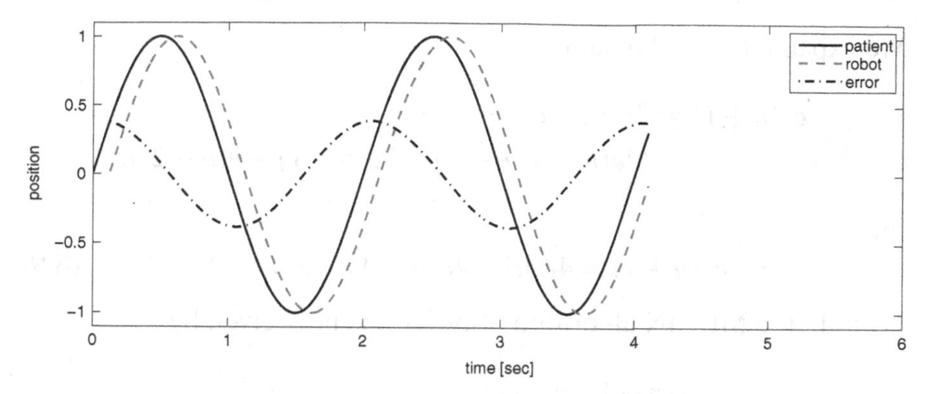

Fig. 8.5: Prediction error (*dotted curve*)

To predict the error curve, we must compute a value for $e(n+1) = p(n+1) - r(n+1)$ from the past history, i.e. from $p(n), r(n)$ etc.
In the same way as above, we can estimate

$$e(n+1) = e(n) + [e(n) - e(n-1)]. \tag{8.3}$$

This is the same as

$$e(n+1) = p(n) - r(n) + [p(n) - r(n) - (p(n-1) - r(n-1))]. \tag{8.4}$$

The right hand side can be rewritten to

$$2[p(n) - r(n)] - [p(n-1) - r(n-1)]. \tag{8.5}$$

Overall, we obtain a MULIN-algorithm of order 1 by setting

$$p(n+1) = p(n) + 2[p(n) - r(n)] - [p(n-1) - r(n-1)]. \tag{8.6}$$

We can now repeat the same construction to obtain a MULIN algorithm of order 2:
Define a function e^* by setting

$$e^*(n) = 2[p(n) - r(n)] - [p(n-1) - r(n-1)] = 2e(n) - e(n-1). \tag{8.7}$$

To predict the function e^*, we set as above

$$e^*(n+1) = e^*(n) + e^*(n) - e^*(n-1). \tag{8.8}$$

We expand this, and obtain

$$e^*(n+1) = 2e(n) - e(n-1) + \\ [2e(n) - e(n-1) - 2e(n-1) + e(n-2)],$$

thus

$$e^*(n+1) = 4e(n) - 4e(n-1) + e(n-2). \tag{8.9}$$

Overall, the MULIN algorithm of order 2 is now given by

$$p(n+1) = \\ p(n) + 4[p(n) - r(n)] - \\ 4[p(n-1) - r(n-1)] + \\ [p(n-2) - r(n-2)]. \tag{8.10}$$

We see that MULIN of higher order looks more deeply into the past of the signal, as it uses the older values $p(n-1)$, $p(n-2)$.
MULIN can be generalized to order k (see Exercise 8.1 at the end of this chapter).
When deriving MULIN, we have always assumed that the value of p for the immediate next time step $p(n+1)$ must be predicted. Thus our prediction horizon was a single time step. However, it may also be necessary to predict several time steps into the future.
To look further into the signal's future, we would predict values

$$p(n+s), p(n+s-1), \ldots, p(n+1) \tag{8.11}$$

from

$$p(n), p(n-1), p(n-2), p(n-3), \ldots. \tag{8.12}$$

Likewise, we could look further into the past by using the values

$$p(n), p(n-s), p(n-2s), p(n-3s), \ldots \tag{8.13}$$

instead of $p(n), p(n-1), p(n-2), p(n-3), \ldots$.
In this case, the parameter s controls how far we look into the past.
Finally, to avoid sudden changes in the values computed by MULIN, we introduce a smoothing parameter μ. Thus, to compute

$$p(n+s) \tag{8.14}$$

we use the same method as above, but we also compute $p^*(n+s-1)$ and then set

$$p^*(n+s) = \mu p(n+s) + (1-\mu)p^*(n+s-1). \tag{8.15}$$

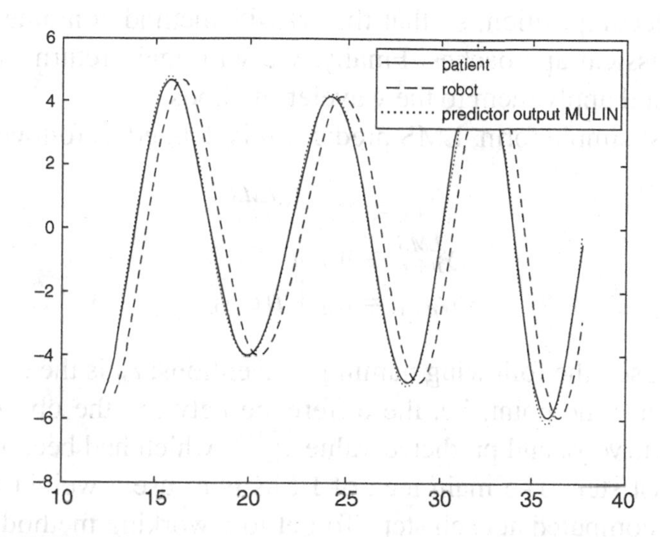

Fig. 8.6: MULIN predictor for a motion signal. *Thick solid line*: patient position. *Dashed line*: robot position, *dotted line*: predictor output for MULIN order two

Figure 8.6 shows an example for MULIN of order two. The dotted line shows the predictor output. Notice that overshooting occurs at the maxima and minima.

8.2 Least Means Square Prediction

Classical methods from signal processing can also be applied to the problem of signal prediction. A number of methods has been developed since the 1960s for this problem. Amongst those methods are LMS-prediction [20], as well as Fourier decomposition, Kalman filtering and newer versions of the LMS prediction, such as nLMS and RLS (see [8] for a survey). Experimentally, none of these methods gives good results for the problem of anatomical motion prediction, since

respiration is far more irregular than typical electronic signals. However, such methods provide a basis for the development of more dedicated methods. We will next describe the LMS method, and extend this method to a wavelet-method which we will call wLMS. Wavelet decomposition can be regarded as an extension and generalization of Fourier decomposition, so that the wLMS method combines several of the classical approaches. Finally, we will again return to support vectors, and apply them to the wavelet methods.
In its most simple form, LMS prediction is defined as follows:

$$e_n = y_n - y_n^{LMS} \tag{8.16}$$
$$y_{n+1}^{LMS} = w_n y_n \tag{8.17}$$
$$w_{n+1} = w_n + \mu e_n y_n \tag{8.18}$$

Here we used the following naming conventions: e_n is the error in the last known time point, i.e. the difference between the observed respiration curve y_n and predicted value y_n^{LMS}, which had been predicted for the last step. The main idea of LMS is to use a weight value w_n which is computed at each step. To get to a working method, the values y_0^{LMS} and w_0 must be initialized. We set $y_0^{LMS} = y_0$ and $w_0 = 1$. The parameter μ controls the step-length.
To understand the definition of the LMS predictor we consider the square of the error e_n.
Thus, set

$$E_{n+1} = \left(y_{n+1} - y_{n+1}^{LMS}\right)^2. \tag{8.19}$$

But by definition,

$$E_{n+1} = (y_{n+1} - w_n y_n)^2. \tag{8.20}$$

We take the derivative of the squared error function E thus defined, with respect to w, and obtain

$$\frac{\mathrm{d}E}{\mathrm{d}w} = 2\,(y_{n+1} - w_n y_n)\,(-y_n) \tag{8.21}$$

thus

$$\frac{\mathrm{d}E}{\mathrm{d}w} = 2\left(y_{n+1} - y_{n+1}^{LMS}\right)(-y_n) = -2e_{n+1}y_n. \tag{8.22}$$

Now, to decrease the error, we subtract $\frac{dE}{dw}$ from w_n to obtain the new estimate for w_{n+1}. This gives

$$w_{n+1} = w_n + \mu e_{n+1} y_n. \tag{8.23}$$

Since we do not yet have a value for e_{n+1}, we will simply use e_n instead, which gives the formula in the definition of the LMS predictor.

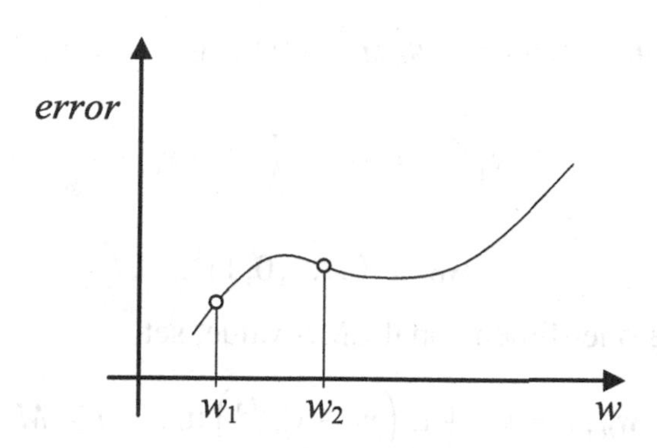

Fig. 8.7: Gradient descent

Notice that LMS performs a gradient descent by taking the derivative of the squared error function. Figure 8.7 illustrates the computation. We compute the local value of the derivative of the (squared) error function. If this gradient is *positive* (value w_1 in the figure), then we know the error will increase if we increase the weight value w, i.e. step to the right of w_1. Likewise, if the gradient is *negative* (value w_2), then our error will decrease, if we increase the value for w. Thus, in both cases, we know in which direction to change our value of w. But we do not know by which amount to change this value. Assume, for example, we have the value w_2 (again compare the figure), so we must step to the right. If the step-length is too big, we will over-step, and actually increase the error. As noted above, the parameter μ controls the step-length of the gradient descent. In practice, it often turns out to be difficult to find a good value for μ. The necessity to choose such a parameter is one of the disadvantages of the LMS algorithm. The figure also shows that the gradient descent performed by LMS will only compute a local minimum for the error function. Notice the difference to the least squares methods used in previous chapters, which actually compute global minima.

One further disadvantage of LMS is the necessity to estimate e_{n+1} (we did this by replacing e_{n+1} by e_n). This resembles the assumption underlying MULIN, namely the assumption that the error will remain constant.
A vector-based version of LMS allows for increasing the depth of the past history M we look at.
We set

$$\mathbf{u}_n = (u_{n,1},\ldots,u_{n,M})^{\mathrm{T}} = (y_{n-M+1},\ldots,y_n)^{\mathrm{T}}, \tag{8.24}$$

and

$$y_1^{LMS} = \cdots = y_M^{LMS} = y_0 \tag{8.25}$$

with

$$\mathbf{w}_0 = (0,\ldots,0,1)^{\mathrm{T}}. \tag{8.26}$$

Similar to the one-dimensional LMS value, set

$$\mathbf{w}_{n+1} = \mathbf{w}_n + \mu \left(y_n - y_n^{LMS} \right) \mathbf{u}_n, \quad n \geq M, \tag{8.27}$$

and

$$y_{n+1}^{LMS} = \mathbf{w}_n^{\mathrm{T}} \mathbf{u}_n. \tag{8.28}$$

A further variant of LMS is nLMS, or the normalized LMS method. It is defined as follows:

$$e_n = y_n - y_n^{nLMS} \tag{8.29}$$

$$y_{n+1}^{nLMS} = w_n y_n \tag{8.30}$$

$$w_{n+1} = w_n + \mu \frac{e_n}{y_n} \tag{8.31}$$

If you compare the definitions in Eqs. Eq. 8.18 and 8.31, you will notice that a multiplication is simply replaced by a division. How can this be right? It may seem astonishing that we can simply replace this, and still obtain a valid definition. And how can this division be a normalization?
The riddle is solved if we look again at the multi-dimensional version of LMS: Here, a multi-dimensional version is obtained by replacing the definition in Eq. 8.27 by

$$\mathbf{w}_{n+1} = \mathbf{w}_n + \frac{\mu \left(y_n - y_n^{nLMS} \right) \mathbf{u}_n}{\|\mathbf{u}_n\|_2^2}, \quad n \geq M. \tag{8.32}$$

Thus, we simply divided by the *square* of the magnitude of our input signal, and this was done to normalize! After normalization, it becomes easier to choose the value μ, especially in cases where the magnitude of our input changes rapidly. Of course, in the one-dimensional-case, the division will cancel out, so that we obtain a derivation for the one-dimensional nLMS method.
Note that it is necessary to add a constant α (typically 10^{-4} or smaller) to the denominators of Eqs. 8.31 and 8.32 to avoid division by zero.
The next section will deal with a principle similar to LMS, applied to the bands of a wavelet decomposition.

8.3 Wavelet-Based LMS Prediction

Wavelet decomposition resembles Fourier transformation, where a given periodic function is written as a sum of sine and cosine waves. However, Fourier transformation requires a periodic input function. Our respiratory functions are not strictly periodic. It is true that the shape of one respiratory cycle resembles the shape of the other cycles. But the resemblance of the cycles can be quite faint, even if the patient breathes normally.
To motivate the use of wavelets in our application, we again look at the example in Fig. 8.6. Here we applied the MULIN predictor to an aperiodic, but nonetheless very smooth signal. MULIN gives good results in this case. However, if the signal is not smooth, problems will arise. Often, anatomical motion data are far from being smooth (Fig. 8.8). If a sudden change in direction occurs near a peak point along the curve (see arrow in Fig. 8.8), then the predictor will assume that the peak has been reached, and initiate a downwards motion, thereby causing errors.
Thus, it is reasonable to apply averaging or smoothing before prediction. However, averaging is difficult in our case. To understand the difficulty here, assume we average over the past k time points during prediction. This would give equal weight to the past k data points including our current point. But the most recent data point is the most critical one, i.e. it carries the most information. Thus we lose a substantial amount of information by averaging. Wavelet methods provide a more

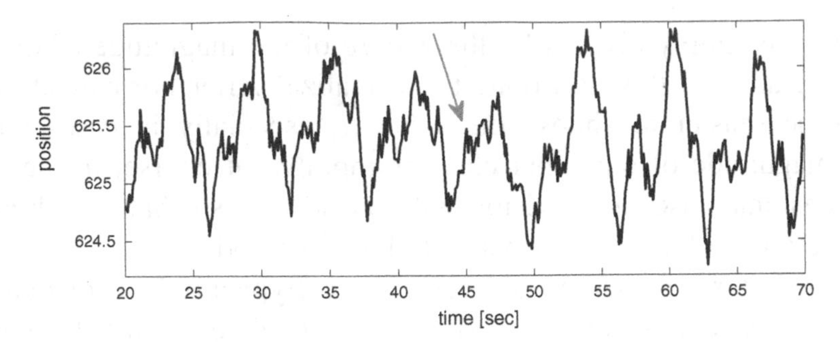

Fig. 8.8: Respiratory motion curve recorded with an infrared tracking system. Maxima and minima along the curve are difficult to predict, due to noise and irregular breathing pattern

systematic way for smoothing data. As an important feature, smoothing can be applied without loss of information. Specifically, we need a method that filters the data into distinct frequency bands, such that the sum of these bands exactly represents the original signal. Instead of filtering out high-frequency noise altogether, we apply prediction to each frequency band separately. Bands which become known to have carried noise in the past can then receive lower weights in the course of prediction. We can then apply machine learning to the individual bands in the wavelet decomposition.
Consider the definitions

$$c_{0,n} = y_n \tag{8.33}$$

$$c_{j+1,n} = \frac{1}{2}\left(c_{j,n-2^j} + c_{j,n}\right), \quad j \geq 0 \tag{8.34}$$

$$W_{j+1,n} = c_{j,n} - c_{j+1,n}, \quad j \geq 0. \tag{8.35}$$

Here y_n is again our signal. To better understand this definition, first notice that Eq. 8.34 simply computes an average between two consecutive values of our original signal.
We now select a positive integer J which will determine the resolution depth up to which we compute the decomposition, i.e. $j = 0, \ldots, J$.
We next illustrate the computation of the c-values. These values are written into a table.

As described in the definition above, we begin by setting $j = 0$, and

$$c_{0,n} = y_n, \quad n = 0,\dots,m. \tag{8.36}$$

This will give the first line of the c-table. I.e. assume $m = 8$, so we have computed the first line, giving

$$c_{0,0}\ c_{0,1}\ c_{0,2}\ c_{0,3}\ c_{0,4}\ c_{0,5}\ c_{0,6}\ c_{0,7}\ c_{0,8}.$$

Having done that, we can compute

$$c_{1,1} = \frac{1}{2}(c_{0,0} + c_{0,1}). \tag{8.37}$$

Next we can compute $c_{1,2}$ from $c_{0,1}$ and $c_{0,2}$. Both latter values are already in the first line of the table:

$$c_{1,2} = \frac{1}{2}(c_{0,1} + c_{0,2}) \tag{8.38}$$

Likewise we now compute $c_{1,3}, c_{1,4}, \dots c_{1,8}$ from the values in the first line of the table. Our table will look like this:

$$\begin{array}{ccccccccc} c_{0,0} & c_{0,1} & c_{0,2} & c_{0,3} & c_{0,4} & c_{0,5} & c_{0,6} & c_{0,7} & c_{0,8} \\ & c_{1,1} & c_{1,2} & c_{1,3} & c_{1,4} & c_{1,5} & c_{1,6} & c_{1,7} & c_{1,8} \end{array}$$

We now compute

$$c_{2,3} = \frac{1}{2}(c_{1,1} + c_{1,3}). \tag{8.39}$$

Likewise we obtain $c_{2,4}, \dots, c_{2,8}$. Finally, we obtain the full c-table (for $J = 3$):

$$\begin{array}{ccccccccc} c_{0,0} & c_{0,1} & c_{0,2} & c_{0,3} & c_{0,4} & c_{0,5} & c_{0,6} & c_{0,7} & c_{0,8} \\ & c_{1,1} & c_{1,2} & c_{1,3} & c_{1,4} & c_{1,5} & c_{1,6} & c_{1,7} & c_{1,8} \\ & & & c_{2,3} & c_{2,4} & c_{2,5} & c_{2,6} & c_{2,7} & c_{2,8} \\ & & & & & & & c_{3,7} & c_{3,8} \end{array}$$

Notice that our c-table is not rectangular, i.e. table entries $c_{1,0}$, $c_{2,0}$, $c_{2,1}$, $c_{2,2}$, $c_{3,0}$ etc. do not exist.

Remember, we set

$$W_{j+1,n} = c_{j,n} - c_{j+1,n} \tag{8.40}$$

for $j = 0, \ldots, J$.
The computation of the W-values proceeds in much the same way.
We obtain the table

$$\begin{array}{cccccccc} W_{1,1} & W_{1,2} & W_{1,3} & W_{1,4} & W_{1,5} & W_{1,6} & W_{1,7} & W_{1,8} \\ & & W_{2,3} & W_{2,4} & W_{2,5} & W_{2,6} & W_{2,7} & W_{2,8} \\ & & & & & & W_{3,7} & W_{3,8}. \end{array}$$

We remain in the above example. For $n = 8$ and $J = 2$ we consider $W_{1,8}$ and $W_{2,8}$.
Then we have

$$W_{1,8} + W_{2,8} + c_{2,8} = c_{0,8} - c_{1,8} + c_{1,8} - c_{2,8} + c_{2,8} \tag{8.41}$$
$$= c_{0,8} \tag{8.42}$$
$$= y_8. \tag{8.43}$$

And more generally,

$$y_n = W_{1,n} + \cdots + W_{J,n} + c_{J,n}. \tag{8.44}$$

We can now illustrate the role of the parameter J. This parameter determines the depth of the decomposition of our signal y. Hence, for $J = 1$, we obtain the results shown in Table 8.1. In the last line of Table 8.1, we see the original signal y_i. Notice that, as a result of Eq. 8.44, each column in Tables 8.1 and 8.2 sums up to one of the signal values y_i.

Table 8.1: Wavelet decomposition with two bands

$W_{1,1}$	$W_{1,2}$	$W_{1,3}$	$\ldots$	$W_{1,n}$
$c_{1,1}$	$c_{1,2}$	$c_{1,3}$	$\ldots$	$c_{1,n}$
y_1	y_2	y_3	$\ldots$	y_n

Each line in the table is called a *band*. For $J = 2$, we obtain three bands (Table 8.2).

Table 8.2: Wavelet decomposition with three bands

$W_{1,3}$	$W_{1,4}$	$W_{1,5}$	$\dots$	$W_{1,n}$
$W_{2,3}$	$W_{2,4}$	$W_{2,5}$	$\dots$	$W_{2,n}$
$c_{2,3}$	$c_{2,4}$	$c_{2,5}$	$\dots$	$c_{2,n}$
y_3	y_4	y_5	$\dots$	y_n

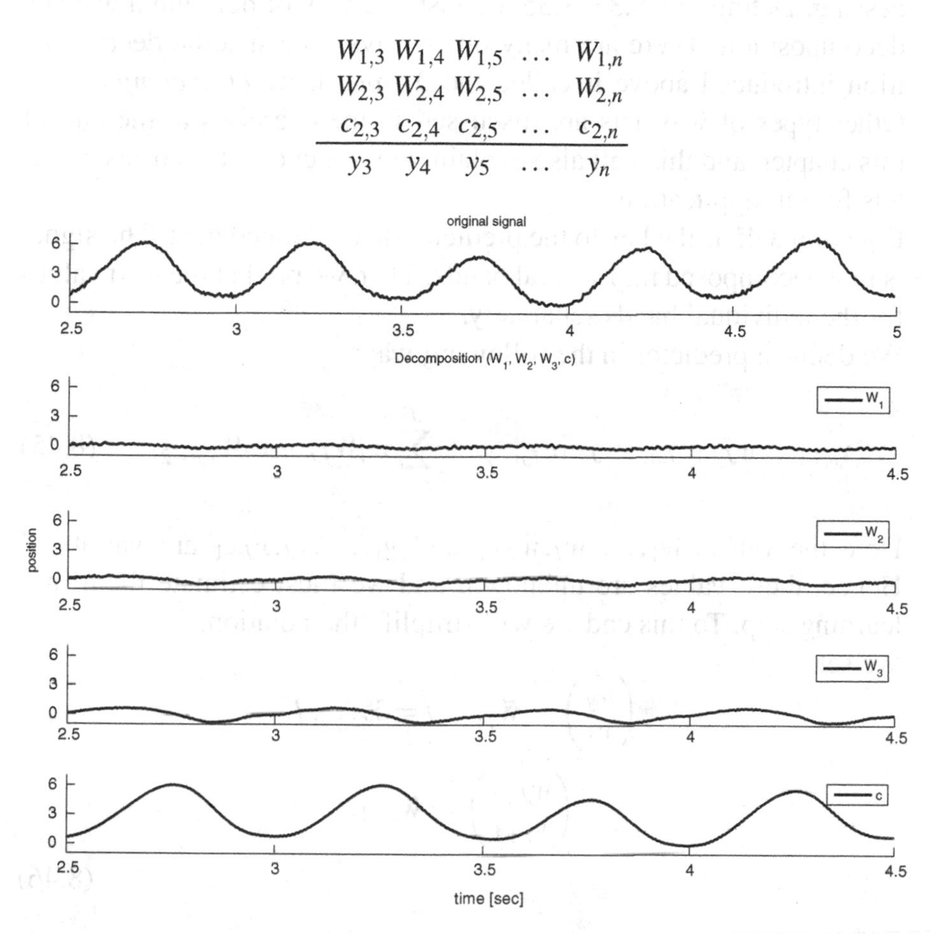

Fig. 8.9: Wavelet decomposition for an input signal (with $J = 3$). *Top row*: input signal. *Bottom rows*: Wavelet bands W_1, W_2, W_3 and c

Overall, vertical summation of the bands gives the original signal. Thus, the tables indeed yield a decomposition of the original signal y_i. The decomposition is graphically illustrated in Fig. 8.9. An input signal (shown in the top row) is decomposed into four bands W_1, W_2, W_3 and c (four bottom rows). Notice that the input signal is noisy when compared to the c-band in the decomposition. Thus, a standard

application of wavelet decomposition is noise removal in signal processing. Definitions 8.33–8.35 are just one way of defining a wavelet decomposition. There are many other ways. The specific decomposition introduced above is called the *à trous wavelet decomposition.* Other types of wavelets are discussed in the exercises at the end of this chapter, and this will also explain why we chose the à trous wavelets for our application.
Equation 8.45 is the key to the predictor, to be defined next. The signal is first decomposed into several bands. Then we predict the next values for the individual bands separately.
We define a predictor in the following way:

$$y_{n+1} = w_{J+1} c_{J,n} + v_{J+1} c_{J,n-2^J} + \sum_{j=1}^{J} w_j W_{j,n} + v_j W_{j,n-2^j} \tag{8.45}$$

Here the values $w_1, \ldots, w_J, w_{J+1}$ and $v_1, \ldots, v_J, v_{J+1}$ are variables! Hence, these values are unknown, and we must estimate them in a learning step. To this end we will simplify the notation.
We set

$$\begin{pmatrix} w_j \\ v_j \end{pmatrix} = \tilde{\mathbf{w}}_j, \quad j = 1, \ldots, J,$$

$$\begin{pmatrix} w_{J+1} \\ v_{J+1} \end{pmatrix} = \tilde{\mathbf{w}}_{J+1}, \tag{8.46}$$

and

$$(W_{j,n}, W_{j,n-2^j}) = \tilde{W}_{j,n}, \tag{8.47}$$

for $j = 1, \ldots, J$ and

$$(c_{J,n}, c_{J,n-2^J}) = \tilde{c}_{J,n}. \tag{8.48}$$

Then we rewrite our above predictor in the following way:

$$y_{n+1} = \tilde{\mathbf{c}}_{J,n} \tilde{\mathbf{w}}_{J+1} + \sum_{j=1}^{J} \tilde{\mathbf{W}}_{j,n} \tilde{\mathbf{w}}_j \tag{8.49}$$

To estimate the values for our variables $w_1, \ldots, w_J, w_{J+1}$ and $v_1, \ldots, v_J, v_{J+1}$ we set up a matrix B, by defining:

$$B = \begin{pmatrix} \tilde{\mathbf{W}}_{1,n-1} & \tilde{\mathbf{W}}_{2,n-1} & \cdots & \tilde{\mathbf{W}}_{J-1,n-1} & \tilde{\mathbf{W}}_{J,n-1} & \tilde{\mathbf{c}}_{J,n-1} \\ \vdots & \vdots & \vdots & \vdots & \vdots & \vdots \\ \tilde{\mathbf{W}}_{1,n-M} & \tilde{\mathbf{W}}_{2,n-M} & \cdots & \tilde{\mathbf{W}}_{J-1,n-M} & \tilde{\mathbf{W}}_{J,n-M} & \tilde{\mathbf{c}}_{J,n-M} \end{pmatrix} \quad (8.50)$$

Note that the entries of the matrix B are themselves vectors, namely 1-by-2 vectors. But this does not change the fact that the following equation is simply a linear system of equations!

$$B \begin{pmatrix} \tilde{\mathbf{w}}_1 \\ \vdots \\ \tilde{\mathbf{w}}_{J+1} \end{pmatrix} = \begin{pmatrix} y_n \\ \vdots \\ y_{n-M+1} \end{pmatrix} \quad (8.51)$$

This system has the $2J+2$ variables $w_1, \ldots, w_{J+1}$ and $v_1, \ldots, v_{J+1}$ and a number M of equations. If M is larger than $2J+2$, then the system is over-determined.

Equation 8.51 is the training equation for $w_1, \ldots, w_{J+1}$ and $v_1, \ldots, v_{J+1}$. Each matrix line in B corresponds to one training sample, and we thus have M training samples. The training samples stem from the signal history $y_0, y_1, \ldots, y_n$. As we go down the matrix lines, we step backwards in the signal history by one sample for each matrix line.

It remains to discuss how the system in Eq. 8.51 should be solved. Naturally, one could use Gaussian elimination. However, over-determined systems of this type can be solved with advantage by normal equations, so here again the method from the previous chapter can be used. This will fit a regression line in the least-mean-square sense to the data points represented by the matrix lines. Obviously, we can also use support vectors for this regression. There are several ways to do this, and we will discuss this possibility below.

But before we do this, we will look at two issues related to the implementation and practical improvements of the wLMS algorithm. Remember that the original version of the LMS algorithm (without wavelets) used a smoothing parameter μ. Indeed we have used such a parameter for MULIN as well.

To emphasize the fact that we had set up the B-matrix from the decomposition data with the indices $n-1,\ldots,n-M$, we will add these indices to the notation. Hence, write

$$B^{(n-1,\ldots,n-M)} \tag{8.52}$$

for the above B-matrix in Eq. 8.51.
Likewise we extend the notation for the weight-vector, giving

$$B^{(n-1,\ldots,n-M)} \begin{pmatrix} \tilde{\mathbf{w}}_1 \\ \vdots \\ \tilde{\mathbf{w}}_{J+1} \end{pmatrix}^{(n-1,\ldots,n-M)} = \begin{pmatrix} y_n \\ \vdots \\ y_{n-M+1} \end{pmatrix}. \tag{8.53}$$

Using the same notation, we can rewrite the predictor equation:

$$B^{(n)} \begin{pmatrix} \tilde{\mathbf{w}}_1 \\ \vdots \\ \tilde{\mathbf{w}}_{J+1} \end{pmatrix}^{(n-1,\ldots,n-M)} = y_{n+1} \tag{8.54}$$

Now to apply the smoothing parameter μ we will use the old weight vector (computed in the preceding step) and the weight vector computed from Eq. 8.53. Hence, we set

$$\begin{pmatrix} \tilde{\mathbf{w}}_1 \\ \vdots \\ \tilde{\mathbf{w}}_{J+1} \end{pmatrix}^{(new)} =$$

$$(1-\mu) \begin{pmatrix} \tilde{\mathbf{w}}_1 \\ \vdots \\ \tilde{\mathbf{w}}_{J+1} \end{pmatrix}^{(n-2,\ldots,n-M-1)} + \mu \begin{pmatrix} \tilde{\mathbf{w}}_1 \\ \vdots \\ \tilde{\mathbf{w}}_{J+1} \end{pmatrix}^{(n-1,\ldots,n-M)}.$$

And we replace Eq. 8.54 by

$$B^{(n)} \begin{pmatrix} \tilde{\mathbf{w}}_1 \\ \vdots \\ \tilde{\mathbf{w}}_{J+1} \end{pmatrix}^{(new)} = y_{n+1}. \tag{8.55}$$

8.3.1 Variable Scale Lengths

In the above description of the wavelet predictor, we have used a minor simplification. This was done to reduce the amount of subscripts in the notation. We return to Eqs. 8.45 and 8.46. In Eq. 8.45, y_{n+1} was obtained from the decomposition data with weight variables $w_1, \ldots, w_J, w_{J+1}$ and $v_1, \ldots, v_J, v_{J+1}$ by

$$y_{n+1} = w_{J+1} c_{J,n} + v_{J+1} c_{J,n-2^J} + \sum_{j=1}^{J} w_j W_{j,n} + v_j W_{j,n-2^j}.$$

Instead of this latter definition, with just two weight variables w and v per value of j, we use a series of such variables (for each j), now called

$$w_j^{(0)}, \ldots, w_j^{(a_j)}.$$

Thus we obtain

$$\begin{aligned} y_{n+1} = \; & w_{J+1}^{(0)} c_{J,n} + w_{J+1}^{(1)} c_{J,n-2^J \cdot 1} + \ldots + \\ & w_{J+1}^{(a_{J+1}-1)} c_{J,n-2^J \cdot (a_{J+1}-1)} + \\ & \sum_{j=1}^{J} w_{J+1}^{(0)} W_{j,n-2^j \cdot 0} + w_j^{(1)} W_{j,n-2^j \cdot 1} + \ldots + \\ & w_j^{(a_j-1)} W_{j,n-2^j \cdot (a_j-1)}. \end{aligned} \tag{8.56}$$

The necessary extensions to Eq. 8.46 are straightforward, i.e. we now have

$$\begin{pmatrix} w_j^{(0)} \\ \vdots \\ w_j^{(a_j-1)} \end{pmatrix} = \tilde{\mathbf{w}}_j, j = 1, \ldots, J$$

$$\begin{pmatrix} w_{J+1}^{(0)} \\ \vdots \\ w_{J+1}^{(a_{J+1}-1)} \end{pmatrix} = \tilde{\mathbf{w}}_{J+1}$$

instead of Eq. 8.46.

8.4 Support Vectors for Prediction

SVR methods, as described in the previous chapter, can also be applied to respiration prediction [7]. To obtain a model for inhale-exhale motion, we can proceed as follows: Training samples are pairs $(t_1, y(t_1)), \ldots, (t_m, y(t_m))$, where $y(t_i)$ denotes the position of some target point at time t_i. During production, we compute the value $y(t_m + \delta_t)$. However, our signal is non-stationary. The depth of inhalation varies over time. Types of curves thus obtained are individual, and may vary considerably between patients. In particular, resting phases of varying lengths between respiratory cycles occur. The slope of inhalation and exhalation is different and time-varying in many cases. The following approach addresses these problems.
Instead of samples of the form $(t_i, y(t_i))$ we use a series of values

$$y(t_1), y(t_2), \ldots, y(t_s), y(t_{s+k})$$

as a single training sample.
Notice that the entire series $y(t_1), y(t_2), \ldots, y(t_s), y(t_{s+k})$ is one single sample, whereas $y(t_1), y(t_2), \ldots, y(t_s)$ is our production sample. Here we require that the time points $t_1, t_2, \ldots, t_s, t_{s+k}$ have equidistant spacing. The parameter k controls the prediction horizon. As noted above, there are other ways to use support vectors for our application, one of which combines wavelets and support vectors. The next section prepares this alternative.

8.4.1 Online Regression and AOSVR

Respiration prediction is time-critical, and we must keep computing time to a minimum. Online support vector algorithms have been developed [13] to shorten computing time.
In linear programming, so-called warm-start methods have been developed. Such methods incrementally compute a solution of the input LP problem for a given data set. That is, given a solution for the first m inequality constraints, one can quickly update this solution when a single new constraint is added. This can be done without starting the entire computation from scratch. This is often of advantage since, in

many cases, the new constraint does not even restrict the feasible region any further, and this condition can be tested readily. But even if it does further restrict the feasible region, then an updated solution can be obtained very quickly from the solution for the original problem. Such warm-start methods have been extended to support vector machines, called AOSVR. In this case, it is necessary to be able to learn the training data after a new sample has been added. It may also be necessary to "un-learn" single samples.

8.4.2 Combining Support Vectors and Wavelets

In Chap. 7, we investigated correlation methods. We used a very simple strategy based on normal equations to find a regression line amidst data points in the plane. In this case we had input values x_i and desired output values y_i. Very much the same situation occurred in the estimation of our weight values for wavelet-based prediction (see Eq. 8.51). This equation computes a linear least mean square fit to the data. Obviously, it is possible to apply support vector methods to the training data in Eq. 8.51. Each line of this matrix equation corresponds to one training sample, giving a total of M training samples. Specifically, a sample of the form

$$(\tilde{\mathbf{W}}_{1,n-1}, \ldots, \tilde{\mathbf{W}}_{J,n-1}, \tilde{\mathbf{c}}_{J,n-1}, y_n) \tag{8.57}$$

is one single training sample for this SVR.
To obtain a full set of samples, we again use the matrix lines in Eq. 8.51, giving:

$$\begin{gathered}(\tilde{\mathbf{W}}_{1,n-1}, \ldots, \tilde{\mathbf{W}}_{J,n-1}, \tilde{\mathbf{c}}_{J,n-1}, y_n) \\ \vdots \\ (\tilde{\mathbf{W}}_{1,n-M}, \ldots, \tilde{\mathbf{W}}_{J,n-M}, \tilde{\mathbf{c}}_{J,n-M}, y_{n-M+1})\end{gathered}$$

Then the production sample has the form

$$(\tilde{\mathbf{W}}_{1,n}, \ldots, \tilde{\mathbf{W}}_{J,n}, \tilde{\mathbf{c}}_{J,n}). \tag{8.58}$$

We thus obtain a combination of wavelet methods and support vector methods, which will be called wSVR.

8.5 Fast-Lane Methods and Performance Measures

Motion prediction is about forecasting the future. It is well-known that this can be arbitrarily difficult. If the given signal data are sufficiently evil, then prediction will fail. Luckily, respiration and cardiac motion data are mostly regular, so that prediction algorithms provide a substantial gain of accuracy. Today, motion prediction is used in routine clinical practice in robotic radiosurgery. However, no single one of the above methods works best for all patients. Rather, wLMS is best in *nearly* all cases. But in some cases, SVR methods provide improvements which cannot be achieved with wLMS. Finally, MULIN is a simple and robust method, and sometimes gives the best results. This gives rise to the following idea: the patient data are measured for a while before treatment, and data are recorded. We can run all known algorithms in parallel, and then decide which algorithm to use for this patient. But then we can also keep all other methods running during treatment, and switch whenever one of the other methods, currently not used, improves over the current method. This approach will be called the fast-lane method [4]. To implement such an approach, we will need methods for measuring performance.
A simple measure is the RMS error between the signal and the predicted curve:

$$\mathrm{RMS}(y, y^{PRED}) = \sqrt{\frac{1}{N}\sum_{i=1}^{N} \left\| y_i - y_i^{PRED} \right\|^2} \tag{8.59}$$

The RMS error thus gives an average over the squared distances between the signal itself and the value returned by the predictor. N is the total number of time steps.
This simple measure provides an absolute error, but does not allow for much comparison. Thus, normalization is needed. In order to normalize the RMS error, we divide by the error which would have occurred if we had not applied any prediction at all. Stated in simpler terms, we compute the RMS-distance between the patient curve and the predicted curve (Fig. 8.6), then the RMS-distance between the patient

curve and the delayed curve, then divide the two values. This yields the relative RMS error. With y_δ denoting the delayed curve:

$$\mathrm{RMS}(y, y_\delta) = \sqrt{\frac{1}{N}\sum_{i=1}^{N} \|y_i - y_{\delta,i}\|^2} \tag{8.60}$$

Now dividing gives the relative RMS error:

$$\mathrm{RMS}_{\mathrm{rel}} = \frac{\mathrm{RMS}(y, y^{PRED})}{\mathrm{RMS}(y, y_\delta)} \tag{8.61}$$

In this way, the improvement obtained by prediction can be expressed as a percentage of reduction in terms of RMS error. Thus, if successful, prediction reduces RMS error by a certain percentage.
Relative RMS error is not the only measure for evaluating motion prediction for robots. Maximum absolute error can be an important measure as well. For technical reasons, it is often useful to limit the so-called jitter of the predictor output signal. The jitter measures distances between two consecutive (discrete) points along the signal:

$$\mathfrak{J}(y^{PRED}) = \frac{1}{N}\frac{1}{\Delta t}\sum_{i=0}^{N} \|y_i^{PRED} - y_{i+1}^{PRED}\| \tag{8.62}$$

Here, the factor $\frac{1}{\Delta t}$ normalizes with respect to the spacing between the samples. Thus the jitter value $\mathfrak{J}$ measures the average distance (per second) traveled by the robot following the predictor output.
Notice that the measures just described may be in conflict with one another. Respiration patterns vary considerably among patients. For patients with large lung tumors, the patterns can become very irregular. Unfortunately, for lung tumors, the respiratory motion excursion is particularly large. As noted above, no single algorithm works best for all patients. For further empirical evaluation, and for the implementation of a fast-lane method, histograms are very useful. Given a data base of test cases, a histogram plots the number of data base cases (x-axis) versus the percentage gains (relative RMS) obtained with the individual algorithm (y-axis). An example of such a histogram for a

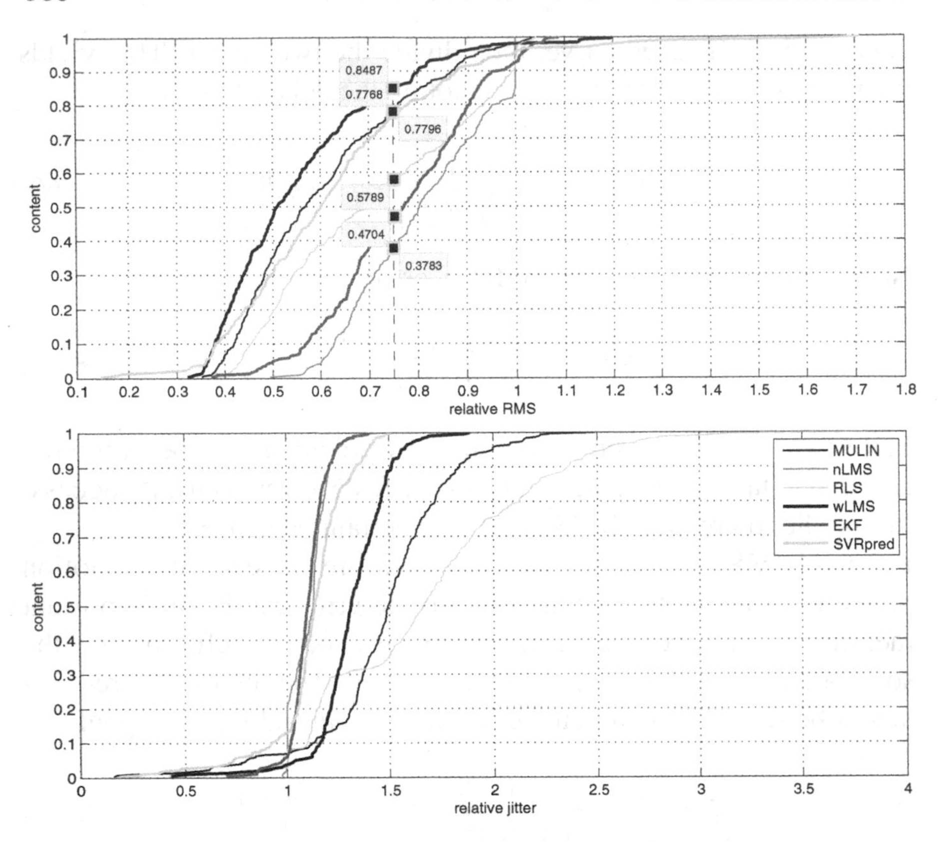

Fig. 8.10: Histograms for evaluating predictor output

number of predictors is shown in Fig. 8.10. The figure shows both, RMS error and jitter. Here six algorithms are shown. The RLS method is a variant of the LMS method, whereas EKF denotes the extended Kalman filter [8, 14], applied to motion prediction.

Table 8.3 states results of relative RMS errors for a large database of respiratory traces from patient treatments, containing data from 304 full treatment sessions [3].

It turns out that wLMS gives the best results in terms of RMS for over 60 % of the data base cases. MULIN gives best results on 28 % of the cases. However, for a small number of cases, SVR is capable of removing over 80 % of the residual error. This is not possible for the other methods. For SVR and wSVR, the computing time is longer than

Table 8.3: Results of relative RMS errors obtained with different prediction methods

wLMS:	RMS_{rel} 56.99 %
MULIN:	RMS_{rel} 64.36 %
SVRpred:	RMS_{rel} 68.32 %
LMS:	RMS_{rel} 76.32 %

for the other methods, but jitter can be reduced with SVR and wSVR in comparison to other methods. It turns out that wSVR can still improve substantially over wLMS in many cases. However, wSVR has the largest number of parameters. Thus it can be difficult to find the optimal set of parameters for wSVR.

We have not discussed the choice of parameters for the algorithms. It is clear that most algorithms will need a good choice of parameters to be practical. But how to choose the parameters? The fast-lane scheme sketched above provides a good background for this discussion. Because not only can we switch between algorithms, but we can also switch between different "versions" of one single algorithm, where we will obtain different versions by supplying the same algorithm with different parameters.

Grid search is a very straight-forward approach for evaluating parameters. We place a fine grid over each axis of parameter space. We then evaluate the algorithm for each point in parameter space thus obtained. An example is shown in Fig. 8.11 for the case of wLMS.

Clearly, grid search is often not feasible in practice. Grid search is limited to situations where a large amount of data is available, the algorithm is fast, and the number of parameters is small. Then the parameters can be optimized for a small sub-sample and the result can be used for the rest of the signal.

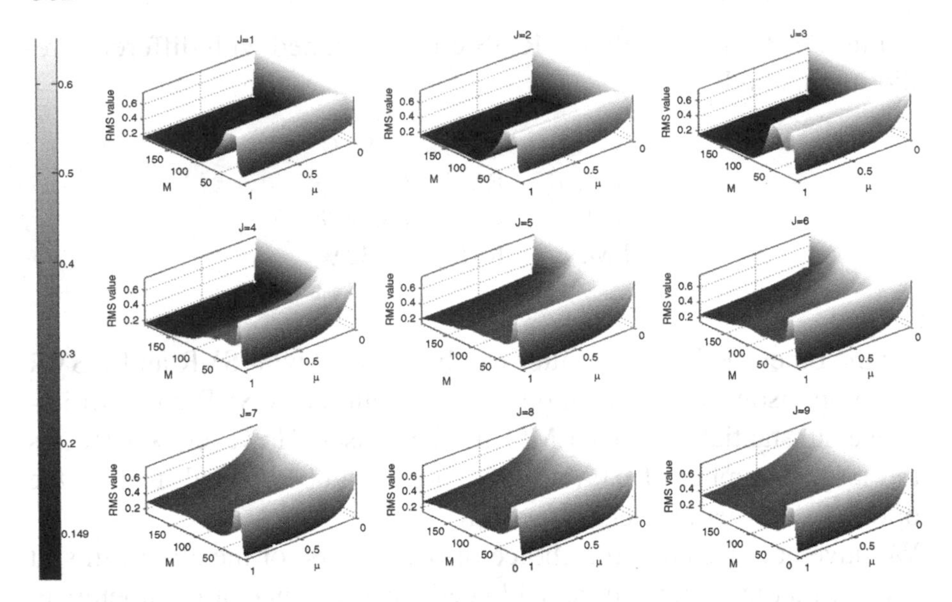

Fig. 8.11: Grid search in parameter space for the wLMS algorithm

Exercises

Exercise 8.1 *MULIN Algorithm*

Show that the general MULIN-algorithm of order n is given by

$$p(k+1) = p(k) + \sum_{i=0}^{n} \frac{(-1)^i 2^{n-i} n!}{i!(n-i)!} [p(k-i) - r(k-i)]. \tag{8.63}$$

Exercise 8.2 *nLMS Algorithm*

In an implementation, compare the LMS and the nLMS algorithms for synthetic inputs, i.e. the function $y = \sin(x)$. Check the convergence radius in both cases, by a grid search with varying parameter μ. Construct a synthetic input function with varying amplitude (such as the one in Fig. 8.6). Evaluate the convergence radius for both cases, again by grid search over the parameter μ.

Exercise 8.3 ***Haar Transform***

Let $(t_1,\ldots,t_m)$ be a list of m equidistant time points. Then a discretized signal curve is given by assigning function values y_i to each time point, i.e. $(y(t_1),\ldots,y(t_m))=(y_1,\ldots,y_m)$. The signal $\mathbf{y}=(y_1,\ldots,y_m)$ can be transformed in the following way [19]: (We assume m is even, otherwise we add a zero element to the end of the string $(y_1,\ldots,y_m)$.) Set

$$a_1=\frac{y_1+y_2}{\sqrt{2}},a_2=\frac{y_3+y_4}{\sqrt{2}},\ldots,a_{m/2}=\frac{y_{m-1}+y_m}{\sqrt{2}} \quad (8.64)$$

and

$$d_1=\frac{y_1-y_2}{\sqrt{2}},d_2=\frac{y_3-y_4}{\sqrt{2}},\ldots,d_{m/2}=\frac{y_{m-1}-y_m}{\sqrt{2}}. \quad (8.65)$$

Let $T(\mathbf{y})=(a_1,\ldots,a_{m/2},d_1,\ldots,d_{m/2})$ denote the transformed signal. The transformation of the signal $\mathbf{y}$ thus obtained is called the Haar transform. The signal $T(\mathbf{y})$ has the same length m as the input signal $\mathbf{y}$.

a) Show that the transformation thus defined is invertible, i.e. there is a mapping $I(\mathbf{y})$, such that $I(T(\mathbf{y}))=\mathbf{y}$.
b) Show that T preserves the energy of the input signal, i.e. the scalar product $\mathbf{yy}$ is equal to $T(\mathbf{y})T(\mathbf{y})$.
c) Define and implement a 'denoising' scheme based on the Haar transform. Your denoiser should work as follows: Transform the signal under T, set to zero all values in $T(\mathbf{y})$ below a fixed threshold γ, then transform the thresholded signal back under I.
d) Define a synthetic signal, add random noise, and derive a threshold γ such that 99.9 percent of the energy of the original signal is preserved.

Exercise 8.4 ***Haar Wavelets***

The Haar transform T was defined in the previous exercise. The definition of Haar wavelets is based on the Haar transform.

a) Iterate the construction leading to the Haar transform T, giving a multi-level transform. Hint: for level 2, assume m is divisible by 4. Construct the second level transform $T^{(2)}$ by transforming only the values $a_1,\ldots,a_{m/2}$, but leaving the values $d_1,\ldots,d_{m/2}$ at the end of the signal $T(\mathbf{y})$ unchanged. This yields a signal $T^{(2)}\mathbf{y} = (\mathbf{a}^{(2)},\mathbf{d}^{(2)},\mathbf{d}^{(1)})$. Here, the lengths of the strings $\mathbf{a}^{(2)}$ and $\mathbf{d}^{(2)}$ are $m/4$, while $\mathbf{d}^{(1)}$ has length $m/2$.
b) Define a component-wise multiplication for signals, i.e. $\mathbf{yz} = (y_1z_1,\ldots,y_mz_m)$. Show that the transform T can be represented by this component-wise multiplication with so-called Haar wavelets and Haar scaling functions. Hint: The Haar wavelets and Haar scaling functions are signals of the same lengths as $\mathbf{y}$. m wavelets and m scaling functions will be needed here. Multiplication of the input signal $\mathbf{y}$ with the first Haar-wavelet gives the value d_1. Multiplication with the first Haar scaling function gives the value a_1. In the same way, multiplication with the remaining wavelets gives the remaining values $d_2,\ldots,d_{m/2}$ and $a_2,\ldots,a_{m/2}$.
c) The computation in Eq. 8.65 uses adjacent values from the original signal to compute new values. Thus, the difference of two adjacent values y_i and y_{i+1} is used to compute d_i. Looking at the computation sequence of the c-values in the definition of the à trous decomposition, discuss the meaning of the term 'à trous'.

Exercise 8.5 *Daubechies Wavelets*

The Daubechies wavelets are defined in much the same way as the Haar wavelets. However, four adjacent values from the original signal are used to compute two values a_i and d_i. Specifically, we have

$$a_1 = y_1\frac{1+\sqrt{3}}{4\sqrt{2}} + y_2\frac{3+\sqrt{3}}{4\sqrt{2}} + y_3\frac{3-\sqrt{3}}{4\sqrt{2}} + y_4\frac{1-\sqrt{3}}{4\sqrt{2}}. \tag{8.66}$$

The values defined in Eqs. 8.33–8.35 resemble the definitions in Eqs. 8.64 and 8.65. In both cases, an average and a difference of two values is used to define the new values. Thus we could rename the à trous method and call it the 'à trous Haar' method. In fact the so-called Haar-function is the basis of both definitions: The definition in Eqs. 8.33–8.35 and the definition in Eqs. 8.64 and 8.65. (The Haar

function is defined as the step function with values -1 in the interval $[0,1/2)$, $+1$ in the interval $[1/2,1)$, and 0 elsewhere.)
Draw a graph of a Daubechies wavelet, and discuss why Daubechies wavelets (although highly effective in signal processing) would seem less adequate for prediction than the à trous scheme in Eqs. 8.33–8.35.

Summary

Motion prediction is used to overcome the time lag required for data and image processing, as well as robot motion time, and collimator motion time. Thus the command sequence sent to the robot will not refer to the current position of the anatomical target, but to its future position. The future position of the target can be extrapolated in time, if the motion is stable and periodic. We obtain a straightforward, yet very practical method simply by adding the error from previous time steps. Classical methods from signal processing attempt to capture unknown characteristics of an incoming signal, and can be applied to signal prediction and feed-forward loops. In practice, the convergence radius of the signal processing methods for our application is rather small, and better results are obtained with more advanced methods, such as wavelet decomposition and support vector regression. Wavelet decomposition filters the input signal into several bands. For each band, a least squares method estimates parameter values for describing the curve corresponding to this band. Support vector regression can be applied in several ways to the problem of prediction. Firstly, we can simply set up samples $(t,y(t))$, or samples containing several points of the form $(t,y(t))$ with equidistant time spacing. But secondly, we can apply support vector regression to the bands in a wavelet decomposition. Finally, fast online methods are particularly suitable for the problem, since typically only a single new sample is added at each time step. Measurements for evaluating predictors can themselves be used in new predictors, which gives rise to a fast-lane scheme.

Notes

Applications of motion prediction arise in radiosurgery, where we compensate for respiratory motion by a robotic arm [17]. As an alternative, we can move the leaves of a multi-leaf collimator (Fig. 6.22) [12], the treatment couch [23] or a gimbaled radiation source [9, 11]. The LMS algorithm was developed in 1960 for signal filtering [20]. nLMS is the normalized version of the LMS algorithm, see also [21]. Kalman filtering and RLS were developed in the same context. [8] is a text book on filtering methods from signal processing. [22] gives a survey of time series prediction.
The combination of correlation and prediction for moving anatomic targets was suggested in 2000 [17]. It is in routine clinical use since 2002 [18]. The MULIN method was specifically developed for respiration tracking [6]. Newer methods for respiration prediction include methods based on kernel adaptive filtering [16].
The wavelet-based predictor is based on the à trous wavelet decomposition [10]. The term à trous refers to the multi-level computation series described in the chapter. The authors in [15] have turned this general decomposer into a predictor, and this was applied to respiration prediction in [5]. [19] is a text book with an introduction to discrete wavelet decomposition.
As we have seen, support vector methods require several external parameters to be chosen beforehand. One can estimate and modify the values of the parameters during the application, via fast-lane methods (see also [4]). Probabilistic methods from machine learning, also based on kernels, can also be applied to estimate the parameters [1, 2].

References

[1] Dürichen, R., Wissel, T., Schweikard, A.: Prediction of respiratory motion using wavelet-based support vector regression. In: Proceedings of the 2012 IEEE International Workshop on Machine Learning for Signal Processing (MLSP), pp. 1–6. IEEE Signal Processing Society (2012). DOI 10.1109/MLSP.2012.6349742

[2] Dürichen, R., Wissel, T., Schweikard, A.: Optimized order estimation for autoregressive models to predict respiratory motion. International Journal of Computer Assisted Radiology and Surgery **8**(6), 1037–1042 (2013). DOI 10.1007/s11548-013-0900-0

[3] Ernst, F.: Compensating for Quasi-periodic Motion in Robotic Radiosurgery. Springer, New York (2011). DOI 10.1007/978-1-4614-1912-9

[4] Ernst, F., Schlaefer, A., Dieterich, S., Schweikard, A.: A fast lane approach to LMS prediction of respiratory motion signals. Biomedical Signal Processing and Control **3**(4), 291–299 (2008). DOI 10.1016/j.bspc.2008.06.001

[5] Ernst, F., Schlaefer, A., Schweikard, A.: Prediction of respiratory motion with wavelet-based multiscale autoregression. In: N. Ayache, S. Ourselin, A. Maeder (eds.) MICCAI 2007, Part II, *Lecture Notes in Computer Science*, vol. 4792, pp. 668–675. MICCAI, Springer, Brisbane, Australia (2007). DOI 10.1007/978-3-540-75759-7_81

[6] Ernst, F., Schweikard, A.: Predicting respiratory motion signals for image-guided radiotherapy using multi-step linear methods (MULIN). International Journal of Computer Assisted Radiology and Surgery **3**(1–2), 85–90 (2008). DOI 10.1007/s11548-008-0211-z

[7] Ernst, F., Schweikard, A.: Forecasting respiratory motion with accurate online support vector regression (SVRpred). International Journal of Computer Assisted Radiology and Surgery **4**(5), 439–447 (2009). DOI 10.1007/s11548-009-0355-5

[8] Haykin, S.: Adaptive Filter Theory, 4th edn. Prentice Hall, Englewood Cliffs, NJ (2002)

[9] Hiraoka, M., Matsuo, Y., Sawada, A., Ueki, N., Miyaba, Y., Nakamura, M., Yano, S., Kaneko, S., Mizowaki, T., Kokubo, M.: Realization of dynamic tumor tracking irradiation with real-time monitoring in lung tumor patients using a gimbaled x-ray head radiation therapy equipment. International Journal of Radiation Oncology, Biology, Physics **84**(3, S1), S560–S561 (2012). DOI 10.1016/j.ijrobp.2012.07.1493

[10] Holschneider, M., Kronland-Martinet, R., Morlet, J., Tchamitchian, P.: A real-time algorithm for signal analysis with the help of the wavelet transform. In: J.M. Combes, A. Grossmann, P. Tchamitchian (eds.) Wavelets: Time-Frequency Methods and Phase Space. Proceedings of the International Conference, pp. 286–297. Springer, Marseille, France (1987)
[11] Kamino, Y., Takayama, K., Kokubo, M., Narita, Y., Hirai, E., Kawada, N., Mizowaki, T., Nagata, Y., Nishidai, T., Hiraoka, M.: Development of a four-dimensional image-guided radiotherapy system with a gimbaled X-ray head. International Journal of Radiation Oncology, Biology, Physics **66**(1), 271–278 (2006). DOI 10.1016/j.ijrobp.2006.04.044
[12] Keall, P.J., Sawant, A., Cho, B.C., Ruan, D., Wu, J., Poulsen, P.R., Petersen, J., Newell, L.J., Cattell, H., Korreman, S.: Electromagnetic-guided dynamic multileaf collimator tracking enables motion management for intensity-modulated arc therapy. International Journal of Radiation Oncology, Biology, Physics **79**(1), 312–320 (2011). DOI 10.1016/j.ijrobp.2010.03.011
[13] Ma, J., Theiler, J., Perkins, S.: Accurate on-line support vector regression. Neural Computation **15**(11), 2683–2703 (2003). DOI 10.1162/089976603322385117
[14] Ramrath, L., Schlaefer, A., Ernst, F., Dieterich, S., Schweikard, A.: Prediction of respiratory motion with a multi-frequency based Extended Kalman Filter. In: Proceedings of the 21st International Conference and Exhibition on Computer Assisted Radiology and Surgery (CARS'07), *International Journal of CARS*, vol. 2, pp. 56–58. CARS, Berlin, Germany (2007). DOI 10.1007/s11548-007-0083-7. URL http://www.cars-int.org/
[15] Renaud, O., Starck, J.L., Murtagh, F.: Wavelet-based combined signal filtering and prediction. IEEE Transactions on Systems, Man and Cybernetics, Part B: Cybernetics **35**(6), 1241–1251 (2005)
[16] Ruan, D., Keall, P.J.: Online prediction of respiratory motion: multidimensional processing with low-dimensional feature learning. Physics in Medicine and Biology **55**(11), 3011–3025 (2010). DOI 10.1088/0031-9155/55/11/002

[17] Schweikard, A., Glosser, G., Bodduluri, M., Murphy, M.J., Adler Jr., J.R.: Robotic Motion Compensation for Respiratory Movement during Radiosurgery. Journal of Computer-Aided Surgery **5**(4), 263–277 (2000). DOI 10.3109/10929080009148894
[18] Schweikard, A., Shiomi, H., Adler Jr., J.R.: Respiration tracking in radiosurgery. Medical Physics **31**(10), 2738–2741 (2004). DOI 10.1118/1.1774132. Motion Compensation in Radiosurgery
[19] Walker, J.S.: A Primer on Wavelets and Their Scientific Applications, 2nd edn. Studies in Advanced Mathematics. Chapman & Hall/CRC, Boca Raton, London, New York (2008)
[20] Widrow, B., Hoff, M.E.: Adaptive switching circuits. In: IRE WESCON Convention Record, vol. 4, pp. 96–104 (1960)
[21] Widrow, B., Stearns, S.D.: Adaptive Signal Processing. Prentice Hall Signal Processing Series. Prentice Hall, Upper Saddle River, NJ (1985)
[22] Wiener, N.: Extrapolation, Interpolation, and Smoothing of Stationary Time Series, *M.I.T. Press Paperback Series*, vol. 9. The MIT Press, Cambridge, MA (1964)
[23] Wilbert, J., Meyer, J., Baier, K., Guckenberger, M., Herrmann, C., Hess, R., Janka, C., Ma, L., Mersebach, T., Richter, A., Roth, M., Schilling, K., Flentje, M.: Tumor tracking and motion compensation with an adaptive tumor tracking system (ATTS): system description and prototype testing. Medical Physics **35**(9), 3911–3921 (2008). DOI 10.1118/1.2964090

Chapter 9
Motion Replication

In Chaps. 7 and 8 we saw two aspects of motion learning: motion correlation and motion prediction. In both cases, the motions were anatomical. We now look at more complex motions occurring during surgery. Suppose we record the motion of the surgeon, i.e. with optical tracking. We will see three types of motion in our data: intentional motion, tremor, and noise. But which is which? Clearly, this is a learning problem. We must classify the different types of motion. As an application, we consider robotic systems for motion replication. Such systems replicate the motion of the surgeon, e.g. in microsurgery.

Systems for motion replication consist of two robots: the first robot is moved by the human operator (here the surgeon), the second robot moves the (surgical) instrument. Thus, the surgeon moves a passive master robot, and an active replicator robot performs the same motions at a remote site. The scenario is illustrated in Fig. 9.1.

It is immediately clear why such a system is of advantage in surgery. Delicate motions can be 'scaled'. Thus, we can command that any motion of 1 cm, as performed by the surgeon, should be scaled to a smaller motion, i.e. 0.1 cm. Systems for prostatectomy and cardiac valve surgery, relying on this robotic scaling paradigm, are now in wide-spread clinical use.

But beyond motion scaling, we can filter the natural tremor of the surgeon. This means that we transmit any regular motion of the surgeon to the replicator robot, but not the tremor. Advanced classification methods, such as support vector classification (see Chap. 7) can

A. Schweikard, F. Ernst, *Medical Robotics*,
DOI 10.1007/978-3-319-22891-4_9

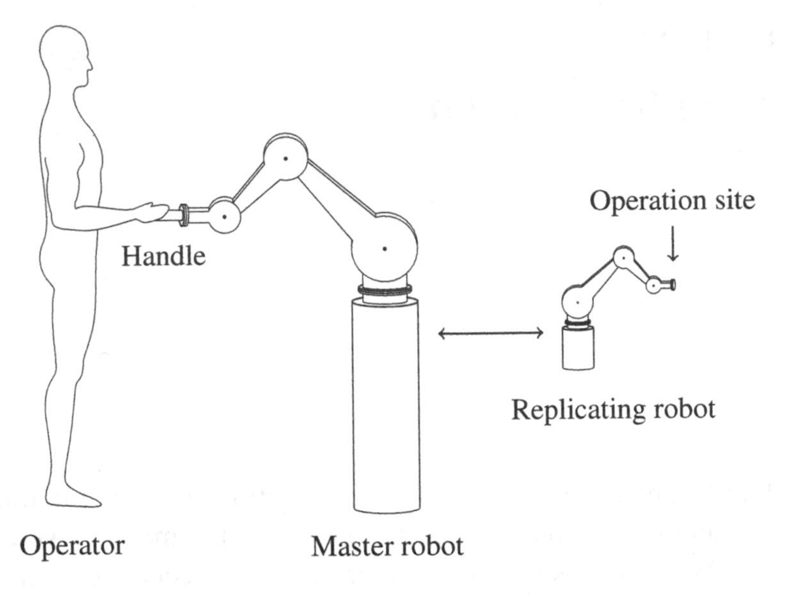

Fig. 9.1: Motion replication

be used to classify between involuntary and intended motion, so that dexterity can be improved.
Likewise, we can detect and compensate for motion at the other end of the system. Namely, for a very delicate operation, e.g. near the heart, pulsatory motion can be disturbing. Thus the replicator robot can actively compensate for such motion. Again, as in Chap. 8, it can be useful to predict periodic motion.
Finally, surgical training is a major issue in this context. A variety of scenarios for rehearsing complex surgical procedures can be based on systems for motion replication. If manual motion is replicated by robot motion, then motion paths can be recorded and compared. Thus, training based on animal models can be avoided.
The kinematics of the two robots in Fig. 9.1 are clearly not optimal. Firstly, it is useful to replicate the motion of both hands. Thus we will need a two-arm construction for the master robot, and for the replicator as well. Secondly, the kinematics of each individual arm of the master can be optimized to suit the application.

Replication of motion includes the replication of static forces. Thus, in this chapter, we will look at how to compute the joint torques needed to apply a force at the tool. Conversely, we will need to find the forces resulting from given joint torques. For both cases, the geometric Jacobian matrix derived in Chap. 4 will be useful.

9.1 Tremor Filtering

Figure 9.2 shows the x-position of a hand-held optical marker held by a test person. The subject was asked not to move, and to suppress motion as much as possible. Small motions were then recorded. Three types of displacements can be distinguished in the curve. There is a periodic tremor, and on top of the tremor, a drift in the position is visible. Finally, measurement noise is visible. The tremor has a fixed frequency, which can be seen in the curve. It would seem possible for the surgeon to suppress the drift, if there is some close visual feedback, e.g. an instrument is held in close vicinity to a target structure. Then the drift can be recognized and suppressed. However, the surgeon cannot suppress the tremor.

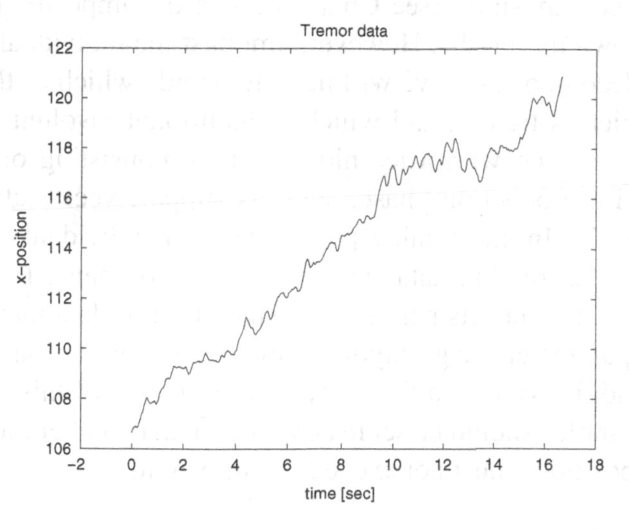

Fig. 9.2: Tremor data recorded with infrared tracking

Our goal is to detect and suppress the tremor automatically. A number of methods can be developed on the basis of the techniques described in the preceding chapters. In particular, we could simply fit a regression curve to the motion curve shown in Fig. 9.2. Support vector machines give us a very powerful tool for addressing this problem. Thus, we would use the following three-step procedure:

1. Perform an online support vector regression on the past k position samples.
2. Based on step one, predict the next position value.
3. Command this position value for the replicator robot, as long as the master's motion in the current time step does not exceed a fixed threshold δ. If δ is exceeded, go to the current position commanded by the master robot.

Here, simple thresholding is used to detect the intended motion of the surgeon. The procedure thus sketched has several drawbacks. In step three, we must retrain the machine in case δ is exceeded. Thus we will not have any filtering during the training time. However, we could detect the frequency of the tremor in the data, but have not used this possibility.
A frequency-oriented decomposition can be obtained with the Ã trous wavelet decomposition (see Chap. 8). The decomposition of tremor data is shown in Fig. 9.3. However, amongst the individual bands in a wavelet decomposition, we will have to decide which of the bands is noise, which is tremor, and which is additional involuntary motion. This can be done with a learning method, consisting of a training phase and a production phase, such as support vector classification (see Chap. 7). In the training phase, data for individual subjects are recorded. The training data can be classified by hand. It is useful to record several data sets per subject, since tremor data may vary with external parameters (e.g. daytime, stress, temperature and other external conditions). Given the safety requirements of this application, small thresholds should be set in advance, such that alterations in commanded positions must not exceed the thresholds.

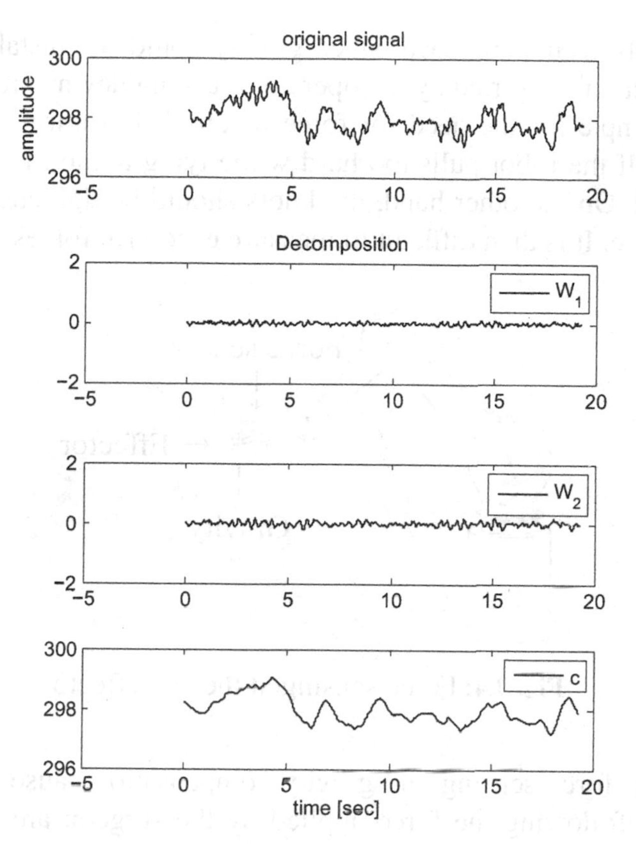

Fig. 9.3: Wavelet decomposition of tremor data, original signal in the top row, recorded with infrared tracking

9.2 Forces

The simple kinematic construction in Fig. 9.1 has a major drawback. The master robot is an industrial robot, designed for repeating small motion sequences in manufacturing procedures. In order to use such robots for motion replication, forces applied by the operating surgeon must be measured continuously. If the operator exerts a force onto the robot's end effector, the robot must actively follow the force. The robot must then calculate the direction of the motion intended by the measured force, and after this comply with the acting force by moving to a new position (Fig. 9.4). During this process, we must compensate

for gravity from a payload, since gravity could be mistaken by the robot as a force exerted by the operator, pushing downwards.
One example for the need for force feedback is suturing in cardiac surgery. If the robot pulls too hard while tying a knot, tissue can be damaged. On the other hand, the knots should be tightened as much as possible. It is then difficult to measure excessive forces.

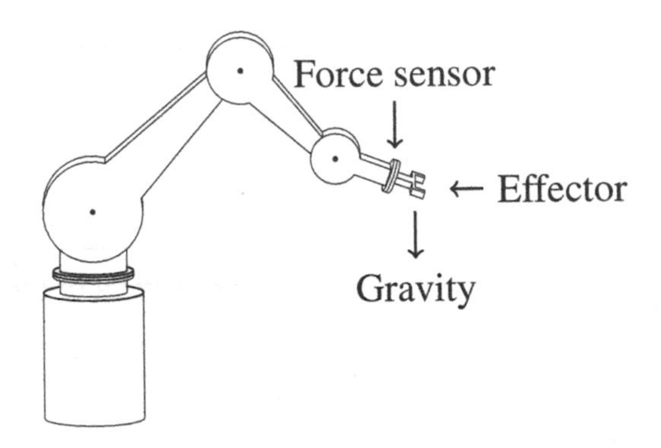

Fig. 9.4: Force sensing at the end effector

However, force sensing and gravity compensation cause a time lag. Motions following the force applied by the surgeon are not carried out immediately, but after a time delay. This delay is noticeable for the user, and will act as a barrier. To overcome the temporal barrier, an inexperienced user will apply more forces than necessary. This will often result in an undesirably large robot reaction. An alternative to force sensors is to use light-weight cable-driven passive arms for the master robot, specifically designed for the application. Such arms can be moved with negligible forces, and friction of the cable construction acts as a natural barrier towards drift caused by gravity.
Figure 9.5 shows a five-joint kinematic construction for a master robot arm. The shoulder of the master arm is positioned close to the shoulder of the operator. The total arm length of this master arm roughly corresponds to the length of an adult human arm, such that small motions can be replicated in a natural way.

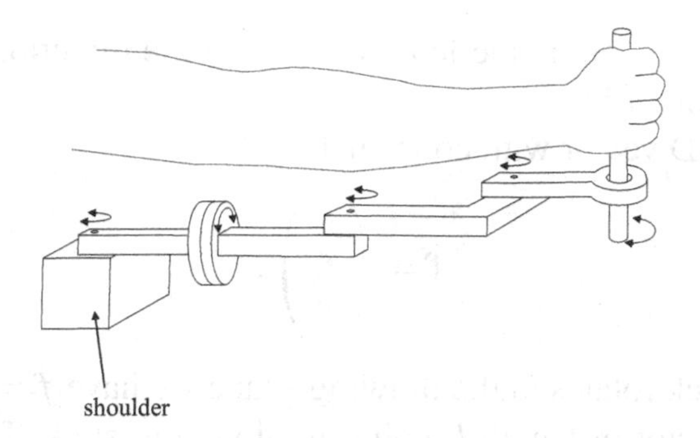

Fig. 9.5: Five-joint kinematics for a cable-driven master robot arm

Suppose our goal is to apply a specific force at the tool tip of the replicator robot. What are the torques needed a the individual joints of the robot?

Clearly, in practice, we would need sensors in this application. Nonetheless, it is useful to understand the connection between forces applied at the tip of the robot, and torques acting on the joints. We again consider the planar two-link manipulator (with revolute joints), in Fig. 4.1 and we again assume equal link lengths, i.e. $l_1 = l_2 = 1$. Before we begin, we must define the term joint torque.

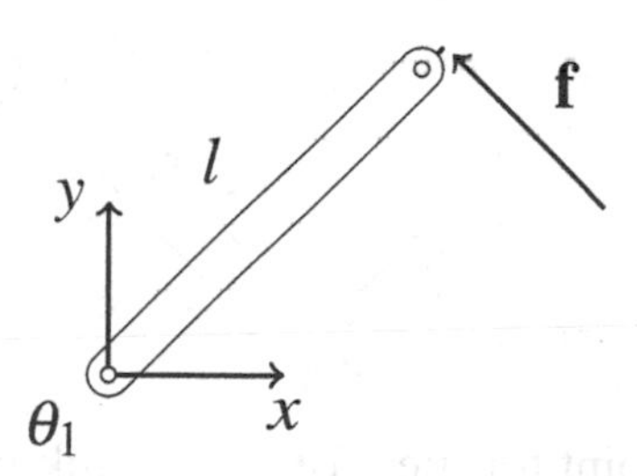

Fig. 9.6: Definition of joint torque. A stick is attached to a base with a revolute joint (joint angle θ_1). A force vector **f** acts at the tip of a stick. The force applied pushes the stick towards the y-axis

We thus assume we have a stick, attached to a base (Fig. 9.6). The stick can rotate about the joint, but will remain in the drawing plane. We denote by l the length of the stick. A force, applied to the stick, is simply a vector. The vector **f** in Fig. 9.6 illustrates this. The magnitude

of the force is given by the length of **f**, and the direction of the force is the direction of **f**.
Here, **f** is a 3D vector with coordinates

$$\mathbf{f} = \begin{pmatrix} f_x \\ f_y \\ f_z \end{pmatrix}. \tag{9.1}$$

Since our stick rotates in the drawing plane we have $f_z = 0$.
Let **r** be a vector of length l, pointing along our stick. Then applying a force **f** to the tip of the stick will result in a torque at the joint. We define the joint torque **t** by

$$\mathbf{t} = \mathbf{r} \times \mathbf{f}. \tag{9.2}$$

Hence, **t** is simply defined as the cross-product of **r** and **f**. Since **r** and **f** are in the drawing plane, **t** will be orthogonal to the drawing plane. Hence, **t** coincides with the axis of rotation. The length τ of **t** is the magnitude of our torque, i.e.

$$\tau = ||\mathbf{t}||. \tag{9.3}$$

Our next goal is to analyze the two-link manipulator with respect to forces and joint torques.

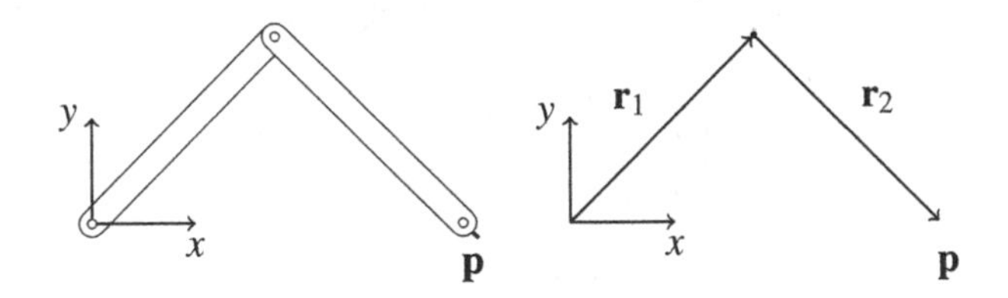

Fig. 9.7: Joint torques for a two-link manipulator

Place vectors $\mathbf{r}_1$ and $\mathbf{r}_2$ along the two links, as shown in Fig. 9.7.
Then,

$$\mathbf{r}_1 = \begin{pmatrix} \cos(\theta_1) \\ \sin(\theta_1) \end{pmatrix}, \tag{9.4}$$

and

$$\mathbf{r}_2 = \begin{pmatrix} \cos(\theta_1 + \theta_2) \\ \sin(\theta_1 + \theta_2) \end{pmatrix}. \tag{9.5}$$

We apply a force to the tip (point $\mathbf{p}$). Following our definition of joint torque, the torque at joint 2 is then simply given by

$$\mathbf{t}_2 = \mathbf{r}_2 \times \mathbf{f}. \tag{9.6}$$

The tip $\mathbf{p}$ of our robot is obtained simply by adding the two vectors $\mathbf{r}_1$ and $\mathbf{r}_2$.
We now think of the vector $\mathbf{r}_1 + \mathbf{r}_2$ as a single stick (in the sense of our above definition of torque). This stick connects the origin and the point $\mathbf{p}$. Thus the joint torque at joint 1, caused by $\mathbf{f}$, is simply

$$\mathbf{t}_1 = (\mathbf{r}_1 + \mathbf{r}_2) \times \mathbf{f}. \tag{9.7}$$

This last equation again follows directly from our definition of joint torques.
Now both vectors $\mathbf{t}_1$ and $\mathbf{t}_2$ are orthogonal to our robot plane (i.e. the x-y-plane), hence they are of the form

$$\mathbf{t} = \begin{pmatrix} 0 \\ 0 \\ \tau \end{pmatrix}. \tag{9.8}$$

Again τ denotes the magnitude of our torque. We consider the magnitudes of the two torques (acting at joints 1 and 2) separately, and we will call these magnitudes τ_1 and τ_2. Inserting our definitions for $\mathbf{r}_1$ and $\mathbf{r}_2$, we see that

$$\begin{aligned} \tau_1 &= (c_1 + c_{12}) f_y - (s_1 + s_{12}) f_x, \\ \tau_2 &= c_{12} f_y - s_{12} f_x. \end{aligned} \tag{9.9}$$

We put the equations for τ_1 and τ_2 into a matrix:

$$\tau = \begin{pmatrix} \tau_1 \\ \tau_2 \end{pmatrix} = \begin{pmatrix} -s_1 - s_{12} & c_1 + c_{12} \\ -s_{12} & c_{12} \end{pmatrix} \begin{pmatrix} f_x \\ f_y \end{pmatrix} \tag{9.10}$$

We had assumed that $l_1 = l_2 = 1$. This is not a necessary assumption, but it simplifies our notation. If we repeat the same calculations for arbitrary values of l_1 and l_2, then our result extends to:

$$\tau = \begin{pmatrix} \tau_1 \\ \tau_2 \end{pmatrix} = \begin{pmatrix} -l_1 s_1 - l_2 s_{12} & l_1 c_1 + l_2 c_{12} \\ -l_2 s_{12} & l_2 c_{12} \end{pmatrix} \begin{pmatrix} f_x \\ f_y \end{pmatrix} \tag{9.11}$$

Notice that we have expressed **f** in terms of the base coordinate system B. To reflect this fact, we write Eq. 9.11 as

$$\tau = \mathbf{A} \cdot {}^{B}\mathbf{f}, \tag{9.12}$$

where

$$\mathbf{A} = \begin{pmatrix} -l_1 s_1 - l_2 s_{12} & l_1 c_1 + l_2 c_{12} \\ -l_2 s_{12} & l_2 c_{12} \end{pmatrix}. \tag{9.13}$$

We see that the joint torques are directly proportional to the arm lengths. Thus, typically, for a six-joint robot, the torques for joints 2 and 3 are the dominant torques.

Remark 9.1

The matrix **A** in Eq. 9.13 looks familiar. It is the transpose of the Jacobi-matrix in Eq. 4.27, see Chap. 4. We will discuss this observation in the next section.

(End of Remark 9.1)

Remark 9.2

In the above discussion, we had assumed that the force vector **f** is given in terms of the base coordinate system. In an application, we often have the forces given at the tool. We must thus transform **f**, in order to specify forces in the tool coordinate system. To this end, we simply multiply by the forward kinematic matrix for the two-link manipulator. But notice, since **f** is a vector, we do not need the translational part of our matrices. We can thus simply multiply with the orientation part of the matrix alone, and obtain

$${}^{B}\mathbf{f} = \begin{pmatrix} c_{12} & -s_{12} \\ s_{12} & c_{12} \end{pmatrix} \cdot {}^{E}\mathbf{f}. \tag{9.14}$$

Inserting this into Eq. 9.12, we see that

$$\tau = \mathbf{A} \cdot \begin{pmatrix} c_{12} & -s_{12} \\ s_{12} & c_{12} \end{pmatrix} \cdot {}^{E}\mathbf{f}. \tag{9.15}$$

We now evaluate the product

$$\mathbf{A} \cdot \begin{pmatrix} c_{12} & -s_{12} \\ s_{12} & c_{12} \end{pmatrix} \tag{9.16}$$

and obtain

$$\mathbf{A} \cdot \begin{pmatrix} c_{12} & -s_{12} \\ s_{12} & c_{12} \end{pmatrix} = \begin{pmatrix} l_1 s_2 & l_2 + l_1 c_2 \\ 0 & l_2 \end{pmatrix}. \tag{9.17}$$

Overall, given a force vector $\mathbf{f}$ (with respect to the effector coordinate system), we have joint torques of

$$\tau = \begin{pmatrix} l_1 s_2 & l_2 + l_1 c_2 \\ 0 & l_2 \end{pmatrix} \cdot {}^E\mathbf{f}. \tag{9.18}$$

(End of Remark 9.2)

We have derived a matrix relating forces at the end effector to joint torques, for the two-link manipulator. The general case will be discussed in the next section.

9.3 Joint Torques and Jacobi-Matrices

In our definition of the joint torque, we set $\mathbf{t} = \mathbf{r} \times \mathbf{f}$, where $\mathbf{r}$ is a vector along the link, and $\mathbf{f}$ is a planar force vector. The torque $\mathbf{t}$ is thus a vector. Here, $\mathbf{t}$ is aligned with $\mathbf{z} = z_0$, the axis of the joint.
In Eq. 9.8 we computed the magnitude τ of the torque $\mathbf{t}$, simply by taking the scalar product, i.e. $\tau = \mathbf{tz}$. This was possible, since $\mathbf{z} = z_0 = (0,0,1)^{\mathrm{T}}$ in this case, and $\mathbf{f}$ was a planar force (Fig. 9.8).
What if $\mathbf{f}$ is not planar? In this case, $\mathbf{t}$ is also aligned with the joint axis $\mathbf{z} = z_0$, and its length τ is the length of the projection of $\mathbf{r} \times \mathbf{f}$ onto the joint axis (Fig. 9.9).
Thus,

$$\tau = (\mathbf{r} \times \mathbf{f})\mathbf{z} \tag{9.19}$$

and

$$\mathbf{t} = ((\mathbf{r} \times \mathbf{f})\mathbf{z})\mathbf{z}. \tag{9.20}$$

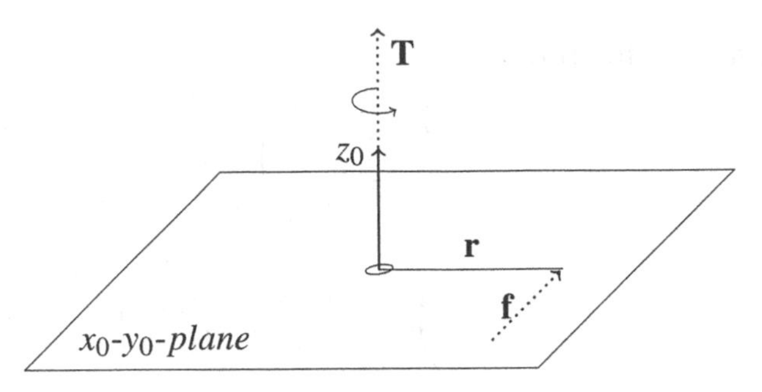

Fig. 9.8: Joint torque

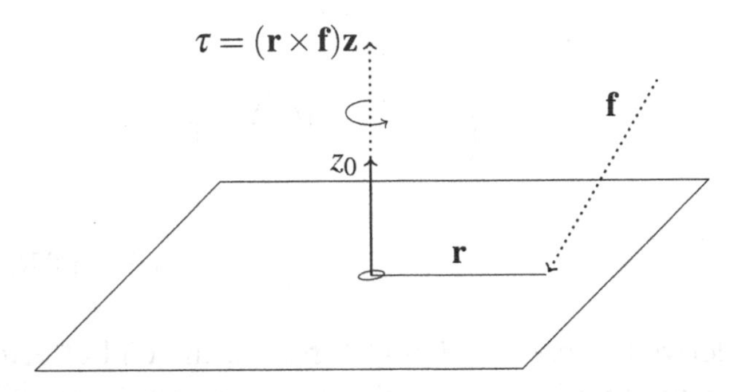

Fig. 9.9: Non-planar force

In Eq. 9.10 we set up a matrix relating the force **f** to the joint torques τ_1 and τ_2, for the planar two-link manipulator.
In the following theorem, we will do the same for the general case of n revolute joints and three-dimensional forces.

Theorem 9.1

We consider a robot with n revolute joints. Let **f** be a force vector, expressed in base coordinates. Let $\mathbf{p}_{i-1}$ be the origin of the coordinate system for joint i. Likewise, $\mathbf{z}_{i-1}$ is the **z**-vector of this coordinate system. Then the torques $\tau_1, \ldots, \tau_n$ induced by **f** at the n joints are given by

$$\begin{pmatrix} \tau_1 \\ \vdots \\ \tau_n \end{pmatrix} = \begin{pmatrix} \mathbf{z}_0 \times (\mathbf{p}_n - \mathbf{p}_0) \\ \vdots \\ \mathbf{z}_{n-1} \times (\mathbf{p}_n - \mathbf{p}_{n-1}) \end{pmatrix} \cdot \mathbf{f} \tag{9.21}$$

Proof:

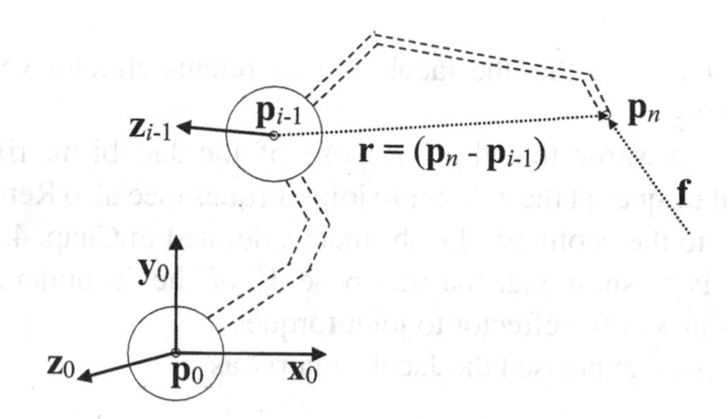

Fig. 9.10: Proof of Theorem 9.1

We must show that

$$\tau_i = [\mathbf{z}_{i-1} \times (\mathbf{p}_n - \mathbf{p}_{i-1})]\mathbf{f}. \tag{9.22}$$

According to our definition in Eq. 9.19, we have $\tau = (\mathbf{r} \times \mathbf{f})\mathbf{z}$. Then $(\mathbf{p}_n - \mathbf{p}_{i-1})$ takes the role of $\mathbf{r}$, and $\mathbf{z}_{i-1}$ takes the role of $\mathbf{z}$.
Thus

$$\tau_i = [(\mathbf{p}_n - \mathbf{p}_{i-1}) \times \mathbf{f}]\mathbf{z}_{i-1}. \tag{9.23}$$

But now,

$$\tau_i = \mathbf{z}_{i-1}[(\mathbf{p}_n - \mathbf{p}_{i-1}) \times \mathbf{f}]. \tag{9.24}$$

For arbitrary 3-vectors **a**, **b**, **c** we have

$$\mathbf{a}(\mathbf{b} \times \mathbf{c}) = (\mathbf{a} \times \mathbf{b})\mathbf{c}. \tag{9.25}$$

We apply this to Eq. 9.24 and obtain:

$$\tau_i = [\mathbf{z}_{i-1} \times (\mathbf{p}_n - \mathbf{p}_{i-1})]\mathbf{f} \tag{9.26}$$

(End of proof)

Remark 9.3

In Chap. 4 we saw that the Jacobi-matrix relates effector velocity to joint velocity.
We will now show that the transpose of the Jacobi-matrix relates forces and torques at the effector to joint torques (see also Remark 9.1).
We return to the geometric Jacobi-matrix defined in Chap. 4.
Our goal is to show that the transpose $\mathbf{J}^{\mathrm{T}}$ of the Jacobian $\mathbf{J}$ relates forces/torques at the effector to joint torques.
In Eq. 4.53 we expressed the Jacobi-matrix as

$$\mathbf{J} = \begin{pmatrix} \mathbf{J}_v \\ \mathbf{J}_\omega \end{pmatrix}, \tag{9.27}$$

where

$$\mathbf{J}_v = \begin{pmatrix} \mathbf{z}_0 \times (\mathbf{p}_n - \mathbf{p}_0) & \mathbf{z}_1 \times (\mathbf{p}_n - \mathbf{p}_1) & \dots & \mathbf{z}_{n-1} \times (\mathbf{p}_n - \mathbf{p}_{n-1}) \end{pmatrix}, \tag{9.28}$$

and

$$\mathbf{J}_\omega = \begin{pmatrix} \mathbf{z}_0 & \mathbf{z}_1 & \dots & \mathbf{z}_{n-1} \end{pmatrix}. \tag{9.29}$$

Thus

$$\mathbf{J}_v^{\mathrm{T}} = \begin{pmatrix} \mathbf{z}_0 \times (\mathbf{p}_n - \mathbf{p}_0) \\ \mathbf{z}_1 \times (\mathbf{p}_n - \mathbf{p}_1) \\ \vdots \\ \mathbf{z}_{n-1} \times (\mathbf{p}_n - \mathbf{p}_{n-1}) \end{pmatrix}. \tag{9.30}$$

Comparing this to Eq. 9.21 we see that indeed

$$\begin{pmatrix} \tau_1 \\ \vdots \\ \tau_n \end{pmatrix} = \begin{pmatrix} \mathbf{z}_0 \times (\mathbf{p}_n - \mathbf{p}_0) \\ \vdots \\ \mathbf{z}_{n-1} \times (\mathbf{p}_n - \mathbf{p}_{n-1}) \end{pmatrix} \cdot \mathbf{f} = \mathbf{J}_v^{\mathrm{T}} \mathbf{f}. \tag{9.31}$$

(End of Remark 9.3)

We can thus express the relationship between forces at the effector and torques at the joints by the transpose of the upper part of the geometric Jacobian. The following remark shows that the lower part $\mathbf{J}_\omega$ of the geometric Jacobian allows for computing joint torques from torques acting upon the effector.

Remark 9.4

We can not only apply a force to the effector, but we can also apply torque to the effector. Thus, we can induce joint torque in two different ways: (1) A force is applied to the effector. (2) A torque acts on the effector.
In case (1) we push the effector with a finger tip. In case (2) we grasp and twist the effector. Both cases result in joint torque.
Let $\mathbf{m} = (m_x, m_y, m_z)^{\mathrm{T}}$ be a torque, applied to the effector. Then the induced joint torque is

$$\mathbf{t} = (\mathbf{mz})\mathbf{z}. \tag{9.32}$$

The length of $\mathbf{t}$ is again the magnitude τ of the torque

$$\tau = \mathbf{mz}. \tag{9.33}$$

As a result of this definition, we obtain $\mathbf{t}$ as an orthogonal projection of the effector torque vector $\mathbf{m}$ onto $\mathbf{z} = z_0$ (see Fig. 9.11).
From Eq. 9.27 we see that

$$\mathbf{J}^{\mathrm{T}} = (\mathbf{J}_v^{\mathrm{T}}, \mathbf{J}_\omega^{\mathrm{T}}). \tag{9.34}$$

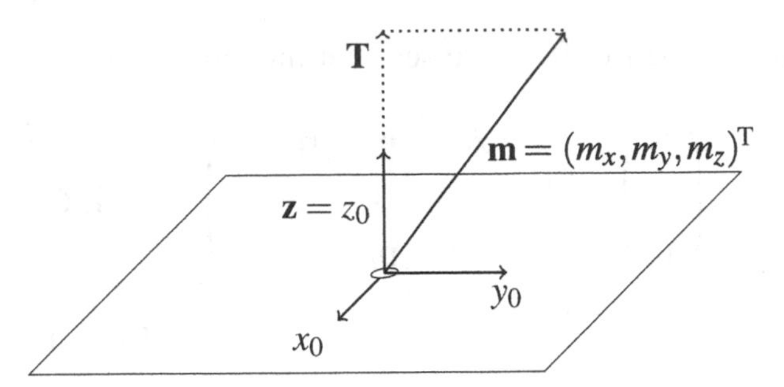

Fig. 9.11: Joint torque **T** resulting from an effector torque **m**

According to Eq. 9.29 we have

$$\mathbf{J}_{\omega}^{\mathrm{T}} = \begin{pmatrix} \mathbf{z}_0 \\ \vdots \\ \mathbf{z}_{n-1} \end{pmatrix}. \tag{9.35}$$

Now Eq. 9.33 shows that

$$\begin{pmatrix} \tau_1 \\ \vdots \\ \tau_n \end{pmatrix} = \mathbf{J}_{\omega}^{\mathrm{T}} \mathbf{m}. \tag{9.36}$$

We add the two types of joint torques according to Eqs. 9.21 and 9.36, and obtain

$$\begin{pmatrix} \tau_1 \\ \vdots \\ \tau_n \end{pmatrix} = \mathbf{J}^{\mathrm{T}} \begin{pmatrix} \mathbf{f} \\ \mathbf{m} \end{pmatrix}. \tag{9.37}$$

(End of Remark 9.4)

The geometric Jacobian **J** for arbitrary robots was defined in Chap. 4. With the result in Eq. 9.37, we can now compute the joint torques necessary for applying a given tool force. We also see how to find thresholds for joint torques, given limits for applicable forces and torques.

Example 9.1

Suppose we have a grid of unit vectors. We call these vectors $\mathbf{f}_1, \ldots, \mathbf{f}_n$. The vectors represent directions of forces, which we apply to the end effectors of a six-joint robot and a seven-joint robot (Chap. 3). We will apply the force vectors sequentially, and determine the maximum joint torques resulting from the forces $\mathbf{f}_i$.
Now assume we scale each vector $\mathbf{f}_i$ to a magnitude of 50 N. We saw that geometric Jacobians relate forces to joint torques. To compute the joint torques resulting from $\mathbf{f}_i$, we must set up the geometric Jacobians for both robots. Appendix C does just this, namely deriving the geometric Jacobians for the six- and seven-joint robots from Chap. 3. Joint torques are position-dependent. This means that they will vary with the joint settings of the robot. In the comparison, we can select corresponding positions for the two robots, or positions from a grid.

Table 9.1: Maximum joint torques (in Nm) for a force vector $\mathbf{f}$ of 50N acting at the effector. Positions of the effector ranging over a point grid in the work space, and directions of $\mathbf{f}$ defined as grid points on a hemisphere

Joint	Six-joint case	Seven-joint case
J1	38.42	31.33
J2	39.07	32.29
J3	22.45	19.35
J4	3.70	19.49
J5	3.70	7.99
J6	0	8.00
J7		0

Table 9.1 lists the maximum joint torques at each joint. We see that the torques at the last joint (joint six for the six-joint robot and joint seven for the seven-joint robot) are always zero. This is due to the orientation of the last joint, and to the fact that we do not apply torque to the effector. To allow for comparison, we adjusted the DH-parameters in such a way that the total arm length is the same for both robots (1251 mm). The DH-parameters are the same as in Table 3.3.

In practice, gear ratios should be as small as possible. For typical small-size and light-weight motors, the maximum motor torques range between 0.5 *Nm* and 1.2 *Nm*. Thus, from Table 9.1 we see that a gear ratio of 1:60 suffices for forces of up to 50 *N*, depending on the maximum motor torque.

(End of Example 9.1)

Exercises

Exercise 9.1

Extend the static force equation in Eq. 9.10 for the planar two-link manipulator to a planar three-link manipulator. Compare to the force equation obtained by transposing the Jacobian.

Exercise 9.2

Extend the result in Theorem 1 above to the case of prismatic joints, following the extended definition of the Jacobian in Chap. 4. Confirm your result in a small example.

Summary

Systems for motion replication allow for down-scaling motion in complex microsurgical applications. Four-arm systems (two master arms, and two replicator arms) passively replicate motion of the operating surgeon. The master arms are often light-weight arms driven by cables.
In addition to motion-scaling, tremor compensation is possible with motion replicators. To detect tremor, motions are recorded and analyzed by signal processing methods. Both wavelet decomposition and support vector methods can be applied in this context.

Time is a critical resource for most surgical interventions (due to the increase of hemorrhage, and the increase of infection risk with operating time). Thus the motion replication process should not increase operating time. Repetitive tasks can often be automatized. Thus, to save operating time, small sutures can be tied autonomously by the robot.

Realistic haptic and tactile feedback, as well as autonomous methods for repetitive tasks (such as suturing) are research topics in the context of motion replication systems. If the transformation between torques at joints and forces at the effector is known, we can give force feedback to the surgeon. The geometric Jacobian provides this force transformation through the equation:

$$\begin{pmatrix} \tau_1 \\ \vdots \\ \tau_n \end{pmatrix} = \mathbf{J}^{\mathrm{T}} \begin{pmatrix} \mathbf{f} \\ \mathbf{m} \end{pmatrix}.$$

where $\tau_1, \ldots, \tau_n$ denote the joint torques, and $\mathbf{f}$ and $\mathbf{m}$ are the forces and moments acting at the effector.

Notes

Equation 9.37 is the main equation of the chapter. We saw that it follows directly from the scalar triple product equation $\mathbf{a}(\mathbf{b} \times \mathbf{c}) = (\mathbf{a} \times \mathbf{b})\mathbf{c}$. In [2], Eq. 9.37 is proven via the concept of *virtual work* (see also [6]).

Robotic motion replicator systems for surgery are in routine clinical use for prostate surgery and cardiac surgery since 2002 [1]. During the first year following regulatory clearance, more than 5000 operations were performed [4]. The number and type of surgical applications are expanding very rapidly. Early methods for motion scaling were described in [8]. While the original system (da Vinci system, Intuitive Surgical, Sunnyvale, USA) uses no force feedback (tools are disposable, which presents a difficulty towards integrating complex force sensing), several methods for including such feedback have been described in the literature (see [4] for a survey).

Active tremor compensation for microsurgery has been addressed in a number of contributions (see [5] for a survey). Beyond the context of motion replication, tremor compensation can be applied to typical hand-held surgical instruments as well [7].
To reduce operating time, new generations of instruments, specifically designed for motion replicator systems, were introduced [3].

References

[1] R. J. Cerfolio, A. S. Bryant, L. Skylizard, and D. J. Minnich. Initial consecutive experience of completely portal robotic pulmonary resection with 4 arms. *The Journal of Thoracic and Cardiovascular Surgery*, **142**(4):740–746, 2011. DOI 10.1016/j.jtcvs.2011.07.022.
[2] J. J. Craig. *Introduction to Robotics: Mechanics and Control.* Prentice Hall, 3rd edition, 2005.
[3] G.-P. Haber, M. A. White, R. Autorino, P. F. Escobar, M. D. Kroh, S. Chalikonda, R. Khanna, S. Forest, B. Yang, F. Altunrende, R. J. Stein, and J. H. Kaouk. Novel robotic da Vinci instruments for laparoendoscopic single-site surgery. *Urology*, **76**(6):1279–1282, 2010. DOI 10.1016/j.urology.2010.06.070.
[4] A. M. Okamura. Methods for haptic feedback in teleoperated robot-assisted surgery. *Industrial Robot: An International Journal*, **31**(6):499–508, 2004. DOI 10.1108/01439910410566362.
[5] C. N. Riviere, W.-T. Ang, and P. K. Khosla. Toward active tremor canceling in handheld microsurgical instruments. *IEEE Transactions on Robotics and Automation*, **19**(5):793–800, 2003. DOI 10.1109/tra.2003.817506.
[6] M. W. Spong, S. Hutchinson, and M. Vidyasagar. *Robot Modeling and Control*. John Wiley & Sons, Inc., New York, 1st edition, 2005.

[7] K. C. Veluvolu and W. T. Ang. Estimation and filtering of physiological tremor for real-time compensation in surgical robotics applications. *The International Journal of Medical Robotics and Computer Assisted Surgery*, **6**(3):334–342, 2010. DOI 10.1002/rcs.340.

[8] J. Yan and S. E. Salcudean. Teleoperation controller design using h_∞-optimization with application to motion-scaling. *IEEE Transactions on Control Systems Technology*, **4**(3):244–258, 1996. DOI 10.1109/87.491198.

Chapter 10
Applications of Surgical Robotics

In Chap. 1, we described several applications for surgical robotics. Having discussed the building blocks for such systems in the preceding chapters, we will now return to the applications. In many cases, robotic systems were developed to improve existing surgical procedures, and not for new types of interventions. Thus, we must adapt robotic systems to the needs of the application, to bring out the benefits. For the sample applications considered here (radiosurgery, orthopedic surgery, cardiac surgery, urologic surgery, neurosurgery and neurology) we give some additional background.

10.1 Radiosurgery

In 1949, Lars Leksell constructed a metal frame to rigidly fix a patient's head in space [15]. The frame is directly bolted to the skull bone under local anesthesia. With this frame, Leksell was able to irradiate targets in the head with very high precision. The term stereotaxic radiosurgery was then introduced to describe this new method.
With the advent of tomography, a first full method for navigation was developed. Similar to stereotaxic navigation in neurosurgery, it consists of the following steps (see Fig. 1.14):

Step 1. The frame is attached to the patient's skull.

Step 2. Tomographic images are taken (CT or MR image data with 30–50 slices).

A. Schweikard, F. Ernst, *Medical Robotics*,
DOI 10.1007/978-3-319-22891-4_10

Step 3. The relative position of the tumor with respect to the frame coordinates is calculated from the tomography.

Step 4. The frame base remains attached to the patient's head, and is additionally attached to the irradiation device.

Step 5. With the double attachment from step 4, we find the exact spatial reference. The patient couch is repositioned such that the target is centered at the isocenter of the treatment beams (typically beams of photon radiation).

Step 6. Treatment

There are two types of radiosurgical systems:

- static beam systems (GammaKnife)
- moving beam systems (LINAC systems, Fig. 10.1)

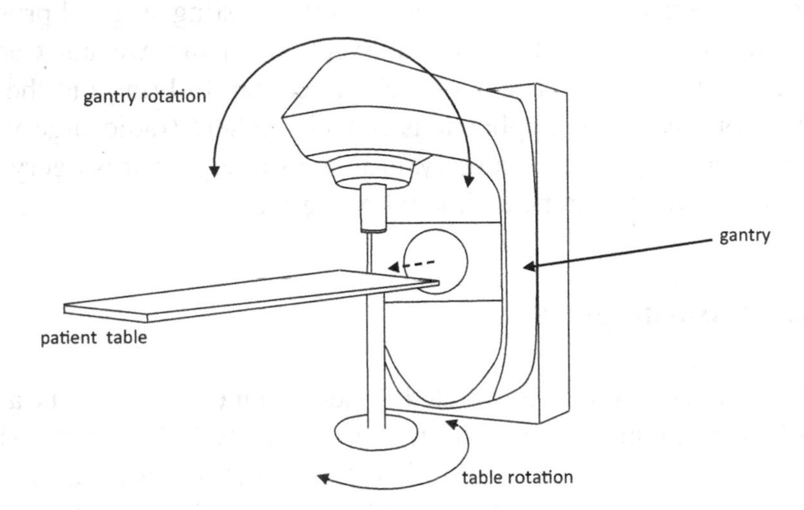

Fig. 10.1: Five-joint kinematics for a LINAC radiosurgery system. The dashed arrow shows the axis of the gantry rotation. The patient couch has three built-in translation axes

For the first type (Gamma Knife), beams are placed in a helmet, and do not move during treatment. Thus the frame is attached to the patient's head, and also to the treatment couch. We thus have a static spatial relationship between target and the radiation source(s). By contrast, LINAC systems move the radiation beam along circular arcs in

space, while the target is at the center of rotation. By moving the patient couch, different angles can be reached. Initially, radiosurgery was limited to the head, due to organ motion in the chest or abdomen.
Robotic radiosurgery with a six-joint robot was introduced in 1995 to obviate the need for attaching a head frame, and to obtain more kinematic flexibility for beam motion paths [1]. Inverse treatment planning with linear programming (see Chap. 6) computes beam directions and beam weights [19]. Planning for multi-leaf collimators is different when compared to planning for cylinder collimators, but the general principles are similar: beam directions for the multi-leaf collimator are chosen in the same way as for cylindrical collimators. It is then necessary to partition the cross-section of each beam into smaller subsections to protect critical tissue in the vicinity of the target. As for the case of beam selection, this is done by a randomized search. Random geometric sub-patterns for beam cross-sections are generated, and a large set of 'beam-lets' thus chosen is submitted to linear programming for weight computation. In the weighting step, a large number of sub-patterns will receive weight zero. Such patterns are removed, so that a re-sampling scheme is obtained for inverse planning [22]. The registration procedure relies on stereo X-ray imaging and digitally reconstructed radiographs (DRRs) (see Chap. 5). Thus, no frame is needed. An on-line position correction is performed after periodic X-ray imaging.
Respiratory motion compensation (based on motion correlation) was then added to existing robotic radiosurgery systems [20]. This procedure is called stereotaxic body radiosurgery (SBRS). Fast-lane methods for motion prediction improve the accuracy of motion tracking in the chest and abdomen. For correlation-based tracking, 1–5 gold markers are implanted near the target. Marker-less treatment for lung tumors uses the following procedure for image registration: Digitally reconstructed radiographs are matched to live images (stereo X-ray image pairs). The X-ray images of the target region are partitioned into small patches. Typically, a 5×5 array of patches is used. Registration match coefficients based on cross-correlation are evaluated for each pair of patches. Pairs of patches giving poor matches are discarded, while small adjustments of relative patch positions are permitted. We can

thus address small deformations between CT image acquisition and treatment.
Before the introduction of SBRS, there was the implicit assumption that respiratory motion in the pancreas is negligible. However, it turned out that there is substantial respiratory motion in this case as well. This observation led to new clinical developments, amongst them stereotaxic procedures for renal tumors, and modifications to standard protocols for liver tumors, lung tumors and prostate tumors. Since then, real-time imaging and tracking have much improved, and are now in routine clinical use.

10.2 Orthopedic Surgery

An early robotic system is the Robodoc system described in [25]. The system burs the implant cavity for hip replacement surgery (Fig. 10.2). In this case, the registration procedure is stereotaxic. Thus, the bone must be attached rigidly to the patient couch, while the position of the couch with respect to the robot remains fixed. The cavity is burred by the robot without user interaction.

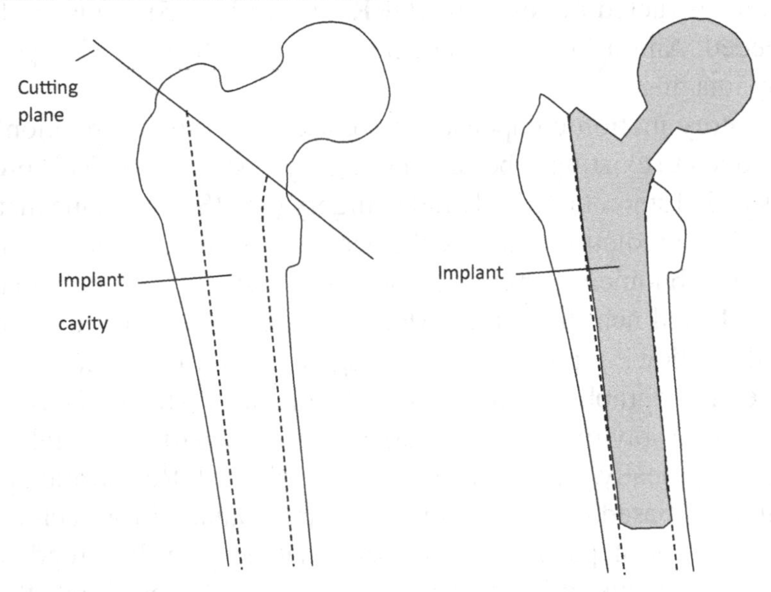

Fig. 10.2: Total hip replacement surgery

Knee replacement is now the most common robotic intervention in orthopedic surgery. In conventional knee replacement surgery, the surface of the knee joint is removed with a surgical saw (Fig. 10.3). Typically, three to five cuts are made along different angles for the distal femur. Likewise, a single cut is made on the proximal tibia head. A recent development obviates the need for rigid bone fixation during robotic knee surgery, and allows for improved user interaction [3, 12]. It is also possible to replace only parts of the knee surface (Fig. 10.4). The distal end of the femur bone consists of two condyles. In conventional knee replacement, the entire end of the femur is replaced (see Fig. 10.3). However, if only a single condyle is damaged, then it is of advantage to replace only this condyle. This unicondylar implant should be manufactured to fit the individual anatomy (Fig. 10.4).

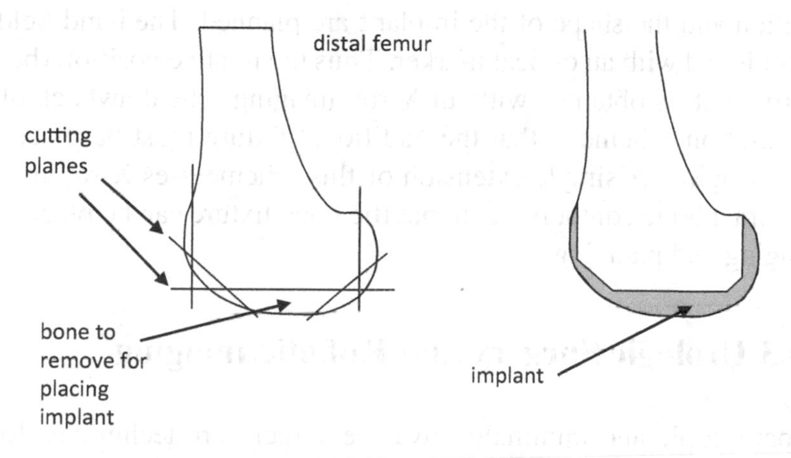

Fig. 10.3: Cutting planes for knee replacement surgery

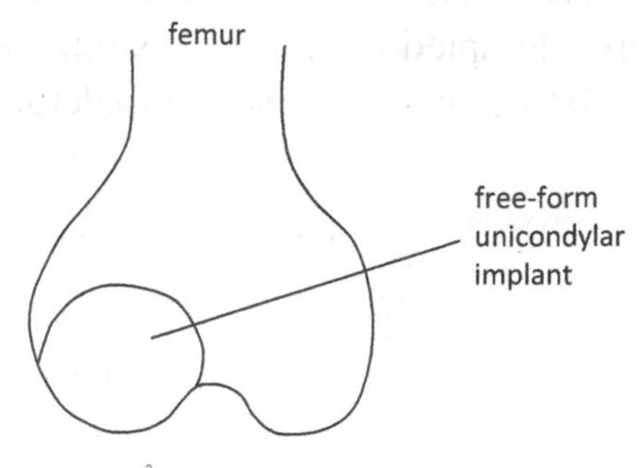

Fig. 10.4: Femur condyles and free-form implant

Placing such free-form implants requires improved navigation and tools for planning the implant shape and position [12]. Thus, an implant shape is planned before treatment, taking into account biomechanical constraints, while allowing for small posture corrections. The intervention now proceeds as follows: a surgical bur ablates bony tissue from the surface. The navigation is semi-active, i.e. the surgeon performs the actual burring. With the shape of the implant matching allowed motions for the bur, the robot creates a so-called virtual wall for guiding the surgery. The registration is based on optical tracking. A fixture for holding an optical marker is attached to the bone in a separate procedure before tomographic imaging. The position of the bone relative to this attached marker is known and will remain fixed throughout the entire treatment, although the bone itself is free to move. After extracting the bone surface from a CT image, the intervention and the shape of the implant are planned. The hand-held bur is equipped with an optical marker. Thus the relative position (bone to instrument) is obtained without X-ray imaging. The drawback of this registration scheme is that the additional fixture must be placed before imaging. A simple extension of this scheme uses X-ray imaging to extract bone contours, such that the bone fixture can be placed after imaging and planning.

10.3 Urologic Surgery and Robotic Imaging

Laparoscopic and minimally invasive surgery are techniques for reducing recovery time and surgical trauma. Both techniques were developed in the 1980s. Soon after the introduction of laparoscopic surgery, researchers attempted to replace instrument holders, laparoscopes and camera fixtures by actuated manipulators [13].

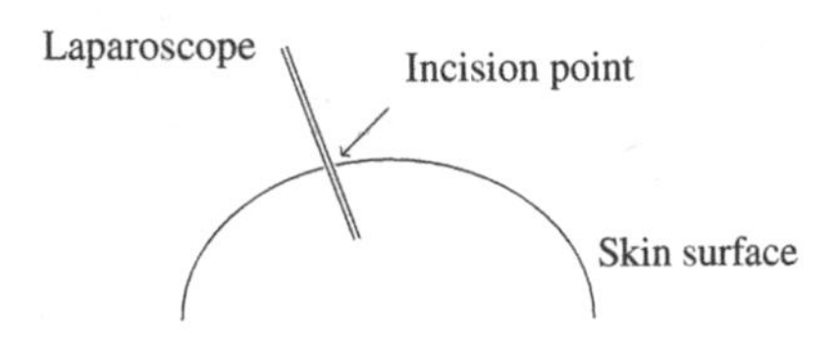

Fig. 10.5: Laparoscopy: reversal of motion direction at the skin incision point

The da Vinci system [8] was designed for robotic telesurgery, partly to address shortcomings of laparoscopic surgery. The laparoscope is a long instrument inserted into a small skin incision. The incision point constrains the possible motion of the laparoscope. In addition to constraining the motion, user interaction and visualization is not intuitive. Thus, the incision point is a pivot point, and a leftward motion of the upper end of the laparoscope results in a rightward motion of the lower end (Fig. 10.5). By contrast, a robotic system can produce a reversal-free mapping of motion directions and a more intuitive user interface.

The da Vinci system consists of two units: a control unit (console), operated by the surgeon, and a patient side cart. The console unit consists of a screen display, two passive serial link arms, the surgeon user interface and the controller system. The patient side cart comprises a manipulator arm for moving the endoscope, two robotic motion replicator arms (tool manipulators), as well as an additional user interface for a surgical assistant.

The passive arms are equipped with grippers and can thus transmit grip commands to the replicator arms. The screen display projects a virtual image plane over the motion range of the passive arms. In this display, the current position of the two replicator arms is visible, so that both arms can be moved under direct control of the surgeon. Additional means are provided to move the endoscope from the control unit. Several different instruments (scalpels, grippers) can be attached to the replicator arms, and act as end effectors. The range of operations now performed with the da Vinci system is not limited to urologic surgery, but also includes a wide variety of other applications, e.g. colorectal surgery, hysterectomy, appendectomy and hernia repair.

Robotic C-arms are now in clinical use. Three different concepts have been proposed: (1) The joints of a conventional C-arm are actuated. Here the four-joint version from Chap. 3 is used. (2) The source and the detector are mounted to two separate six-joint robots. (3) The C-shaped source-detector assembly is mounted to a single large robot [24].

10.4 Cardiac Surgery

Atrial fibrillation is a condition characterized by irregular conduction of electrical impulses in the heart. A surgical treatment of this condition is the so-called Maze procedure [4]. Cuts in the heart wall and the resulting scars can block the irregular flow of current (Fig. 10.6). The cuts are produced with a catheter, guided by external imaging. Catheter steering can be improved by an external robotic arm, similar to the da Vinci procedure [18]. An alternative to this procedure is proposed in [23]. Here, external robotic radiosurgery produces the scars, along the paths indicated by the dashed lines in Fig. 10.6. Active motion compensation is needed to address cardiac and respiratory motion. The advantage is that no catheter is required, which shortens treatment time.

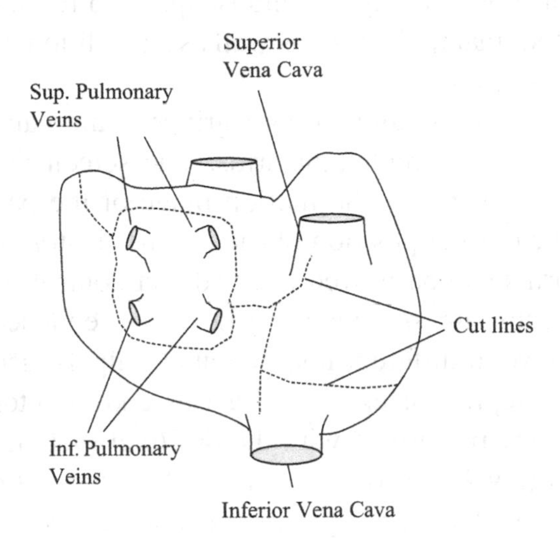

Fig. 10.6: Maze procedure for treating atrial fibrillation

10.5 Neurosurgery

We saw that precise localization of the head is a main element of neurosurgical procedures. Two methods for localization were described above: stereotaxic fixation and X-ray image guidance. Both methods are in routine clinical use.

X-ray guidance directly tracks the bony skull. However, taking continuous X-ray images for frame-less treatment is not always possible. To address this problem, near-infrared methods have been developed [6]. We project a thin laser beam onto the skin surface of the forehead. By analyzing the laser spot on the skin with high resolution cameras, we determine the skin thickness at this point. Repeating this for a large number of points, we obtain an estimate for the skull position via ICP registration (see Chap. 5).
Furthermore, robotic methods can improve the localization in the following ways [10]: The needle is carried by a jointed mechanism, and the joints can be equipped with motors and position sensors. Force sensing can detect forces acting on the needle. In this way it becomes possible to control needle insertion with higher precision and repeatability. Force measurements and tomographic data provide position information for the needle tip.

10.6 Control Modes

Above we have listed exemplary fields of application. We can derive five motion control modes from these examples.

1. Stereotaxic: The anatomy is rigidly fixed, and the robot moves along a pre-planned trajectory during the intervention. Stereotaxis is mostly used in radiosurgery for the head and neck and in neurosurgery.

2. Image-guided with intermittent imaging: An example for this control mode is frame-less radiosurgery. The patient's head is free to move, or only lightly immobilized with a head rest or a head mask. Imaging is used to check for correct alignment at fixed time intervals. The robot adjusts the position of the instrument in case of misalignment beyond a fixed threshold.

3. Motion compensation/predictive motion compensation: Respiratory and/or cardiac motion is determined by appropriate sensors. A robot moving a surgical instrument autonomously tracks this

motion. To overcome latencies, motion prediction for fixed time lags is used. Predictive motion compensation is used for radiosurgical targets in the chest and abdomen.

4. Virtual wall: In a planning phase, the shape of tissue to be removed is determined. During surgery, the surgeon moves a passive arm holding the instrument. The arm restricts the motion of the instrument such that the shape of the tissue area to be removed matches the planned shape. Markers attached to the target allow for tracking any relative motion of the target. This method is most frequently used in orthopedic surgery.

5. Motion replication: As in mode four, the surgeon moves a passive robot arm. The motion is replicated by a second (often smaller) arm. This allows for motion scaling and high precision surgery. Two-arm or multiple-arm kinematics are used. Typical areas of application are urology and cardiac surgery.

The control modes can be combined with one another to provide advantages for specific applications.
There is one more control mode, not yet in clinical use, but desirable in some applications. In this control mode, the robot acts autonomously, based on real-time imaging. We sketch a potential application for this autonomous control mode in neurosurgery. Neurosurgeons describe one of the difficulties in surgery as follows: 'Protect a wet noodle embedded in concrete, while removing the concrete around it'. Here the wet noodle is a healthy structure (e.g. the optic nerve), whereas the concrete is the tumor. Clearly, it would be helpful to be able to see into the tissue by some small distance (1–2 mm) during surgery. Several new image modalities can address this problem, such that we can obtain an in situ endoscopic image [17]. If it was possible to classify healthy cells versus tumor cells in such modalities, and if an appropriate robotic instrument was available, the following method for robotic tumor removal with minimal user interaction would become realistic: Via a small skin incision or opening, we approach the target. The instrument and the endoscopic camera are mounted to a snake-robot. Having reached the target, we step through the cell array in the vicinity of the target, where small regions are classified by

imaging. Tumor cells are removed step by step, while the instrument plans a path around healthy cells. The control mode for this scheme is more autonomous than the above scheme and is based on real-time endoscopic imaging.

Summary

Five motion control paradigms for surgical robots were introduced in the past two decades. The control paradigms are: stereotaxic, image-guided, motion compensated, virtual-wall guidance and motion replication. The control paradigms were designed to improve the accuracy of the surgical intervention, and to facilitate navigation. Each paradigm has a specific area of application. The main areas are: orthopedic surgery, radiosurgery, urologic surgery and minimally invasive surgery, cardiovascular surgery and neurosurgery. However, some of the paradigms have recently been applied outside their original area of application, and it is likely that other, new motion control paradigms and new areas of application will arise.

Notes

A survey of early methods in robotic surgery is given in [16]. The first robotic systems for neurosurgery were introduced in 1985 [13, 14]. Here, a biopsy needle for brain tumors was inserted under robot guidance. The Probot system was designed for transurethral resection of the prostate [9], and introduced in 1997. Positioning an endoscope during surgery with a robotic arm was described in [11], and the underlying system (AESOP) can be considered a predecessor of the da Vinci system. This positioning system was later used in the development of the Zeus system [7], in the context of a telesurgery paradigm similar to the da Vinci system. The CyberKnife system was originally developed to provide frameless radiosurgery in the head [2]. It included an inverse planning system based on linear programming, and first patients were treated with the system in 1994. It was later extended to incorporate full body radiosurgery and robotic motion compensation [21]. Recently, other radiosurgical systems were equipped with respiration tracking based on correlation and prediction, so that robotic methods are now available for conventional radiation therapy as well [5].

References

[1] J. R. Adler, Jr., A. Schweikard, R. Tombropoulos, and J.-C. Latombe. Image-Guided Robotic Radiosurgery, pages 460–470 in H. Bunke, T. Kanade, and H. Noltemeier, editors, *Modelling and Planning for Sensor-based Intelligent Robot Systems*, volume 21 of *Series in Machine Perception and Artificial Intelligence*. World Scientific Publishers Co., 1995. DOI 10.1142/9789812797773_0028.

[2] J. R. J. Adler, M. J. Murphy, S. D. Chang, and S. L. Hancock. Image-guided robotic radiosurgery. *Neurosurgery*, **6**(44): 1299–1306, 1999.

[3] G. Brisson, T. Kanade, A. DiGioia, and B. Jaramaz. Precision freehand sculpting of bone. In C. Barillot, D. R. Haynor, and P. Hellier, editors, *MICCAI 2004, Part II*, Rennes & Saint-Malo, France. MICCAI, Springer. Published in *Lecture Notes in Computer Science*, **3217**:105–112, 2004. DOI 10.1007/978-3-540-30136-3_14.

[4] J. L. Cox, R. B. Schuessler, H. D'Agostino, Jr, C. M. Stone, B. C. Chang, M. E. Cain, P. B. Corr, and J. P. Boineau. The surgical treatment of atrial fibrillation. III. development of a definitive surgical procedure. *Journal of Thoracic and Cardiovascular Surgery*, **101**(4):569–583, 1991.

[5] T. Depuydt, K. Poels, D. Verellen, B. Engels, C. Collen, C. Haverbeke, T. Gevaert, N. Buls, G. van Gompel, T. Reynders, M. Duchateau, K. Tournel, M. Boussaer, F. Steenbeke, F. Vandenbroucke, and M. de Ridder. Initial assessment of tumor tracking with a gimbaled linac system in clinical circumstances: a patient simulation study. *Radiotherapy and Oncology*, **106**(2): 236–240, 2013. DOI 10.1016/j.radonc.2012.12.015.

[6] F. Ernst, R. Bruder, T. Wissel, P. Stüber, B. Wagner, and A. Schweikard. Real time contact-free and non-invasive tracking of the human skull—first light and initial validation. In *Applications of Digital Image Processing XXXVI*. Published in *Proceedings of SPIE*, **8856**:88561G–1 – 88561G–8, 2013. DOI 10.1117/12.2024851.

[7] M. Ghodoussi, S. E. Butner, and Y. Wang. Robotic surgery - the transatlantic case. In *Proceedings of the IEEE International Conference on Robotics and Automation, 2002 (ICRA '02)*, 2002, pages 1882–1888. DOI 10.1109/robot.2002.1014815.

[8] G. S. Guthart and J. Salisbury, J. The Intuitive^{TM} telesurgery system: overview and application. In *Proceedings of the IEEE International Conference on Robotics and Automation, 2000. (ICRA '00)*, 2000, pages 618–621. DOI 10.1109/robot.2000.844121.

[9] S. J. Harris, F. Arambula-Cosio, Q. Mei, R. D. Hibberd, B. L. Davies, J. E. Wickham, M. S. Nathan, and B. Kundu. The Probot—an active robot for prostate resection. *Proceedings of the Institution of Mechanical Engineers, Part H: Journal of Engineering in Medicine*, **211**(4):317–325, 1997.

[10] M. Heinig, M. F. Govela, F. Gasca, C. Dold, U. G. Hofmann, V. Tronnier, A. Schlaefer, and A. Schweikard. Mars - motor assisted robotic stereotaxy system. In *Proceedings of the 5th International IEEE EMBS Conference on Neural Engineering*, 2011, pages 334–337.

[11] L. K. Jacobs, V. Shayani, and J. M. Sackier. Determination of the learning curve of the AESOP robot. *Surgical Endoscopy*, **11**(1): 54–55, 1997. DOI 10.1007/s004649900294.

[12] B. Jaramaz and C. Nikou. Precision freehand sculpting for unicondylar knee replacement: design and experimental validation. *Biomedizinische Technik (Biomedical Engineering)*, **57**(4): 293–299, 2012. DOI 10.1515/bmt-2011-0098.

[13] Y. S. Kwoh, J. Hou, E. A. Jonckheere, and S. Hayati. A robot with improved absolute positioning accuracy for CT guided stereotactic brain surgery. *IEEE Transactions on Biomedical Engineering*, **35**(2):153–160, 1988. DOI 10.1109/10.1354.

[14] S. Lavallee, J. Troccaz, L. Gaborit, P. Cinquin, A. L. Benabid, and D. Hoffmann. Image guided operating robot: a clinical application in stereotactic neurosurgery. In *Proceedings of the IEEE International Conference on Robotics and Automation, 1992. (ICRA'92)*, 1992, pages 618–624. DOI 10.1109/robot.1992.220223.

[15] L. Leksell. A stereotaxic apparatus for intracerebral surgery. *Acta Chirurgica Scandinavica*, **99**:229–233, 1949.

[16] M. J. H. Lum, D. C. W. Friedman, G. Sankaranarayanan, H. King, K. Fodero, R. Leuschke, B. Hannaford, J. Rosen, and M. N. Sinanan. The RAVEN: Design and validation of a telesurgery system. *The International Journal of Robotics Research*, **28** (9):1183–1197, 2009. DOI 10.1177/0278364909101795.

[17] C. Otte, G. Hüttmann, G. Kovács, and A. Schlaefer. Phantom validation of optical soft tissue navigation for brachytherapy. In W. Birkfellner, J. R. McClelland, S. Rit, and A. Schlaefer, editors, *MICCAI Workshop on Image-Guidance and Multimodal Dose Planning in Radiation Therapy*. MICCAI, 2012, pages 96–100.

[18] C. V. Riga, A. Rolls, R. Rippel, C. Shah, M. Hamady, C. Bicknell, and N. Cheshire. Advantages and limitations of robotic endovascular catheters for carotid artery stenting. *Journal of Cardiovascular Surgery*, **53**(6):747–753, 2012.

[19] A. Schweikard, M. Bodduluri, R. Tombropoulos, and J. R. Adler, Jr. Planning, calibration and collision-avoidance for image-guided radiosurgery. In *Proceedings of the IEEE/RSJ/GI International Conference on Intelligent Robots and Systems (IROS'94)*, 1994, pages 854–861. DOI 10.1109/iros.1994.407492.

[20] A. Schweikard, G. Glosser, M. Bodduluri, M. J. Murphy, and J. R. Adler, Jr. Robotic Motion Compensation for Respiratory Movement during Radiosurgery. *Journal of Computer-Aided Surgery*, **5**(4):263–277, 2000. DOI 10.3109/10929080009148894.

[21] A. Schweikard, H. Shiomi, and J. R. Adler, Jr. Respiration tracking in radiosurgery. *Medical Physics*, **31**(10):2738–2741, 2004. DOI 10.1118/1.1774132.

[22] A. Schweikard, A. Schlaefer, and J. R. Adler, Jr. Resampling: An optimization method for inverse planning in robotic radiosurgery. *Medical Physics*, **33**(11):4005–4011, 2006. DOI 10.1118/1.2357020.

[23] A. Sharma, D. Wong, G. Weidlich, T. Fogarty, A. Jack, T. Sumanaweera, and P. Maguire. Noninvasive stereotactic radiosurgery (CyberHeart) for creation of ablation lesions in the atrium. *Heart Rhythm*, **7**(6):802–810, 2010. DOI 10.1016/j.hrthm.2010.02.010.

[24] N. Strobel, O. Meissner, J. Boese, T. Brunner, B. Heigl, M. Hoheisel, G. Lauritsch, M. Nagel, M. Pfister, E.-P. Röhrnschopf, B. Scholz, B. Schreiber, M. Spahn, M. Zellerhoff, and K. Klingenbeck-Regn. 3D imaging with flat-detector C-arm systems. In M. F. Reiser, C. R. Becker, K. Nikolaou, and G. Glazer, editors, *Multislice CT*, Medical Radiology, pages 33–51. Springer Berlin Heidelberg, 2009. DOI 10.1007/978-3-540-33125-4_3.

[25] R. H. Taylor, L. Joskowicz, B. Williamson, A. Guéziec, A. Kalvin, P. Kazanzides, R. V. Vorhis, J. Yao, R. Kumar, A. Bzostek, A. Sahay, M. Börner, and A. Lahmer. Computer-integrated revision total hip replacement surgery: concept and preliminary results. *Medical Image Analysis*, **3**(3):301–319, 1999. DOI 10.1016/s1361-8415(99)80026-7.

Chapter 11
Rehabilitation, Neuroprosthetics and Brain-Machine Interfaces

Most stroke patients need rehabilitation training and physiotherapy. For example, it is possible that a stroke patient can move the left, but not the right hand. Then a very simple training device can help. This device is a tendon-driven hand support, controlled via two commands: grasp and release. The patient can switch between the two states with the healthy hand, and then learn simple tasks requiring both hands. Frequent use of the device in daily routine can improve the results of physiotherapy, e.g. strengthen the right arm, and even help the right hand. An improved version of this device offers more commands, i.e. moving the index finger, so that the patient can type on a keyboard or dial phone numbers.
But there is an even simpler application in this context: passive finger motion can help in the rehabilitation process. Thus, actuators move the fingers of the patient in pre-defined patterns.

11.1 Rehabilitation for Limbs

As an example for robotics in rehabilitation, the end-effector of a small robot arm (typically a three-joint robot) is connected to the fore-arm of the patient. The robot guides the motion of the patient's arm, and force/torque sensors record data. During training, the robot first moves to a pre-defined position. At this position, the patient is asked

A. Schweikard, F. Ernst, *Medical Robotics*,
DOI 10.1007/978-3-319-22891-4_11

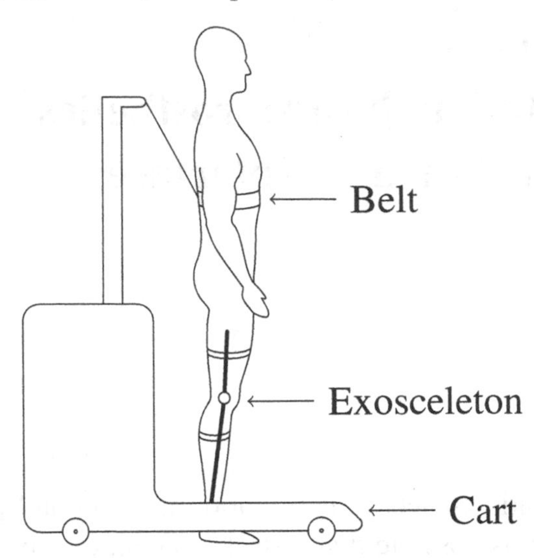

Fig. 11.1: Exoskeleton and mobile cart for gait training

to apply a force or torque. The process is then repeated for a series of different arm positions. We can add a computer screen to this set-up. On the screen, the patient's arm motions are replicated by motions of a cursor. In this case, the robot arm is passive. The patient can now steer a point on the screen while solving small animated puzzles generated by the interface [9, 14].

Likewise, an exoskeleton can be attached at several points along the arm. Both principles (end-effector or exoskeleton) have their advantages with respect to cost and flexibility [3, 11].

A device for leg rehabilitation is shown in Fig. 11.1. The patient's upper body is held by a mobile platform with wheels. The platform can follow the patient. An exoskeleton generates motion patterns for the legs. The device shown in the figure is limited to walking patterns on even floors. For uneven terrains and stairs, the platforms must be equipped with additional sensors and actuators [15, 16].

11.2 Brain-Machine Interfaces

A cochlea implant consists of a small microphone with a signal processing unit. The signal processing unit collects external auditory signals, and stimulates the patient's auditory nerve. Auditory brainstem implants use the same technology as cochlea implants, but directly stimulate the brain stem of the patient. Cochlea implants are in routine use, and demonstrate the potential of brain-machine interfaces.
In general, a brain-machine interface (BMI) records signals from the brain to control external actuators. However, for most applications, the control of external devices alone is not sufficient, and 'upstream' sensory feedback is needed. Four types of BMIs can be distinguished:

- electrodes
- electromyography (EMG)
- spectroscopy
- imaging

For electrodes, several invasive and non-invasive methods have been investigated. The earliest (and one of the least invasive) of such methods is EEG (electro-encephalography). The EEG signal arises from the joint activity of millions of neurons close to the brain surface. It is acquired on the scalp surface by macroscopic electrodes. EEG signals are in the frequency range of DC to 200 Hz with an amplitude of some 10 μV pp. EEG measurements from up to 64 points on the scalp are the standard in neurological diagnostics. The main tool for EEG analysis is visual inspection by the neurologist. To the untrained eye, the signal looks like noise. Nonetheless, some of the typical signals can be used in brain-machine interfaces. One of the most robust signal stems from the so-called 'readiness-potential': some hundred milliseconds before the onset of a typical bodily action, the potential of both brain hemispheres differs by a measureable amount. Likewise, the content within certain frequency bands changes in response to internal or external events. This so called 'Event Related Desynchronization/Synchronization' (ERDS) or micro-Rhythm Modulation can often be recognized by signal processing and machine learning methods. Another recognizable signal stems from the motor cortex as a result of imaginary movements ('Motor Imaginary Paradigm'). It is possible to replace the electrical recordings by near-infrared monitoring of the surface brain tissue, and thereby measure hemodynamic processes. Although EEG-based brain-machine interfaces suffer from a number of shortcomings (low signal bandwidth, low information transfer rates, high response times and low specificity), they have an established place as a communication channel for patients with the locked-in syndrome (patients unable to even move their eyes).

A	B	C	D	E	F
G	**H**	**I**	**J**	**K**	**L**
M	N	O	P	Q	R
S	T	U	V	W	X
Y	Z	1	2	3	4
5	6	7	8	9	

Fig. 11.2: Speller matrix [5]

The so-called speller matrix (Fig. 11.2) further illustrates the use, but also the limitations of EEG for BMIs [10]. The matrix contains the letters of the alphabet and the numbers 0,...,9 in a quadratic table. There are six rows and columns. The matrix is equipped with a small light source for each letter and number. With the light sources, we can highlight either an entire row of the matrix, or a column, as illustrated in the figure. Assume a subject (or patient) wears a cap with EEG electrodes. Our goal is to establish communication between the subject and a second person in another room, solely via the EEG signals. We do this letter by letter.

Suppose now the subject wishes to transmit the letter 'P'. We highlight the rows and columns of the matrix in a random pattern. Thus, for example, row 1 flashes for several seconds. After this, column 3 would flash. The target letter 'P' is neither contained in row 1 nor in column 3. However, when we activate column 4 (containing 'P'), we obtain a detectable reaction in the EEG. More specifically, mismatch and match conditions in visual tasks are typical data extractable from EEG signals.

Similar EEG-based interfaces have been developed for wheel-chairs and avatars in virtual reality environments. Here, EEG analysis detects directional intention (left-right, forward-reverse) [17]. It should be noted that EEG analysis for this application is difficult, and long training phases are needed for each individual patient. For example, the EEG signal will look very different if the patient simply closes the eyes. To address such difficulties, an EEG must be combined with a system for artifact correction, e.g. an electro-oculogram (EOG) for recording eye movement.

The inherent limitations of EEG raise the requirements for the control intelligence of the robotic exoskeleton. One further shortcoming of EEG in this context is the lack of an upstream sensory feedback path.

EMG

Several other control channels such as speech control, eye tracking, micro joysticks and tongue pads have been developed for controlling prostheses. One of the most widely used methods is EMG. In this case, electrical signals are produced in healthy or leftover muscle tissue. In a long established method for upper limb amputees, electrodes are placed in the socket of the anatomical prosthesis. By changing muscular tension in the remaining part of the limb (and with it the electrical output of muscles), prostheses can be triggered to run pre-programmed grip routines. This so-called electromyographic signal (EMG signal) can be acquired with macroscopic electrodes from all superficial muscles by thresholding the filtered and amplified signal. Since only big and superficial muscles give good EMG signals, the number and resolution of control channels is limited and does not match the state of the art hand prostheses. No force or haptic feedback is given to the user, other than visual confirmation of position in space.
A major improvement of myographic control was achieved in 2005 (Fig. 11.3). The procedure is called 'Targeted Muscle Re-Innervation' (TMR). Patients undergo a surgical procedure, which rewires leftover, but now unused arm nerves like the median, ulnar, and radial nerves to

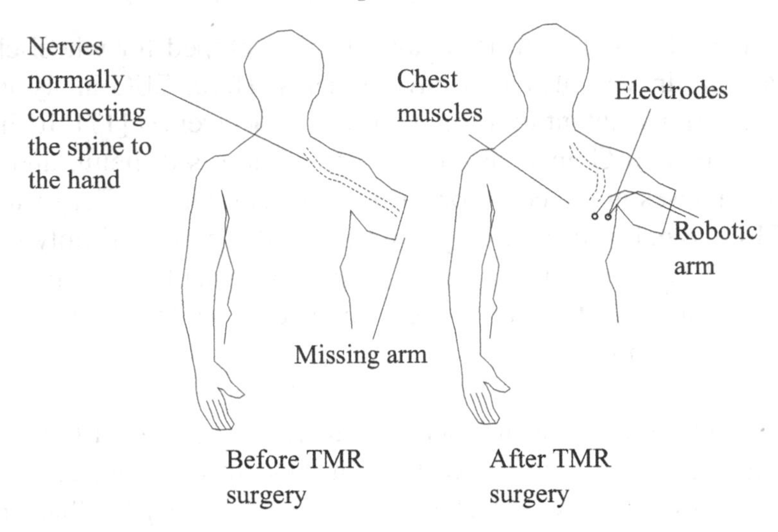

Fig. 11.3: Targeted muscle re-innervation (TMR)

the big pectoral muscle in the chest [12]. Thus larger muscle masses become accessible for high resolution EMG recordings.
With this method, patients can control robotic hand-arm prostheses [13], even for two arms. Although the surgical procedure is not without risk, it has a major advantage: It can provide upstream sensory paths by electrically stimulating the afferent nerve fibers through the skin. In this way, during motion of the prosthesis, a motion feedback can be given back to the patient. For a robotic arm with a large number of degrees of freedom, successful TMR can produce dozens of separable electrical control signals, which enables the bearer to use a highly complex hand-arm prosthesis. The American electrician Jesse Sullivan lost both arms in a work accident in 2004, and was one of the first patients to receive a complete two-arm robotic prosthesis. After TMR-surgery, he was able to perform complex two-arm tasks, such as grasping an empty glass and a bottle of water and pouring water into the glass. One of the research goals in this field is to minimize learning on the side of the patient, and incorporate most of the motion learning into the robotic system.
We count TMR (after the initial surgery) amongst the non-invasive recording methods. More invasively, electrodes can be attached to the

exposed surface of the brain (electrocorticography, ECoG) or inserted into the deep brain (multielectrode arrays, MEAs).
MEAs in the deep brain require invasive interfacing to neurons on a cellular level by microelectrodes. This may seem impossible, given the number of cells, and the complexity of the information processing. Several major discoveries helped to find a path towards this goal. In the 1950s, Hubel and Wiesel showed that the activation of one single cell in a frog's visual system was sufficient to trigger its tongue-reflex to shoot for a target [7]. It was also shown that different cells are sensitive for different, extremely detailed pieces of information stemming from the visual field [8]. One cell might be sensitive to a dark spot moving on bright background (possibly a flying insect), another cell is most sensitive to a pattern moving over a visual scene (a flock of birds). Cells can be tuned to a particular input: specific stimulation patterns correspond to maximal action potentials. To acquire meaningful control signals from a mass of cells, one would need to find the right cell for the particular control task—clearly impossible given the number of cells. In the late 1990s it was discovered that by integrating over the tuning curve of many neurons, it is possible to predict limb movement. This information code of the brain is now called the neuronal population code [2]. Based on this, BMIs were implemented for the control of a robot arm [6, 18].
Clearly, electrical recording is the most widely used method for obtaining information from the brain. However, information processing in the brain not only relies on electrical signals, but also on chemical processes. For spectroscopy, we do not read electrical signals from neurons, but detect changes in local neurotransmitter concentrations. There are several technical approaches to do this, the most common of which are MRI spectroscopy and micro-dialysis. MRI spectroscopy is a variant of MRI imaging, where local concentrations of GABA and glutamate can be measured. For micro-dialysis, a thin catheter is placed in the brain. In this case, measurements for several neurotransmitters including GABA and glutamate, serotonin and dopamine can be taken.

Finally, we can also listen to the local signal processing in the brain via imaging. The first such method is fMRI. Here, the patient or subject must be inside an MRI scanner, i.e. cannot walk around. A second method is optical coherence tomography (OCT). It is capable of detecting local morphology in tissue to a depth of 1–2 mm with very high resolution. We conjecture [1] that neuronal activity is associated with small morphologic changes, i.e. neurons move or contract when they fire. OCT allows for several extensions, which can be of help here. Firstly, it is possible to combine OCT with microscopy, giving a technique called OCM (optical coherence microscopy). Secondly, OCT and OCM devices can be miniaturized and placed at the tip of a thin needle, giving a technique called endoscopic OCM.

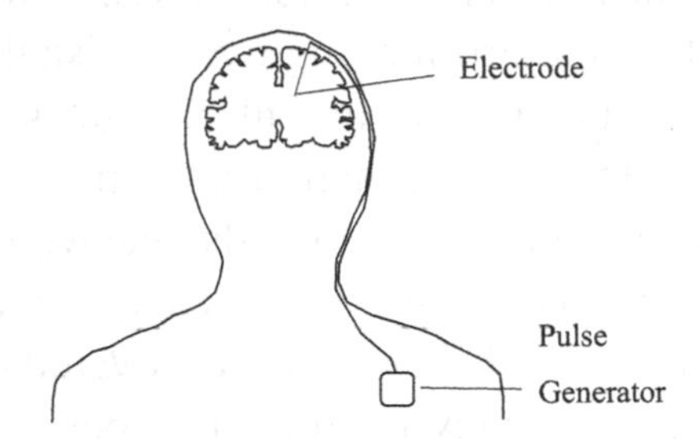

Fig. 11.4: Deep brain stimulation

11.3 Steerable Needles

Tissue damage in the brain (after injury, disease, or stroke) can cause cognitive deficits and movement disorders. For example, Parkinson's disease can be treated with deep brain stimulation (DBS), if medication does not or no longer help (Fig. 11.4). With DBS, electrodes are implanted into the deep brain, targeting specific nuclei responsible for the symptoms. A pulse generator is implanted in the chest and connected to the electrode. The electrode thus stimulates the affected neurons directly. Besides Parkinson's disease, epilepsy, depression, or obsessive compulsive disorders are treated with DBS.

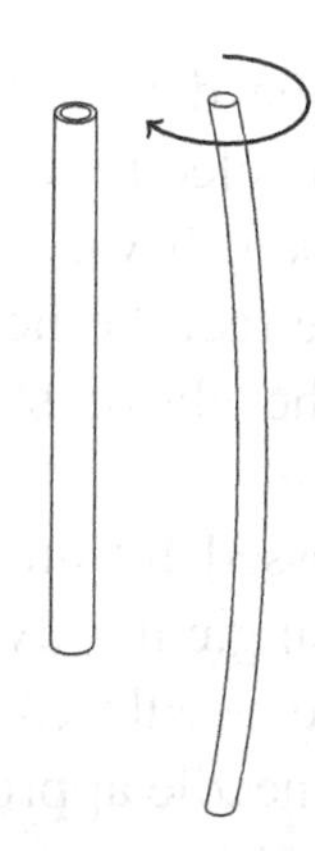

Fig. 11.5: Needle steering

Typically, electrodes are placed with needle-based stereotaxic methods (see Chaps. 1 and 10). The insertion process can be improved if the needle-system is steerable. This means we bend the needle appropriately while inserting it, to avoid critical regions in the brain. The insertion path will then no longer be a straight line, but a curve.

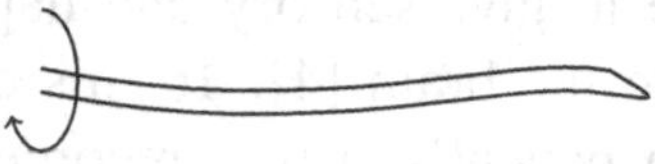

Fig. 11.6: Needle with bevel tip

Several kinematic principles for needle-steering have been developed in recent years. As an example, we consider a system with two needles, one of which is hollow, while the other is much thinner, and bent (Fig. 11.5). We insert the second needle into the first. Since the second needle is bent, it will come out at the bottom end of the first needle on a curved path. When inserting the second needle into the first, we can also rotate it. In this way, we can reach a range of three-dimensional positions with the needle tip, along curved paths. By taking more than two such needles, we can produce more complex curvature patterns.

The neurosurgeon controls the position of the needle tip via acoustic signals. The firing patterns of individual regions of the brain

are characteristic. This can be detected acoustically during needle insertion, by reading from the electrodes at the tip of the needle and sending the signals to a speaker. If we notice a slight deviation from the path, we would have to retract the needle pair and insert it again. This is a disadvantage of the above steering method with hollow needles.
This difficulty can be addressed by an alternative steering scheme (Fig. 11.6). Here we have a single highly flexible needle with a bevel tip. The bevel tip causes the needle to move into the tissue along curved paths. By rotating the needle appropriately during the inserting process, we can steer the tip [19].

As noted above, MEAs can record signals from the deep brain. To apply MEAs, we need to place the electrodes into the appropriate location in the deep brain. Similarly, in the future, endoscopic imaging (e.g. OCT or OCM imaging) may be capable of recording such signals from individual neurons. The goal of OCM in this case is to read the entire firing pattern of three-dimensional clusters of neurons, which would not be possible with MEAs [1].
Finally, it is possible to give sensory and haptic feedback from an artificial hand back to the brain [4]. To this end the activity of the peripheral nerve of a patient's arm is recorded with flexible micro electrode arrays. This enables the patient not only to send control signals to a prosthetic hand, but also to use the afferent nerve structures to obtain shape information via the artificial hand.

Exercises

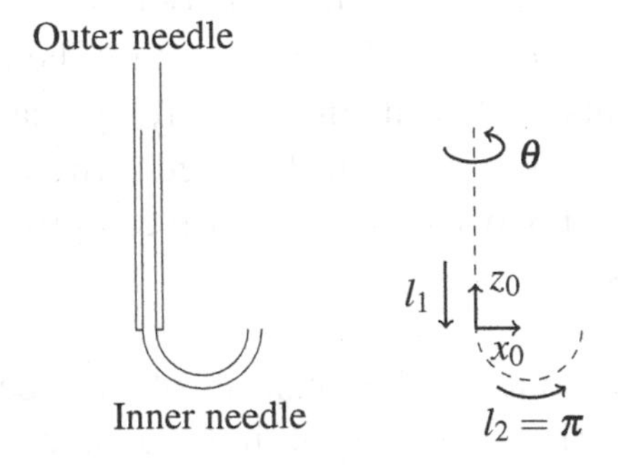

Fig. 11.7: Needle kinematics

Exercise 11.1

a) Derive forward and inverse kinematic equations for needle steering with two needles as shown in Fig. 11.5. Assume the inner needle has the shape of a walking stick, i.e. a half-circle mounted to a straight top (Fig. 11.7) and the curvature radius is 1.
The position of the tip is determined by three parameters θ, l_1 and l_2. Assume the needle is always inserted along the negative $\mathbf{z}_0$-axis. l_1 (and l_2) are the insertion depths of the outer (and inner) needle. At $l_2 = \pi$, the inner needle is fully inserted, and the tip of the inner needle is at the position $(2,0,0)^\mathrm{T}$. At $l_2 = 0$ the tip is at the origin.
b) Generalize the result from part a) to the case of an inner needle with elliptic curvature.

References

[1] R. Ansari, C. Myrtus, R. Aherrahrou, J. Erdmann, A. Schweikard, and G. Hüttmann. Ultrahigh-resolution, high-speed spectral domain optical coherence phase microscopy. *Optics Letters*, **39**(1):45–47, 2014. DOI 10.1364/ol.39.000045.
[2] J. K. Chapin, K. A. Moxon, R. S. Markowitz, and M. A. L. Nicolelis. Real-time control of a robot arm using simultaneously recorded neurons. *Nature Neuroscience*, **2**(7):664–670, 1999. DOI 10.1038/10223.
[3] R. Colombo, F. Pisano, S. Micera, A. Mazzone, C. Delconte, M. C. Carrozza, P. Dario, and G. Minuco. Robotic techniques for upper limb evaluation and rehabilitation of stroke patients. *IEEE Transactions on Neural Systems and Rehabilitation Engineering*, **13**(3):311–324, 2005. DOI 10.1109/tnsre.2005.848352.
[4] G. S. Dhillon and K. W. Horch. Direct neural sensory feedback and control of a prosthetic arm. *IEEE Transactions on Neural Systems and Rehabilitation Engineering*, **13**(4):468–472, 2005. DOI 10.1109/tnsre.2005.856072.

[5] L. A. Farwell and E. Donchin. Talking off the top of your head: toward a mental prosthesis utilizing event-related brain potentials. *Electroencephalography and Clinical Neurophysiology*, **70** (6):510–523, 1988. DOI 10.1016/0013-4694(88)90149-6.

[6] L. R. Hochberg, D. Bacher, B. Jarosiewicz, N. Y. Masse, J. D. Simeral, J. Vogel, S. Haddadin, J. Liu, S. S. Cash, P. van der Smagt, and J. P. Donoghue. Reach and grasp by people with tetraplegia using a neurally controlled robotic arm. *Nature*, **485** (7398):372–375, 2012. DOI 10.1038/nature11076.

[7] D. H. Hubel and T. N. Wiesel. Receptive fields of single neurones in the cat's striate cortex. *The Journal of Physiology*, **148** (3):574–591, 1959. DOI 10.1113/jphysiol.1959.sp006308.

[8] D. H. Hubel and T. N. Wiesel. Receptive fields, binocular interaction and functional architecture in the cat's visual cortex. *The Journal of Physiology*, **160**(1):106–154, 1962. DOI 10.1113/jphysiol.1962.sp006837.

[9] C. H. Hwang, J. W. Seong, and D.-S. Son. Individual finger synchronized robot-assisted hand rehabilitation in subacute to chronic stroke: a prospective randomized clinical trial of efficacy. *Clinical Rehabilitation*, **26**(8):696–704, 2012. DOI 10.1177/0269215511431473.

[10] P.-J. Kindermans, D. Verstraeten, and B. Schrauwen. A Bayesian model for exploiting application constraints to enable unsupervised training of a P300-based BCI. *PLoS ONE*, **7**(4):e33758, 2012. DOI 10.1371/journal.pone.0033758.

[11] H. I. Krebs, B. T. Volpe, D. Williams, J. Celestino, S. K. Charles, D. Lynch, and N. Hogan. Robot-aided neurorehabilitation: A robot for wrist rehabilitation. *IEEE Transactions on Neural Systems and Rehabilitation Engineering*, **15**(3):327–335, 2007. DOI 10.1109/tnsre.2007.903899.

[12] T. A. Kuiken, G. A. Dumanian, R. D. Lipschutz, L. A. Miller, and K. A. Stubblefield. The use of targeted muscle reinnervation for improved myoelectric prosthesis control in a bilateral shoulder disarticulation amputee. *Prosthetics and Orthotics International*, **28**(3):245–253, 2004. DOI 10.3109/03093640409167756.

[13] T. A. Kuiken, G. Li, A. Lock, R. D. Lipschutz, L. A. Miller, K. A. Stubblefield, and K. B. Englehart. Targeted muscle reinnervation for real-time myoelectric control of multifunction artificial arms. *JAMA*, **301**(6):619–628, 2009. DOI 10.1001/jama.2009.116.

[14] P. S. Lum, C. G. Burgar, and P. C. Shor. Evidence for improved muscle activation patterns after retraining of reaching movements with the MIME robotic system in subjects with post-stroke hemiparesis. *IEEE Transactions on Neural Systems and Rehabilitation Engineering*, **12**(2):186–194, 2004. DOI 10.1109/tnsre.2004.827225.

[15] Y.-L. Park, B.-r. Chen, D. Young, L. Stirling, R. J. Wood, E. Goldfield, and R. Nagpal. Bio-inspired active soft orthotic device for ankle foot pathologies. In *2011 IEEE/RSJ International Conference on Intelligent Robots and Systems (IROS)*, 2011, pages 4488–4495. DOI 10.1109/iros.2011.6094933.

[16] R. Riener, L. Lunenburger, S. Jezernik, M. Anderschitz, G. Colombo, and V. Dietz. Patient-cooperative strategies for robot-aided treadmill training: first experimental results. *IEEE Transactions on Neural Systems and Rehabilitation Engineering*, **13**(3):380–394, 2005. DOI 10.1109/tnsre.2005.848628.

[17] G. Vanacker, J. d. R. Millán, E. Lew, P. W. Ferrez, F. G. Moles, J. Philips, H. Van Brussel, and M. Nuttin. Context-based filtering for assisted brain-actuated wheelchair driving. *Computational Intelligence and Neuroscience*, **2007**:25130, 2007. DOI 10.1155/2007/25130.

[18] M. Velliste, S. Perel, M. C. Spalding, A. S. Whitford, and A. B. Schwartz. Cortical control of a prosthetic arm for self-feeding. *Nature*, **453**(7198):1098–1101, 2008. DOI 10.1038/nature06996.

[19] R. J. Webster, J. S. Kim, N. J. Cowan, G. S. Chirikjian, and A. M. Okamura. Nonholonomic modeling of needle steering. *The International Journal of Robotics Research*, **25**(5-6): 509–525, 2006. DOI 10.1177/0278364906065388.

Appendix A
Image Modalities and Sensors

The main modalities applicable to medical navigation are: X-ray, fluoroscopy, ultrasound, infrared tracking, magnetic tracking, computed tomography (CT) and magnetic resonance imaging (MRI). A number of newer modalities are also used: positron emission tomography (PET), single photon emission computed tomography (SPECT), diffusion tensor imaging (DTI), optical coherence tomography (OCT) and photo-acoustic tomography (PAT). Further methods are variants and extensions of the basic methods. They include: four-dimensional CT and MRI, optical coherence microscopy (OCM), functional modalities such as functional MRI (fMRI) and magnetic particle imaging (MPI).
We briefly summarize characteristics of these modalities and sensors with respect to navigation and robotics.

X-Ray Imaging and CT

Radiologic navigation is based on X-ray imaging with a C-arm. This method is described in Chap. 1. Typical domains of application are cardiac surgery and orthopedic surgery. By moving the C-arm along an arc in space, we can acquire CT-images. The process of reconstructing a 3D CT from a series of C-arm images is discussed in exercise 1.2. Standard CT scanners are sometimes used directly during surgery. However, CT image data from CT scanners mostly serves as

A. Schweikard, F. Ernst, *Medical Robotics*,
DOI 10.1007/978-3-319-22891-4

preoperative reference, and is often registered to intra-operative C-arm images. For older C-arms, the images must be calibrated, i.e. we must place a calibration phantom into the beam path. The geometry of the phantom is assumed to be known and we can thus determine the projection geometry and distortion features.

MRI

In MRI, a strong magnetic field (B_0-field) is generated together with gradient fields. The gradient fields allow for selectively measuring a tissue response to an external pulse. Selective measurement means that only the response of points in tissue within a certain region (e.g. a plane in space) determines the measurement. By repeating the measurement with modified parameters, this region can be moved. This generates an equation system which can be solved in a reconstruction process. The solution of the reconstruction yields a correlation to the proton density at points in a three-dimensional grid within the anatomy. MR-imaging was originally developed for diagnostics. To use MR-imaging in navigation, images must be calibrated. Distortions in MR images are difficult to correct, for the following reasons. Anatomic tissue is susceptible to magnetization. Thus the B_0-field will cause a magnetization of the tissue. Different types of tissue (bone, soft tissue, air cavities) are more or less susceptible to such magnetization. This results in small inhomogeneities in the B_0-field, causing distortions. Notice that we cannot use calibration phantoms here. An ad hoc method for calibrating MR images for navigation is described in [2]. In this ad hoc method, no registration to other imaging modalities and no calibration phantoms are used. Instead, the effects of the magnetization caused by the B_0-field are simulated in an equation system, using a table of different magnetic susceptibilities of tissue types. A forward calculation on the (distorted) image will then cause additional distortion. This additional distortion is inverted, giving an approximation vector field for correcting the original distortion.
If we compare the images in Fig. 1.6 (CT image and MR image of the same anatomy), it becomes clear that MR images show better contrast in the soft tissue. However, the bone can be segmented easily

in the CT image, e.g. by thresholding. Likewise, CT imaging is the modality of choice in a number of applications in radiation therapy and radiosurgery. Here it is necessary to compute dose distributions for radiation treatments. Tissues with different absorption coefficients can be directly differentiated in a CT image.

Four-Dimensional Imaging

In most cases, CT and MR are used in single image mode. This means that a single image stack is taken at a fixed point in time. Breathing artifacts can be reduced with respiratory gating. An alternative is four-dimensional CT or MR imaging. A four dimensional respiratory CT data set consists of 10 image stacks, where each stack corresponds to one single time point in the respiratory cycle [6]. Applications of four-dimensional imaging (e.g. in radiosurgery and cardiology) are discussed in Chap. 7.

Ultrasound

Ultrasound is non-invasive, and can provide functional information (Doppler ultrasound). However, images are distorted, (often more than MR-images) and they contain speckle noise and artifacts. For distortion correction, ultrasound images can be registered to CT or MR images. Here, three-dimensional ultrasound is of advantage. Ultrasound distortions are in the range between 2 and 7 % of the distance between the target and the ultrasound camera. The ultrasound camera is placed directly onto the skin surface, so that this distance estimate becomes meaningful. It is possible to estimate the distortions in an ultrasound image directly, using a table of Hounsfield values for different types of tissue. Thus assume a CT image of the anatomical target region is given. Hounsfield values are derived from the CT image, and the values can be mapped to acoustic properties of the individual tissue types via a table look-up. We then map Hounsfield values to the acoustic

impedance of the tissue type, and to the acoustic speed in that tissue type. With this information, the distortions can be corrected [1].
Furthermore, it is possible to compute an optimized viewing window for the ultrasound camera. After simulating the acoustic properties of the tissue between camera and target, one can compute the optimal camera window from the CT image. The ultrasound camera can thus be positioned by a robot arm to track moving targets.
In laparoscopic surgery (also called keyhole surgery), surgical instruments are inserted via a small incision while the operation process is displayed on a computer monitor. Thus, the surgeon cannot directly see the operation site. Ultrasound imaging is now a standard imaging modality for laparoscopy. Endoscopes, laparoscopic instruments and laparoscopic ultrasound must be navigated to allow for registering images from different modalities.

Infrared Tracking

An infrared tracking system computes the position and orientation of one or more probes in real time. Current infrared tracking systems generate position/orientation data with up to 4000 Hz. Typically, the output is: x-, y-, z-values for the probe tip and a quaternion for probe orientation. Several types of systems can be distinguished. Two-camera systems compute the position of spherical markers on the probe by triangulation. Thus the cameras take an image pair showing the scene from two distinct viewing directions, with known relative positions of the cameras. The stereo view allows for determining the exact position of each marker in space. The geometry of the arrangement of markers is known in advance. Three camera-systems for infrared tracking do not use triangulation. Instead the position of the markers on the probe is computed from three images. Here, each camera is a line camera (Fig. A.1). The marker position is computed in the following way: each line camera reports the position of a flashing marker as the brightest point along the camera line. This brightest point will identify a plane in space, which must contain the marker. Intersecting these three planes gives the spatial position of the marker.

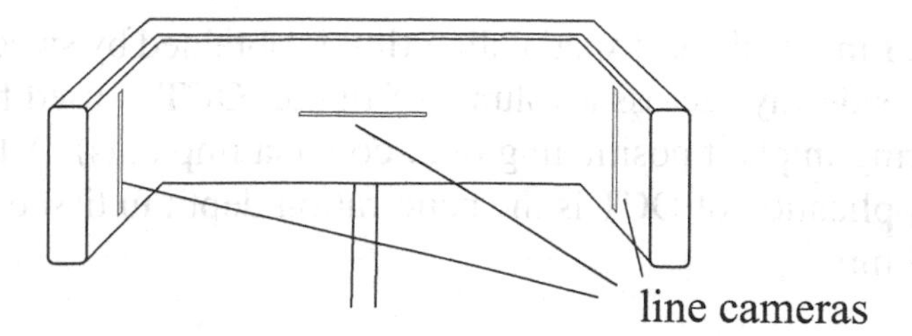

Fig. A.1: Three-camera system for infrared tracking

Magnetic Tracking

The physical principle for magnetic tracking is very different from infrared tracking. The position of small active coils is computed from readings of a magnetic sensor array. The advantage of magnetic tracking over infrared tracking is the following: the marker (coil) does not have to be visible in a camera image. Thus magnetic tracking is suitable for navigating laparoscopic instruments, endoscopes and biopsy needle tips. However, the coil must be connected to the host unit by a cable. In surgical applications, the cable must be sterile. Newer systems use small cable-less electromagnetic transponders, which can be implanted into the target region before the operation, and will then serve as landmarks during the operation.

Optical Coherence Tomography

Optical coherence tomography (OCT) generates 3D images in realtime. The physical principle is the following: light is projected onto the anatomic target. The reflected light is compared to the projected light with respect to run-time, via spectrometry [4]. Thus, OCT is sometimes called 'ultrasound with light'. If the light path is a single line, orthogonal to the tissue surface, the resulting scan is called an A-scan. Thus an A-scan collects information about a series of voxels along a short line segment. Likewise, sweeping this line segment along the tissue gives information on all voxels in a small rectangle, perpendicular to the tissue surface. This acquisition sequence is called a B-scan. Finally, the last spatial direction is obtained by sweeping this rectangle sideways across a volume of tissue. OCT is used for navigation during implant positioning (e.g. cochlea implants). A limitation for the application of OCT is the penetration depth in tissue, which is at most 2 mm.

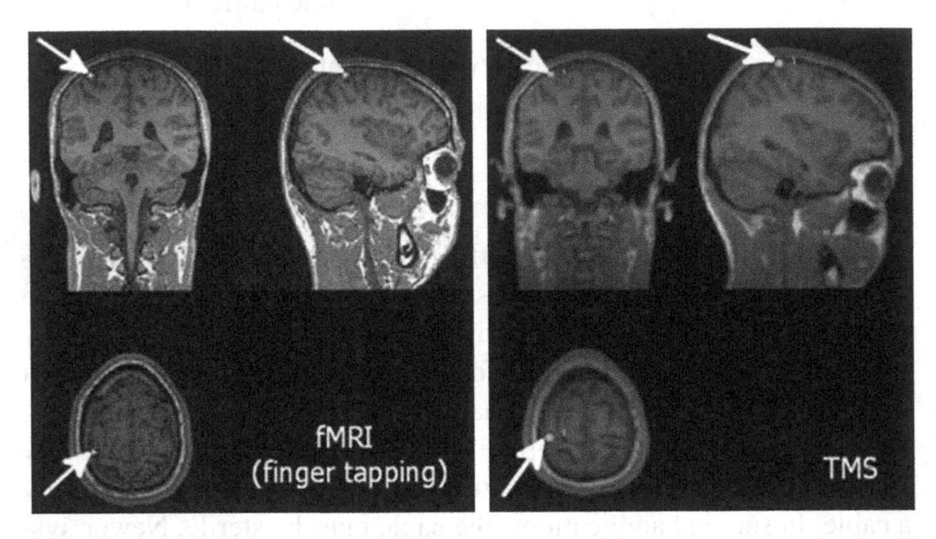

Fig. A.2: Motor cortex mapping with fMRI (*left*), and robotic TMS (*right*)

fMRI

Functional MRI (fMRI) images are taken directly in the MR-scanner, using a special driver software. Magnetic properties of hemoglobin change with the oxygen level of the blood [5]. For navigation, it is useful to register an fMRI image to a morphological MRI image. Thus, one can obtain a functional map for the motor cortex (e.g. before a neurosurgical operation). Figure A.2 (left) shows an example: a subject is asked to tap with the little finger, while fMRI images are taken. For comparison, the right part of the figure shows the result of motor cortex mapping with transcranial magnetic stimulation (TMS). Here, a robot moves the TMS coil. We activate the coil at the points of a fine grid close to the subject's head. At each grid point, the motor evoked potential (MEP) at the finger is measured. The figure shows the interpolated grid position producing peak MEP.

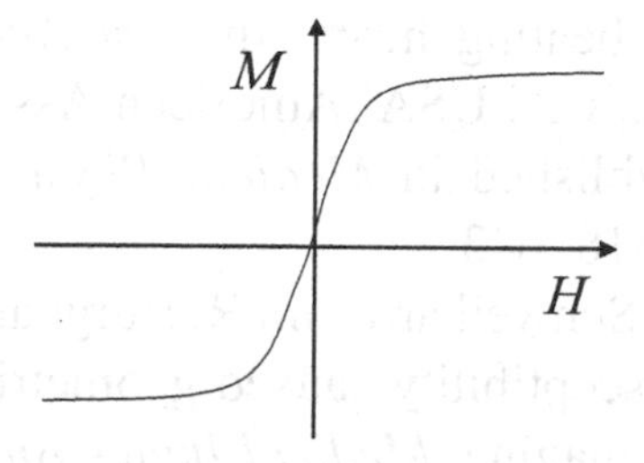

Fig. A.3: Magnetization curve for supraparamagnetic iron oxide particles

Magnetic Particle Imaging

Magnetic particle imaging (MPI) is a functional modality, and shows the diffusion of a contrast agent in the blood vessel tree. In MPI, a field-free point (within a strong static field) is generated by an appropriate spatial arrangement of magnetic coils. The key observation is the following [3]: superparamagnetic nanoparticles have a non-linear magnetization curve, implying that a saturation point can be reached (Fig. A.3). Beyond the saturation point, increasing the field strength will only cause a very small increase in magnetization of the particles. Particles outside the field-free point are under a strong external field, have thus reached magnetic saturation, and will not react to external pulses. Thus, the particles at the field-free point produce an isolated reaction to an external pulse, and this reaction can be measured externally. By adapting currents in the external coils, the field-free point can be moved over an anatomical field of view. MPI thus allows for determining the spatial distribution of the nanoparticles in real-time.

References

[1] R. Bruder, F. Ernst, A. Schlaefer, and A. Schweikard. TH-C-304A-07: Real-time tracking of the pulmonary veins in 3D ultrasound of the beating heart. In *51st Annual Meeting of the AAPM*, Anaheim, CA, USA. American Association of Physicists in Medicine. Published in *Medical Physics*, **36**(6):2804, 2009. DOI 10.1118/1.3182643.

[2] S. Burkhardt, A. Schweikard, and R. Burgkart. Numerical determination of the susceptibility caused geometric distortions in magnetic resonance imaging. *Medical Image Analysis*, **7**(3):221–236, 2003. DOI 10.1016/S1361-8415(02)00109-3.

[3] B. Gleich and J. Weizenecker. Tomographic imaging using the nonlinear response of magnetic particles. *Nature*, **435**(7046): 1214–1217, 2005. DOI 10.1038/nature03808.

[4] D. Huang, E. Swanson, C. Lin, J. Schuman, W. Stinson, W. Chang, M. Hee, T. Flotte, K. Gregory, C. Puliafito, and J. G. Fujimoto. Optical coherence tomography. *Science*, **254**(5035): 1178–1181, 1991. DOI 10.1126/science.1957169.

[5] N. K. Logothetis, J. Pauls, M. Augath, T. Trinath, and A. Oeltermann. Neurophysiological investigation of the basis of the fMRI signal. *Nature*, **412**(6843):150–157, 2001. DOI 10.1038/35084005.

[6] D. A. Low, M. Nystrom, E. Kalinin, P. Parikh, J. F. Dempsey, J. D. Bradley, S. Mutic, S. H. Wahab, T. Islam, G. Christensen, D. G. Politte, and B. R. Whiting. A method for the reconstruction of four-dimensional synchronized CT scans acquired during free breathing. *Medical Physics*, **30**(6):1254–1263, 2003. DOI 10.1118/1.1576230.

Appendix B
Selected Exercise Solutions

Solution for Exercise 1.3

d) Assume $\mathbf{x}^{(n)}$ is not in the plane $\mathbf{a}_i\mathbf{x} - b_i = 0$. We must show that (1) $\mathbf{x}^{(n+1)}$ is in this plane, and (2) the vector $\mathbf{x}^{(n+1)} - \mathbf{x}^{(n)}$ is a non-zero multiple of the normal vector $\mathbf{a}_i$, i.e. $\mathbf{x}^{(n+1)} - \mathbf{x}^{(n)} = \lambda \mathbf{a}_i$, with $\lambda \neq 0$. For (1), we directly find that $\mathbf{a}_i\mathbf{x}^{(n+1)} - b_i = 0$, by inserting the definition of $\mathbf{x}^{(n+1)}$. For (2), we see from the definition of $\mathbf{x}^{(n+1)}$ that $\lambda = -\frac{\mathbf{a}_i\mathbf{x}^{(n)} - b_i}{\mathbf{a}_i^2}$.

Solution for Exercise 2.3

b) For

$$\mathbf{M} = \begin{pmatrix} n_x & o_x & a_x & p_x \\ n_y & o_y & a_y & p_y \\ n_z & o_z & a_z & p_z \\ 0 & 0 & 0 & 1 \end{pmatrix} \tag{B.1}$$

the inverse is given by

$$\mathbf{M}^{-1} = \begin{pmatrix} n_x & n_y & n_z & -\mathbf{np} \\ o_x & o_y & o_z & -\mathbf{op} \\ a_x & a_y & a_z & -\mathbf{ap} \\ 0 & 0 & 0 & 1 \end{pmatrix} \tag{B.2}$$

A. Schweikard, F. Ernst, *Medical Robotics*,
DOI 10.1007/978-3-319-22891-4

Solution for Exercise 2.5

There are several equivalent ways to find the YPR-angles given a rotation matrix. One is the following:
Start from equation

$$\mathbf{R} = \mathbf{R}(z,\gamma)\mathbf{R}(y,\beta)\mathbf{R}(x,\alpha) = \begin{pmatrix} n_x & o_x & a_x \\ n_y & o_y & a_y \\ n_z & o_z & a_z \end{pmatrix} \tag{B.3}$$

Then insert the elementary rotations (see Eq. 2.17) giving

$$\begin{pmatrix} c_\gamma c_\beta & c_\gamma s_\beta s_\alpha - s_\gamma c_\alpha & c_\gamma s_\beta c_\alpha + s_\gamma s_\alpha \\ s_\gamma c_\beta & s_\gamma s_\beta s_\alpha + c_\gamma c_\alpha & s_\gamma s_\beta c_\alpha - c_\gamma s_\alpha \\ -s_\beta & c_\beta s_\alpha & c_\beta c_\alpha \end{pmatrix} = \begin{pmatrix} n_x & o_x & a_x \\ n_y & o_y & a_y \\ n_z & o_z & a_z \end{pmatrix} \tag{B.4}$$

We thus have

$$s_\beta = -n_z \tag{B.5}$$

We could solve this equation for β using the arcsin-function, i.e. we could simply set $\beta = \arcsin -n_z$. However, arcsin only returns values in the range $[-\pi/2, \pi/2]$. There may be solutions outside this range. We could define a function *asin*2 similar to the *atan*2-function (see Eq. 2.33). Instead we prefer to use *atan*2 since we have already defined it. Since $\sin^2\beta + \cos^2\beta = 1$, we have

$$c_\beta = \pm\sqrt{(1-n_z^2)} \tag{B.6}$$

Given Eqs. B.5 and B.6, we are in a position to apply the function *atan*2, i.e.

$$\beta_{1,2} = \text{atan2}(-n_z, \pm\sqrt{(1-n_z^2)}) \tag{B.7}$$

After having solved for β, we can insert our value into Eq. B.4, and obtain values for α and γ.
From the upper two elements of the first matrix column in Eq. B.4 we obtain the value for γ.

$$\gamma = \text{atan2}\left(\frac{n_y}{c_\beta}, \frac{n_x}{c_\beta}\right) \tag{B.8}$$

The last two elements of the last matrix line in Eq. B.4 give α.

$$\alpha = \text{atan2}\left(\frac{o_z}{c_\beta}, \frac{a_z}{c_\beta}\right) \tag{B.9}$$

Notice that in Eqs. B.8 and B.9 we assume $c_\beta \neq 0$. We must handle the case $c_\beta = 0$ separately. In this case, we have two possibilities:

1. $\beta = \pi/2$ and $s_\beta = 1$,
2. $\beta = -\pi/2$ and $s_\beta = -1$.

For the first possibility, the matrix Eq. B.4 simplifies to

$$\begin{pmatrix} 0 & s_{\alpha-\gamma} & c_{\alpha-\gamma} \\ 0 & c_{\alpha-\gamma} & -s_{\alpha-\gamma} \\ -1 & 0 & 0 \end{pmatrix} = \begin{pmatrix} n_x & o_x & a_x \\ n_y & o_y & a_y \\ n_z & o_z & a_z \end{pmatrix} \tag{B.10}$$

Here we have used the trigonometric addition formulas to simplify expressions (for example: $c_\gamma s_\alpha - s_\gamma c_\alpha$ is written as $s_{\alpha-\gamma}$).
Likewise, for the second possibility we obtain:

$$\begin{pmatrix} 0 & -s_{\alpha+\gamma} & -c_{\alpha+\gamma} \\ 0 & c_{\alpha+\gamma} & -s_{\alpha+\gamma} \\ 1 & 0 & 0 \end{pmatrix} = \begin{pmatrix} n_x & o_x & a_x \\ n_y & o_y & a_y \\ n_z & o_z & a_z \end{pmatrix} \tag{B.11}$$

In both cases the solutions for α and γ can again be found with the *atan*2-function from the matrix Eqs. B.10 and B.11. Notice that in both cases the solutions for γ and α will not be unique. We can only obtain expressions for $\alpha + \gamma$ or $\alpha - \gamma$. The interpretation of this fact is the following: at $s_\beta = 0$, we have a singularity, and the two angles γ and α can compensate each other.

Solution for Exercise 2.7

b) Given the quaternion $\mathbf{q} = (q_1, q_2, q_3, q_4)$, set $\theta = 2\arccos(q_1)$ and $(u_x, u_y, u_z) = \frac{1}{\sin\theta/2}(q_2, q_3, q_4)$ and insert $c = cos\theta$, $s = \sin\theta$ and (u_x, u_y, u_z) into Eq. 2.48.

c) Consider

$$\begin{pmatrix} c+u_x^2(1-c) & u_xu_y(1-c)-u_zs & u_xu_z(1-c)+u_ys \\ u_yu_x(1-c)+u_zs & c+u_y^2(1-c) & u_yu_z(1-c)-u_xs \\ u_zu_x(1-c)-u_ys & u_zu_y(1-c)+u_xs & c+u_z^2(1-c) \end{pmatrix} = \begin{pmatrix} n_x & o_x & a_x \\ n_y & o_y & a_y \\ n_z & o_z & a_z \end{pmatrix} \tag{B.12}$$

From the main diagonal we obtain

$$n_x + o_y + a_z = (1-c)(u_x^2 + u_y^2 + u_z^2) + 3c \tag{B.13}$$

We have $(u_x^2 + u_y^2 + u_z^2) = 1$, hence

$$\theta = \arccos(\frac{n_x + o_y + a_z}{2}) \tag{B.14}$$

Furthermore, from Eq. B.12, we have

$$\begin{aligned} o_z - a_y &= 2su_x \\ a_x - n_z &= 2su_y \\ n_y - a_x &= 2su_z \end{aligned}$$

From this, we can directly derive the vector (u_x, u_y, u_z).

Solution for Exercise 4.8

For part a) we have

$$\theta'(0) = 0 \tag{B.15}$$

$$\theta'(1) = 0 \tag{B.16}$$

$$\theta(0) = a_1 \tag{B.17}$$

$$\theta(1) = b_1 \tag{B.18}$$

and

$$\theta(t) = c_0 + c_1t + c_2t^2 + c_3t^3. \tag{B.19}$$

Taking the derivative with respect to t gives

$$\theta'(t) = c_1 + 2c_2 t + 3c_3 t^2. \tag{B.20}$$

From Eq. B.17, we obtain

$$c_0 = a_1 \tag{B.21}$$

Combining Eq. B.15 and Eq. B.20 we have

$$c_1 = 0 \tag{B.22}$$

Hence

$$\theta(t) = a_1 + c_2 t^2 + c_3 t^3. \tag{B.23}$$

From Eq. B.18 we see that

$$b_1 = a_1 + c_2 + c_3 \tag{B.24}$$

Combining Eq. B.16 and Eq. B.20

$$0 = 2c_2 + 3c_3 \tag{B.25}$$

The last two equations are linear equations for c_2 and c_3, and we find:

$$\begin{aligned} c_0 &= a_1 \\ c_1 &= 0 \\ c_2 &= 3(b_1 - a_1) \\ c_3 &= -2(b_1 - a_1) \end{aligned} \tag{B.26}$$

Solution for Exercise 5.6

Show that $H(A) \geq 0$ for a random variable A.
By definition

$$H(A) = -\sum_a p_A(a) \log p_A(a) \tag{B.27}$$

and

$$0 \leq p_A(a) \leq 1. \tag{B.28}$$

Thus for each a, we have

$$p_A(a)\log(1/p_A(a)) \geq 0 \quad \text{(B.29)}$$

so that

$$H(A) = \sum_a p_A(a)\log(1/p_A(a)) \geq 0. \quad \text{(B.30)}$$

Solution for Exercise 7.2

Looking at only two sample points $\mathbf{x}_1$ and $\mathbf{x}_2$, explain why the quadratic program
Minimize

$$w_1^2 + w_2^2$$

Subject to

$$\begin{aligned} y_1(\mathbf{w}\mathbf{x}_1 + d) &\geq 0 \\ y_2(\mathbf{w}\mathbf{x}_2 + d) &\geq 0 \end{aligned} \quad \text{(B.31)}$$

where $y_1 = 1$ and $y_2 = -1$, computes a maximum margin separator line.
Represent the line by its parameters $(\mathbf{w}, d)$, where $\mathbf{w}$ is the normal vector of the line. Then this representation of a line can be multiplied by a factor λ, without changing the line. Thus $(\lambda\mathbf{w}, \lambda d)$ for non-zero λ is the same line as $(\mathbf{w}, d)$. First show that is suffices to consider only those lines having

$$\begin{aligned} y_1(\mathbf{w}\mathbf{x}_1 + d) &= 1 \\ y_2(\mathbf{w}\mathbf{x}_2 + d) &= 1 \end{aligned} \quad \text{(B.32)}$$

Why is it enough to look at those lines only which can indeed be scaled in this way? The reason for this will be explained next: Since we are looking for a maximum margin separator line, we can safely assume that any line we look at has

$$y_1(\mathbf{w}\mathbf{x}_1 + d) = a$$

where $a > 0$, and

$$y_2(\mathbf{w}\mathbf{x}_2 + d) = b$$

with $b > 0$ as well. Otherwise our line would cross one of the points $\mathbf{x}_1, \mathbf{x}_2$, and then it can certainly not be a maximum margin separator line. But now we can also assume $a = b$. Otherwise, if a were not equal to b for a given line we could simply move this line slightly and obtain a line with a yet bigger margin. But now, since $a = b$, we can scale with a factor λ to have the above form Eq. B.32. But now recall that for any line, we obtain the point-line distance by scaling the normal vector $\mathbf{w}$ to unit length, so that the margin is given by:

$$\frac{\mathbf{w}}{||\mathbf{w}||}\mathbf{x}_1 + \frac{d}{||\mathbf{w}||} \tag{B.33}$$

To see why this is indeed the margin, recall that the distance of the origin from a line with equation $\mathbf{w}\mathbf{x} + d = 0$ is d, if the normal vector $\mathbf{w}$ has unit length, i.e. $||\mathbf{w}|| = 1$. Likewise distances of the points $\mathbf{x}_1, \mathbf{x}_2$ from the given line can be calculated. But Eq. B.33 is the same as

$$\frac{1}{||\mathbf{w}||}(\mathbf{w}\mathbf{x}_1 + d) \tag{B.34}$$

And by Eq. B.32 we have $\mathbf{w}\mathbf{x}_1 + d = 1$. Hence the margin is simply $\frac{1}{||\mathbf{w}||}$. To maximize the margin, we must minimize the length of $\mathbf{w}$.
It may seem strange to minimize the length of a normal vector, since it would appear that a minimal length normal vector would simply be the zero vector. But this is not so, since we look at only those (scaled!) normal vectors satisfying Eq. B.32!

Solution for Exercise 7.3

Show that the system in Eq. 7.16 is actually a quadratic program.

b) Define $2m$ variables $\theta_1, \ldots, \theta_{2m}$ by setting:
   $\theta_i = \alpha_i - \alpha_i'$ for $i = 1, \ldots, m$
   and
   $\theta_{i+m} = \alpha_i'$ for $i = 1, \ldots, m$.

For two sample points $\mathbf{x}_1, \mathbf{x}_2$, i.e. $m = 2$ set

$$\mathbf{H} = \begin{pmatrix} \mathbf{x}_1\mathbf{x}_1 & \mathbf{x}_1\mathbf{x}_2 & 0 & 0 \\ \mathbf{x}_2\mathbf{x}_1 & \mathbf{x}_2\mathbf{x}_2 & 0 & 0 \\ 0 & 0 & 0 & 0 \\ 0 & 0 & 0 & 0 \end{pmatrix}. \tag{B.35}$$

Based on our definition of the variables θ_i, we must define constraints on the variables α_i and α_i'. For example (again in the case $m = 2$), we have $\alpha_1 = \theta_1 + \theta_3$, and thus translate the constraint $\alpha_1 \geq 0$ into $\theta_1 + \theta_3 \geq 0$. To call the Matlab-routine, we must set up a matrix $\mathbf{A}$ and a vector $\mathbf{b}$, such that $\mathbf{A}\theta \leq \mathbf{b}$. To express our constraint as a $\leq$-constraint, we write $-\theta_1 - \theta_3 \leq 0$. Thus the first line in the constraint matrix $\mathbf{A}$ is given by the four entries

$$-1\ 0\ -1\ 0 \tag{B.36}$$

and the first entry of the vector $\mathbf{b}$ is 0.
Now define the constraint matrix $\mathbf{A}$ and the vector $\mathbf{b}$ according to

$$\begin{array}{ccccccc} & \mathbf{A} & & & \mathbf{b} & & \textit{meaning} \\ -1 & 0 & -1 & 0 & 0 & & \alpha_1 \geq 0 \\ 0 & -1 & 0 & -1 & 0 & & \alpha_2 \geq 0 \\ 1 & 0 & 1 & 0 & C & & \alpha_1 \leq C \\ 0 & 1 & 0 & 1 & C & & \alpha_2 \leq C \\ 0 & 0 & -1 & 0 & 0 & & \alpha_1' \geq 0 \\ 0 & 0 & 0 & -1 & 0 & & \alpha_2' \geq 0 \\ 0 & 0 & 1 & 0 & C & & \alpha_1' \leq C \\ 0 & 0 & 0 & 1 & C & & \alpha_2' \leq C \\ 1 & 1 & 0 & 0 & 0 & & (\alpha_1 - \alpha_1') + (\alpha_2 - \alpha_2') \leq 0 \\ -1 & -1 & 0 & 0 & 0 & & (\alpha_1 - \alpha_1') + (\alpha_2 - \alpha_2') \geq 0 \end{array}. \tag{B.37}$$

Notice that the last two lines of the matrix are obtained by resolving the constraint $(\alpha_1 - \alpha_1') + (\alpha_2 - \alpha_2') = 0$.
Finally, we define $\mathbf{f}$ as

$$\mathbf{f} = \begin{pmatrix} \varepsilon - y_1 \\ \varepsilon - y_2 \\ 2\varepsilon \\ 2\varepsilon \end{pmatrix} \tag{B.38}$$

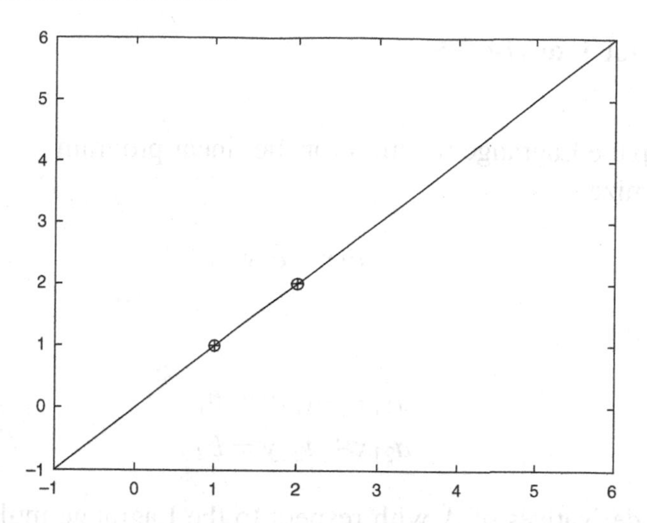

Fig. B.1: Regression with dual quadratic programming, result for two points $x_1 = 1, x_2 = 2, y_1 = 1, y_2 = 2$

Now call $\theta = quadprog(\mathbf{H}, \mathbf{f}, \mathbf{A}, \mathbf{b})$. Your result should look like Fig. B.1.

Solution for Exercise 7.4

Consider the optimization problem
Minimize

$$f(x,y) = x^2 + y^2$$

Subject to

$$g(x,y) = x + y = 2$$

a) Find the Lagrange function for this system.
b) Find the optimum with the help of the Lagrange function.

We have $L(x,y,\alpha) = f(x,y) - \alpha g(x,y) = x^2 + y^2 + \alpha(x+y-2)$.
Taking $\bigtriangledown L = 0$, we have

$$\begin{aligned} x + y &= 2 \\ 2x &= \alpha \\ 2y &= \alpha \end{aligned}$$

This is a linear system with the solution $x = 1, y = 1, \alpha = 2$.

Solution for Exercise 7.5

a) Set up the Lagrange function for the linear program maximize

$$c_1x + c_2y \tag{B.39}$$

subject to

$$\begin{aligned} a_{11}x + a_{12}y &= b_1 \\ a_{21}x + a_{22}y &= b_2 \end{aligned} \tag{B.40}$$

Take derivatives of Λ with respect to the Lagrange multipliers α_i and the primal variables x, y, and set the resulting expressions to zero. Inserting these equations back into L, show that $\Lambda = \mathbf{b}\alpha$, and $\mathbf{A}^{\mathrm{T}}\alpha = \mathbf{c}$.

We have

$$\Lambda = c_1x + c_2y - \alpha_1(a_{11}x + a_{12}y - b_1) - \alpha_2(a_{21}x + a_{22}y - b_2) \tag{B.41}$$

Taking the partial derivatives and setting to zero we obtain

$$\frac{\partial \Lambda}{\partial \alpha_1} = a_{11}x + a_{12}y - b_1 = 0 \tag{B.42}$$

$$\frac{\partial \Lambda}{\partial \alpha_2} = a_{21}x + a_{22}y - b_2 = 0 \tag{B.43}$$

$$\frac{\partial \Lambda}{\partial x} = c_1 - \alpha_1 a_{11} - \alpha_2 a_{21} = 0 \tag{B.44}$$

$$\frac{\partial \Lambda}{\partial y} = c_2 - \alpha_1 a_{12} - \alpha_2 a_{22} = 0 \tag{B.45}$$

From the last two equations, we directly obtain

$$c_1 = \alpha_1 a_{11} + \alpha_2 a_{21} \tag{B.46}$$

$$c_2 = \alpha_1 a_{12} + \alpha_2 a_{22} \tag{B.47}$$

and hence $\mathbf{A}^{\mathrm{T}}\alpha = \mathbf{c}$.

Inserting Eqs. B.42 and B.43 into the expression for Λ, we have

$$\Lambda = c_1 x + c_2 y \tag{B.48}$$

From Eqs. B.46 and B.47 we have

$$\Lambda = (\alpha_1 a_{11} + \alpha_2 a_{21})x + (\alpha_1 a_{12} + \alpha_2 a_{22})y. \tag{B.49}$$

Rearranging and again applying Eqs. B.42 and B.43 gives

$$\Lambda = \alpha_1(a_{11}x + a_{12}y) + \alpha_2(a_{21}x + a_{22}y) = \alpha_1 b_1 + \alpha_2 b_2, \tag{B.50}$$

hence $\Lambda = \alpha\mathbf{b}$.

Solution for Exercise 11.1

We first assume the needle only moves in the $\mathbf{x}_0$- $\mathbf{z}_0$ - plane, i.e. we ignore the rotation of the needle by the angle θ. Thus, our target point is denoted by

$$\mathbf{p} = \begin{pmatrix} p_x \\ p_y \\ p_z \end{pmatrix} = \begin{pmatrix} p_x \\ 0 \\ p_z \end{pmatrix} \tag{B.51}$$

We place a point $\mathbf{q} = (1,0,0)^{\mathrm{T}}$ (Fig. B.2). We have

$$\mathbf{p} = \begin{pmatrix} 0 \\ 0 \\ -l_1 \end{pmatrix} + \mathbf{q} - \begin{pmatrix} \cos(l_2) \\ 0 \\ \sin(l_2) \end{pmatrix} = \begin{pmatrix} 1-\cos(l_2) \\ 0 \\ -l_1 - \sin(l_2) \end{pmatrix} \tag{B.52}$$

We write this in matrix form, i.e. we set up the matrix expressing a purely translational transformation to the needle tip.

$$\mathbf{M}_p = \begin{pmatrix} 1\,0\,0 & 1-\cos(l_2) \\ 0\,1\,0 & 0 \\ 0\,0\,1 & -l_1 - \sin(l_2) \\ 1\,0\,0 & 1 \end{pmatrix} \tag{B.53}$$

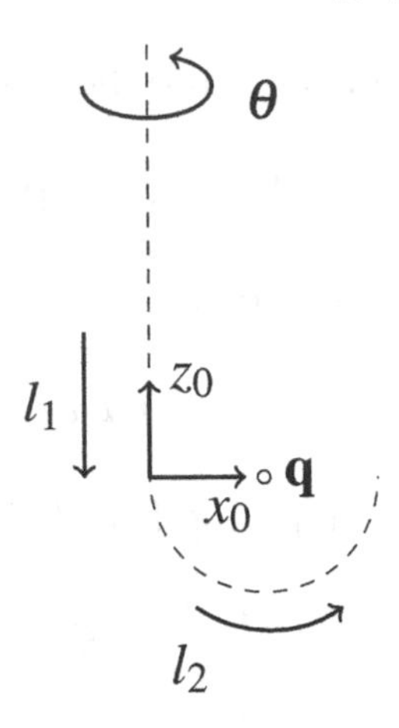

Fig. B.2: Kinematics for needle steering with two needles

To add the rotation by θ, we premultiply this matrix by the 4×4 matrix representing **z**-rotation about the origin. We obtain the product

$$\mathbf{M}_p(\theta) = \begin{pmatrix} \cos(\theta) & -\sin(\theta) & 0 & 0 \\ \sin(\theta) & \cos(\theta) & 0 & 0 \\ 0 & 0 & 1 & 0 \\ 1 & 0 & 0 & 1 \end{pmatrix} \begin{pmatrix} 1 & 0 & 0 & 1-\cos(l_2) \\ 0 & 1 & 0 & 0 \\ 0 & 0 & 1 & -l_1-\sin(l_2) \\ 1 & 0 & 0 & 1 \end{pmatrix} \tag{B.54}$$

Evaluating the matrix product we obtain the forward matrix for the needle tip.

$$\mathbf{M}_p(\theta) = \begin{pmatrix} \cos(\theta) & -\sin(\theta) & 0 & \cos(\theta)(1-\cos(l_2)) \\ \sin(\theta) & \cos(\theta) & 0 & \sin(\theta)(1-\cos(l_2)) \\ 0 & 0 & 1 & -l_1-\sin(l_2) \\ 1 & 0 & 0 & 1 \end{pmatrix} \tag{B.55}$$

From the last column of the matrix, we find the position **p** of the needle tip.

$$\mathbf{p} = \begin{pmatrix} p_x \\ p_y \\ p_z \end{pmatrix} = \begin{pmatrix} \cos(\theta)(1-\cos(l_2)) \\ \sin(\theta)(1-\cos(l_2)) \\ -l_1-\sin(l_2) \end{pmatrix} \tag{B.56}$$

Then (unless $\cos(l_2) = 1$) we have

$$\theta = \text{atan2}(p_y, p_x) \tag{B.57}$$

From first two lines in Eq. B.56 we obtain two cases:
If $\sin^2(\theta) > \varepsilon$, we set

$$l_2 = a\cos(1 - p_y/\sin(\theta)) \tag{B.58}$$

Otherwise

$$l_2 = a\cos(1 - p_x/\cos(\theta)) \tag{B.59}$$

Finally, from the last line in Eq. B.56

$$l_1 = -\sin(l_2) - p_z \tag{B.60}$$

Appendix C
Geometric Jacobian for the Six-Joint Elbow Manipulator

The elbow manipalator with spherical wrist is a six-joint robot with revolute joints (Fig. 3.2). We summarize the results of the forward analysis and derive the geometric Jacobi-matrix for this robot. The DH-table is (Table C.1):

Table C.1: DH-table for the six-joint elbow manipulator with spherical wrist

i	α_i	a_i	d_i	θ_i
1	-90	0	0	θ_1
2	0	a_2	0	θ_2
3	90	0	0	θ_3
4	-90	0	d_4	θ_4
5	90	0	0	θ_5
6	0	0	d_6	θ_6

$$^{i-1}M_i = T(0,0,d_i)R(z,\Theta_i)T(a_i,0,0)R(x,\alpha_i)$$

$$^{i-1}M_i = \begin{bmatrix} \cos(\theta_i) & -\sin(\theta_i)\cos(\alpha_i) & \sin(\theta_i)\sin(\alpha_i) & \cos(\theta_i)\,a_i \\ \sin(\theta_i) & \cos(\theta_i)\cos(\alpha_i) & -\cos(\theta_i)\sin(\alpha_i) & \sin(\theta_i)\,a_i \\ 0 & \sin(\alpha_i) & \cos(\alpha_i) & d_i \\ 0 & 0 & 0 & 1 \end{bmatrix}$$

A. Schweikard, F. Ernst, *Medical Robotics*,
DOI 10.1007/978-3-319-22891-4

DH-Matrices

$$^0M_1 = \begin{bmatrix} c_1 & 0 & -s_1 & 0 \\ s_1 & 0 & c_1 & 0 \\ 0 & -1 & 0 & 0 \\ 0 & 0 & 0 & 1 \end{bmatrix}$$

$$^1M_2 = \begin{bmatrix} c_2 & -s_2 & 0 & c_2 a_2 \\ s_2 & c_2 & 0 & s_2 a_2 \\ 0 & 0 & 1 & 0 \\ 0 & 0 & 0 & 1 \end{bmatrix}$$

$$^2M_3 = \begin{bmatrix} c_3 & 0 & s_3 & 0 \\ s_3 & 0 & -c_3 & 0 \\ 0 & 1 & 0 & 0 \\ 0 & 0 & 0 & 1 \end{bmatrix}$$

$$^3M_4 = \begin{bmatrix} c_4 & 0 & -s_4 & 0 \\ s_4 & 0 & c_4 & 0 \\ 0 & -1 & 0 & d_4 \\ 0 & 0 & 0 & 1 \end{bmatrix}$$

$$^4M_5 = \begin{bmatrix} c_5 & 0 & s_5 & 0 \\ s_5 & 0 & -c_5 & 0 \\ 0 & 1 & 0 & 0 \\ 0 & 0 & 0 & 1 \end{bmatrix}$$

$$^5M_6 = \begin{bmatrix} c_6 & -s_6 & 0 & 0 \\ s_6 & c_6 & 0 & 0 \\ 0 & 0 & 1 & d_6 \\ 0 & 0 & 0 & 1 \end{bmatrix}$$

Forward Kinematics

$$ {}^{0}M_1 = \begin{bmatrix} c_1 & 0 & -s_1 & 0 \\ s_1 & 0 & c_1 & 0 \\ 0 & -1 & 0 & 0 \\ 0 & 0 & 0 & 1 \end{bmatrix} $$

$$ {}^{0}M_2 = \begin{bmatrix} c_1c_2 & -c_1s_2 & -s_1 & c_1c_2a_2 \\ s_1c_2 & -s_1s_2 & c_1 & s_1c_2a_2 \\ -s_2 & -c_2 & 0 & -s_2a_2 \\ 0 & 0 & 0 & 1 \end{bmatrix} $$

$$ {}^{0}M_3 = \begin{bmatrix} c_1\left(-s_2s_3+c_2c_3\right) & -s_1 & c_1\left(c_2s_3+s_2c_3\right) & c_1c_2a_2 \\ s_1\left(-s_2s_3+c_2c_3\right) & c_1 & s_1\left(c_2s_3+s_2c_3\right) & s_1c_2a_2 \\ -s_2c_3-c_2s_3 & 0 & -s_2s_3+c_2c_3 & -s_2a_2 \\ 0 & 0 & 0 & 1 \end{bmatrix} $$

$$ {}^{0}M_4 = \begin{bmatrix} m_{11} & m_{12} & m_{13} & m_{14} \\ m_{21} & m_{22} & m_{23} & m_{24} \\ m_{31} & m_{32} & m_{33} & m_{34} \\ 0 & 0 & 0 & 1 \end{bmatrix} $$

where

$$ \begin{aligned} m_{11} &= -c_1c_4s_2s_3+c_1c_4c_2c_3-s_1s_4 \\ m_{12} &= -c_1\left(c_2s_3+s_2c_3\right) \\ m_{13} &= c_1s_4s_2s_3-c_1s_4c_2c_3-s_1c_4 \\ m_{14} &= c_1\left(d_4c_2s_3+d_4s_2c_3+c_2a_2\right) \end{aligned} $$

$$m_{21} = -s_1c_4s_2s_3 + s_1c_4c_2c_3 + c_1s_4$$
$$m_{22} = -s_1(c_2s_3 + s_2c_3)$$
$$m_{23} = s_1s_4s_2s_3 - s_1s_4c_2c_3 + c_1c_4$$
$$m_{24} = s_1(d_4c_2s_3 + d_4s_2c_3 + c_2a_2)$$

$$m_{31} = -(c_2s_3 + s_2c_3)c_4$$
$$m_{32} = s_2s_3 - c_2c_3$$
$$m_{33} = (c_2s_3 + s_2c_3)s_4$$
$$m_{34} = -d_4s_2s_3 + d_4c_2c_3 - s_2a_2$$

$$^0M_5 = \begin{bmatrix} m_{11} & m_{12} & m_{13} & m_{14} \\ m_{21} & m_{22} & m_{23} & m_{24} \\ m_{31} & m_{32} & m_{33} & m_{34} \\ 0 & 0 & 0 & 1 \end{bmatrix}$$

where

$$m_{11} = -c_5c_1c_4s_2s_3 + c_5c_1c_4c_2c_3 - c_5s_1s_4 - c_1s_5c_2s_3 - c_1s_5s_2c_3$$
$$m_{12} = c_1s_4s_2s_3 - c_1s_4c_2c_3 - s_1c_4$$
$$m_{13} = -s_5c_1c_4s_2s_3 + s_5c_1c_4c_2c_3 - s_5s_1s_4 + c_1c_5c_2s_3 + c_1c_5s_2c_3$$
$$m_{14} = c_1(d_4c_2s_3 + d_4s_2c_3 + c_2a_2)$$

$$m_{21} = -c_5s_1c_4s_2s_3 + c_5s_1c_4c_2c_3 + c_5c_1s_4 - s_1s_5c_2s_3 - s_1s_5s_2c_3$$
$$m_{22} = s_1s_4s_2s_3 - s_1s_4c_2c_3 + c_1c_4$$
$$m_{23} = -s_5s_1c_4s_2s_3 + s_5s_1c_4c_2c_3 + s_5c_1s_4 + s_1c_5c_2s_3 + s_1c_5s_2c_3$$
$$m_{24} = s_1\left(d_4c_2s_3 + d_4s_2c_3 + c_2a_2\right)$$

$$m_{31} = -c_4c_5c_2s_3 - c_4c_5s_2c_3 + s_5s_2s_3 - s_5c_2c_3$$
$$m_{32} = (c_2s_3 + s_2c_3)\, s_4$$
$$m_{33} = -c_4s_5c_2s_3 - c_4s_5s_2c_3 - c_5s_2s_3 + c_5c_2c_3$$
$$m_{34} = -d_4s_2s_3 + d_4c_2c_3 - s_2a_2$$

$$^0M_6 = \begin{bmatrix} m_{11} & m_{12} & m_{13} & m_{14} \\ m_{21} & m_{22} & m_{23} & m_{24} \\ m_{31} & m_{32} & m_{33} & m_{34} \\ 0 & 0 & 0 & 1 \end{bmatrix}$$

where

$$m_{11} = -c_6c_5c_1c_4s_2s_3 + c_6c_5c_1c_4c_2c_3 - c_6c_5s_1s_4 - c_6c_1s_5c_2s_3 - c_6c_1s_5s_2c_3 + s_6c_1s_4s_2s_3 - s_6c_1s_4c_2c_3 - s_6s_1c_4$$
$$m_{12} = s_6c_5c_1c_4s_2s_3 - s_6c_5c_1c_4c_2c_3 + s_6c_5s_1s_4 + s_6c_1s_5c_2s_3 + s_6c_1s_5s_2c_3 + c_6c_1s_4s_2s_3 - c_6c_1s_4c_2c_3 - c_6s_1c_4$$
$$m_{13} = -s_5c_1c_4s_2s_3 + s_5c_1c_4c_2c_3 - s_5s_1s_4 + c_1c_5c_2s_3 + c_1c_5s_2c_3$$
$$m_{14} = -d_6s_5c_1c_4s_2s_3 + d_6s_5c_1c_4c_2c_3 - d_6s_5s_1s_4 + d_6c_1c_5c_2s_3 + d_6c_1c_5s_2c_3 + c_1d_4c_2s_3 + c_1d_4s_2c_3 + c_1c_2a_2$$

$$m_{21} = -c_6c_5s_1c_4s_2s_3 + c_6c_5s_1c_4c_2c_3 + c_6c_5c_1s_4 - c_6s_1s_5c_2s_3 - c_6s_1s_5s_2c_3 + s_6s_1s_4s_2s_3 - s_6s_1s_4c_2c_3 + s_6c_1c_4$$
$$m_{22} = s_6c_5s_1c_4s_2s_3 - s_6c_5s_1c_4c_2c_3 - s_6c_5c_1s_4 + s_6s_1s_5c_2s_3 + s_6s_1s_5s_2c_3 + c_6s_1s_4s_2s_3 - c_6s_1s_4c_2c_3 + c_6c_1c_4$$
$$m_{23} = -s_5s_1c_4s_2s_3 + s_5s_1c_4c_2c_3 + s_5c_1s_4 + s_1c_5c_2s_3 + s_1c_5s_2c_3$$
$$m_{24} = -d_6s_5s_1c_4s_2s_3 + d_6s_5s_1c_4c_2c_3 + d_6s_5c_1s_4 + d_6s_1c_5c_2s_3 + d_6s_1c_5s_2c_3 + s_1d_4c_2s_3 + s_1d_4s_2c_3 + s_1c_2a_2$$

$$m_{31} = -c_6c_4c_5c_2s_3 - c_6c_4c_5s_2c_3 + c_6s_5s_2s_3 - c_6s_5c_2c_3 + s_4s_6c_2s_3 + s_4s_6s_2c_3$$

$$m_{32} = s_6c_4c_5c_2s_3 + s_6c_4c_5s_2c_3 - s_6s_5s_2s_3 + s_6s_5c_2c_3 + s_4c_6c_2s_3 + s_4c_6s_2c_3$$

$$m_{33} = -c_4s_5c_2s_3 - c_4s_5s_2c_3 - c_5s_2s_3 + c_5c_2c_3$$

$$m_{34} = -d_6c_4s_5c_2s_3 - d_6c_4s_5s_2c_3 - d_6c_5s_2s_3 + d_6c_5c_2c_3 - d_4s_2s_3 + d_4c_2c_3 - s_2a_2$$

Geometric Jacobian

$$\mathbf{J} = \begin{bmatrix} \mathbf{J}_v \\ \mathbf{J}_\omega \end{bmatrix}$$

$$\mathbf{J} = \begin{bmatrix} m_{11} & m_{12} & \dots & m_{16} \\ m_{21} & m_{22} & \dots & m_{26} \\ \vdots & \vdots & \ddots & \vdots \\ m_{61} & m_{62} & \dots & m_{66} \end{bmatrix}$$

where

$$m_{11} = d_6s_5s_1c_4s_2s_3 - d_6s_5s_1c_4c_2c_3 - d_6s_5c_1s_4 - d_6s_1c_5c_2s_3 - d_6s_1c_5s_2c_3 - s_1d_4c_2s_3 - s_1d_4s_2c_3 - s_1c_2a_2$$

$$m_{12} = -c_1(d_6c_4s_5c_2s_3 + d_6c_4s_5s_2c_3 + d_6c_5s_2s_3 - d_6c_5c_2c_3 + d_4s_2s_3 - d_4c_2c_3 + s_2a_2)$$

$$m_{13} = -c_1(d_6c_4s_5c_2s_3 + d_6c_4s_5s_2c_3 + d_6c_5s_2s_3 - d_6c_5c_2c_3 + d_4s_2s_3 - d_4c_2c_3)$$

$$m_{14} = s_5(c_1s_4s_2s_3 - c_1s_4c_2c_3 - s_1c_4)d_6$$

$$m_{15} = -d_6(c_5c_1c_4s_2s_3 - c_5c_1c_4c_2c_3 + c_5s_1s_4 + c_1s_5c_2s_3 + c_1s_5s_2c_3)$$

$$m_{16} = 0$$

$$m_{21} = -d_6 s_5 c_1 c_4 s_2 s_3 + d_6 s_5 c_1 c_4 c_2 c_3 - d_6 s_5 s_1 s_4 + d_6 c_1 c_5 c_2 s_3 + d_6 c_1 c_5 s_2 c_3 + c_1 d_4 c_2 s_3 + c_1 d_4 s_2 c_3 + c_1 c_2 a_2$$

$$m_{22} = -s_1 (d_6 c_4 s_5 c_2 s_3 + d_6 c_4 s_5 s_2 c_3 + d_6 c_5 s_2 s_3 - d_6 c_5 c_2 c_3 + d_4 s_2 s_3 - d_4 c_2 c_3 + s_2 a_2)$$

$$m_{23} = -s_1 (d_6 c_4 s_5 c_2 s_3 + d_6 c_4 s_5 s_2 c_3 + d_6 c_5 s_2 s_3 - d_6 c_5 c_2 c_3 + d_4 s_2 s_3 - d_4 c_2 c_3)$$

$$m_{24} = s_5 (s_1 s_4 s_2 s_3 - s_1 s_4 c_2 c_3 + c_1 c_4) d_6$$

$$m_{25} = -d_6 (s_1 s_5 c_2 s_3 + s_1 s_5 s_2 c_3 + c_5 s_1 c_4 s_2 s_3 - c_5 s_1 c_4 c_2 c_3 - c_5 c_1 s_4)$$

$$m_{26} = 0$$

$$m_{31} = 0$$

$$m_{32} = d_6 s_5 c_4 s_2 s_3 - d_6 s_5 c_4 c_2 c_3 - d_6 c_5 c_2 s_3 - d_6 c_5 s_2 c_3 - d_4 c_2 s_3 - d_4 s_2 c_3 - c_2 a_2$$

$$m_{33} = d_6 s_5 c_4 s_2 s_3 - d_6 s_5 c_4 c_2 c_3 - d_6 c_5 c_2 s_3 - d_6 c_5 s_2 c_3 - d_4 c_2 s_3 - d_4 s_2 c_3$$

$$m_{34} = s_5 s_4 (c_2 s_3 + s_2 c_3) d_6$$

$$m_{35} = d_6 (-c_4 c_5 c_2 s_3 - c_4 c_5 s_2 c_3 + s_5 s_2 s_3 - s_5 c_2 c_3)$$

$$m_{36} = 0$$

$$m_{41} = 0$$

$$m_{42} = -s_1$$

$$m_{43} = -s_1$$

$$m_{44} = c_1 (c_2 s_3 + s_2 c_3)$$

$$m_{45} = c_1 s_4 s_2 s_3 - c_1 s_4 c_2 c_3 - s_1 c_4$$

$$m_{46} = -s_5 c_1 c_4 s_2 s_3 + s_5 c_1 c_4 c_2 c_3 - s_5 s_1 s_4 + c_1 c_5 c_2 s_3 + c_1 c_5 s_2 c_3$$

$$m_{51} = 0$$
$$m_{52} = c_1$$
$$m_{53} = c_1$$
$$m_{54} = s_1 \left(c_2 s_3 + s_2 c_3 \right)$$
$$m_{55} = s_1 s_4 s_2 s_3 - s_1 s_4 c_2 c_3 + c_1 c_4$$
$$m_{56} = -s_5 s_1 c_4 s_2 s_3 + s_5 s_1 c_4 c_2 c_3 + s_5 c_1 s_4 + s_1 c_5 c_2 s_3 + s_1 c_5 s_2 c_3$$

$$m_{61} = 1$$
$$m_{62} = 0$$
$$m_{63} = 0$$
$$m_{64} = -s_2 s_3 + c_2 c_3$$
$$m_{65} = \left(c_2 s_3 + s_2 c_3 \right) s_4$$
$$m_{66} = -c_4 s_5 c_2 s_3 - c_4 s_5 s_2 c_3 - c_5 s_2 s_3 + c_5 c_2 c_3$$

Appendix D
Geometric Jacobian for the Seven-Joint DLR-Kuka Robot

The seven-joint robot in Fig. 3.10 is an extension of the six-joint robot, obtained by adding a revolute joint between joints two and three (Table D.1).

DH-Table

Table D.1: DH-table for the seven-joint DLR-Kuka robot

i	α_i	a_i	d_i	θ_i
1	-90	0	d_1	θ_1
2	90	0	0	θ_2
3	-90	0	d_3	θ_3
4	90	0	0	θ_4
5	-90	0	d_5	θ_5
6	90	0	0	θ_6
7	0	0	d_7	θ_7

DH-Matrices

$$
{}^0M_1 = \begin{bmatrix} c_1 & 0 & -s_1 & 0 \\ s_1 & 0 & c_1 & 0 \\ 0 & -1 & 0 & d_1 \\ 0 & 0 & 0 & 1 \end{bmatrix}
$$

A. Schweikard, F. Ernst, *Medical Robotics*,
DOI 10.1007/978-3-319-22891-4

$$^{1}M_2 = \begin{bmatrix} c_2 & 0 & s_2 & 0 \\ s_2 & 0 & -c_2 & 0 \\ 0 & 1 & 0 & 0 \\ 0 & 0 & 0 & 1 \end{bmatrix}$$

$$^{2}M_3 = \begin{bmatrix} c_3 & 0 & -s_3 & 0 \\ s_3 & 0 & c_3 & 0 \\ 0 & -1 & 0 & d_3 \\ 0 & 0 & 0 & 1 \end{bmatrix}$$

$$^{3}M_4 = \begin{bmatrix} c_4 & 0 & s_4 & 0 \\ s_4 & 0 & -c_4 & 0 \\ 0 & 1 & 0 & 0 \\ 0 & 0 & 0 & 1 \end{bmatrix}$$

$$^{4}M_5 = \begin{bmatrix} c_5 & 0 & -s_5 & 0 \\ s_5 & 0 & c_5 & 0 \\ 0 & -1 & 0 & d_5 \\ 0 & 0 & 0 & 1 \end{bmatrix}$$

$$^{5}M_6 = \begin{bmatrix} c_6 & 0 & s_6 & 0 \\ s_6 & 0 & -c_6 & 0 \\ 0 & 1 & 0 & 0 \\ 0 & 0 & 0 & 1 \end{bmatrix}$$

$$^{6}M_7 = \begin{bmatrix} c_7 & -s_7 & 0 & 0 \\ s_7 & c_7 & 0 & 0 \\ 0 & 0 & 1 & d_7 \\ 0 & 0 & 0 & 1 \end{bmatrix}$$

Forward Kinematics

$$
{}^{0}M_1 = \begin{bmatrix} c_1 & 0 & -s_1 & 0 \\ s_1 & 0 & c_1 & 0 \\ 0 & -1 & 0 & d_1 \\ 0 & 0 & 0 & 1 \end{bmatrix}
$$

$$
{}^{0}M_2 = \begin{bmatrix} c_1c_2 & -s_1 & c_1s_2 & 0 \\ s_1c_2 & c_1 & s_1s_2 & 0 \\ -s_2 & 0 & c_2 & d_1 \\ 0 & 0 & 0 & 1 \end{bmatrix}
$$

$$
{}^{0}M_3 = \begin{bmatrix} c_1c_2c_3 - s_1s_3 & -c_1s_2 & -c_1c_2s_3 - s_1c_3 & c_1s_2d_3 \\ s_1c_2c_3 + c_1s_3 & -s_1s_2 & -s_1c_2s_3 + c_1c_3 & s_1s_2d_3 \\ -s_2c_3 & -c_2 & s_2s_3 & c_2d_3 + d_1 \\ 0 & 0 & 0 & 1 \end{bmatrix}
$$

$$
{}^{0}M_4 = \begin{bmatrix} m_{11} & m_{12} & m_{13} & m_{14} \\ m_{21} & m_{22} & m_{23} & m_{24} \\ m_{31} & m_{32} & m_{33} & m_{34} \\ 0 & 0 & 0 & 1 \end{bmatrix}
$$

where

$$
\begin{aligned}
m_{11} &= c_4c_1c_2c_3 - c_4s_1s_3 - c_1s_2s_4 \\
m_{12} &= -c_1c_2s_3 - s_1c_3 \\
m_{13} &= s_4c_1c_2c_3 - s_4s_1s_3 + c_1s_2c_4 \\
m_{14} &= c_1s_2d_3
\end{aligned}
$$

$$m_{21} = c_4 s_1 c_2 c_3 + c_4 c_1 s_3 - s_1 s_2 s_4$$
$$m_{22} = -s_1 c_2 s_3 + c_1 c_3$$
$$m_{23} = s_4 s_1 c_2 c_3 + s_4 c_1 s_3 + s_1 s_2 c_4$$
$$m_{24} = s_1 s_2 d_3$$

$$m_{31} = -s_2 c_3 c_4 - c_2 s_4$$
$$m_{32} = s_2 s_3$$
$$m_{33} = -s_2 c_3 s_4 + c_2 c_4$$
$$m_{34} = c_2 d_3 + d_1$$

$$^0M_5 = \begin{bmatrix} m_{11} & m_{12} & m_{13} & m_{14} \\ m_{21} & m_{22} & m_{23} & m_{24} \\ m_{31} & m_{32} & m_{33} & m_{34} \\ 0 & 0 & 0 & 1 \end{bmatrix}$$

where

$$m_{11} = c_5 c_4 c_1 c_2 c_3 - c_5 c_4 s_1 s_3 - c_5 c_1 s_2 s_4 - s_5 c_1 c_2 s_3 - s_5 s_1 c_3$$
$$m_{12} = -s_4 c_1 c_2 c_3 + s_4 s_1 s_3 - c_1 s_2 c_4$$
$$m_{13} = -s_5 c_4 c_1 c_2 c_3 + s_5 c_4 s_1 s_3 + s_5 c_1 s_2 s_4 - c_5 c_1 c_2 s_3 - c_5 s_1 c_3$$
$$m_{14} = d_5 s_4 c_1 c_2 c_3 - d_5 s_4 s_1 s_3 + d_5 c_1 s_2 c_4 + c_1 s_2 d_3$$

$$m_{21} = c_5 c_4 s_1 c_2 c_3 + c_5 c_4 c_1 s_3 - c_5 s_1 s_2 s_4 - s_5 s_1 c_2 s_3 + s_5 c_1 c_3$$
$$m_{22} = -s_4 s_1 c_2 c_3 - s_4 c_1 s_3 - s_1 s_2 c_4$$
$$m_{23} = -s_5 c_4 s_1 c_2 c_3 - s_5 c_4 c_1 s_3 + s_5 s_1 s_2 s_4 - c_5 s_1 c_2 s_3 + c_5 c_1 c_3$$
$$m_{24} = d_5 s_4 s_1 c_2 c_3 + d_5 s_4 c_1 s_3 + d_5 s_1 s_2 c_4 + s_1 s_2 d_3$$

$$m_{31} = -c_5 s_2 c_3 c_4 - c_5 c_2 s_4 + s_2 s_3 s_5$$
$$m_{32} = s_2 c_3 s_4 - c_2 c_4$$
$$m_{33} = s_5 s_2 c_3 c_4 + s_5 c_2 s_4 + s_2 s_3 c_5$$
$$m_{34} = -d_5 s_2 c_3 s_4 + d_5 c_2 c_4 + c_2 d_3 + d_1$$

$$^0M_6 = \begin{bmatrix} m_{11} & m_{12} & m_{13} & m_{14} \\ m_{21} & m_{22} & m_{23} & m_{24} \\ m_{31} & m_{32} & m_{33} & m_{34} \\ 0 & 0 & 0 & 1 \end{bmatrix}$$

where

$$m_{11} = c_6 c_5 c_4 c_1 c_2 c_3 - c_6 c_5 c_4 s_1 s_3 - c_6 c_5 c_1 s_2 s_4 - c_6 s_5 c_1 c_2 s_3 - \\ c_6 s_5 s_1 c_3 - s_6 s_4 c_1 c_2 c_3 + s_6 s_4 s_1 s_3 - s_6 c_1 s_2 c_4$$
$$m_{12} = -s_5 c_4 c_1 c_2 c_3 + s_5 c_4 s_1 s_3 + s_5 c_1 s_2 s_4 - c_5 c_1 c_2 s_3 - c_5 s_1 c_3$$
$$m_{13} = s_6 c_5 c_4 c_1 c_2 c_3 - s_6 c_5 c_4 s_1 s_3 - s_6 c_5 c_1 s_2 s_4 - s_6 s_5 c_1 c_2 s_3 - \\ s_6 s_5 s_1 c_3 + c_6 s_4 c_1 c_2 c_3 - c_6 s_4 s_1 s_3 + c_6 c_1 s_2 c_4$$
$$m_{14} = d_5 s_4 c_1 c_2 c_3 - d_5 s_4 s_1 s_3 + d_5 c_1 s_2 c_4 + c_1 s_2 d_3$$

$$m_{21} = c_6 c_5 c_4 s_1 c_2 c_3 + c_6 c_5 c_4 c_1 s_3 - c_6 c_5 s_1 s_2 s_4 - c_6 s_5 s_1 c_2 s_3 + \\ c_6 s_5 c_1 c_3 - s_6 s_4 s_1 c_2 c_3 - s_6 s_4 c_1 s_3 - s_6 s_1 s_2 c_4$$
$$m_{22} = -s_5 c_4 s_1 c_2 c_3 - s_5 c_4 c_1 s_3 + s_5 s_1 s_2 s_4 - c_5 s_1 c_2 s_3 + c_5 c_1 c_3$$
$$m_{23} = s_6 c_5 c_4 s_1 c_2 c_3 + s_6 c_5 c_4 c_1 s_3 - s_6 c_5 s_1 s_2 s_4 - s_6 s_5 s_1 c_2 s_3 + \\ s_6 s_5 c_1 c_3 + c_6 s_4 s_1 c_2 c_3 + c_6 s_4 c_1 s_3 + c_6 s_1 s_2 c_4$$
$$m_{24} = d_5 s_4 s_1 c_2 c_3 + d_5 s_4 c_1 s_3 + d_5 s_1 s_2 c_4 + s_1 s_2 d_3$$

$$m_{31} = -c_6 c_5 s_2 c_3 c_4 - c_6 c_5 c_2 s_4 + c_6 s_2 s_3 s_5 + s_6 s_2 c_3 s_4 - s_6 c_2 c_4$$
$$m_{32} = s_5 s_2 c_3 c_4 + s_5 c_2 s_4 + s_2 s_3 c_5$$
$$m_{33} = -s_6 c_5 s_2 c_3 c_4 - s_6 c_5 c_2 s_4 + s_6 s_2 s_3 s_5 - c_6 s_2 c_3 s_4 + c_6 c_2 c_4$$
$$m_{34} = -d_5 s_2 c_3 s_4 + d_5 c_2 c_4 + c_2 d_3 + d_1$$

$$
{}^0M_7 = \begin{bmatrix} m_{11} & m_{12} & m_{13} & m_{14} \\ m_{21} & m_{22} & m_{23} & m_{24} \\ m_{31} & m_{32} & m_{33} & m_{34} \\ 0 & 0 & 0 & 1 \end{bmatrix}.
$$

where

$$
\begin{aligned}
m_{11} = {} & c_7c_6c_5c_4c_1c_2c_3 - c_7c_6c_5c_4s_1s_3 - c_7c_6c_5c_1s_2s_4 - c_7c_6s_5c_1c_2s_3 - \\
& c_7c_6s_5s_1c_3 - c_7s_6s_4c_1c_2c_3 + c_7s_6s_4s_1s_3 - c_7s_6c_1s_2c_4 - \\
& s_7s_5c_4c_1c_2c_3 + s_7s_5c_4s_1s_3 + s_7s_5c_1s_2s_4 - s_7c_5c_1c_2s_3 - s_7c_5s_1c_3 \\
m_{12} = {} & -s_7c_6c_5c_4c_1c_2c_3 + s_7c_6c_5c_4s_1s_3 + s_7c_6c_5c_1s_2s_4 + s_7c_6s_5c_1c_2s_3 + \\
& s_7c_6s_5s_1c_3 + s_7s_6s_4c_1c_2c_3 - s_7s_6s_4s_1s_3 + s_7s_6c_1s_2c_4 - \\
& c_7s_5c_4c_1c_2c_3 + c_7s_5c_4s_1s_3 + c_7s_5c_1s_2s_4 - c_7c_5c_1c_2s_3 - c_7c_5s_1c_3 \\
m_{13} = {} & s_6c_5c_4c_1c_2c_3 - s_6c_5c_4s_1s_3 - s_6c_5c_1s_2s_4 - s_6s_5c_1c_2s_3 - s_6s_5s_1c_3 + \\
& c_6s_4c_1c_2c_3 - c_6s_4s_1s_3 + c_6c_1s_2c_4 \\
m_{14} = {} & d_7s_6c_5c_4c_1c_2c_3 - d_7s_6c_5c_4s_1s_3 - d_7s_6c_5c_1s_2s_4 - d_7s_6s_5c_1c_2s_3 - \\
& d_7s_6s_5s_1c_3 + d_7c_6s_4c_1c_2c_3 - d_7c_6s_4s_1s_3 + d_7c_6c_1s_2c_4 + \\
& d_5s_4c_1c_2c_3 - d_5s_4s_1s_3 + d_5c_1s_2c_4 + c_1s_2d_3
\end{aligned}
$$

$$
\begin{aligned}
m_{21} = {} & c_7c_6c_5c_4s_1c_2c_3 + c_7c_6c_5c_4c_1s_3 - c_7c_6c_5s_1s_2s_4 - c_7c_6s_5s_1c_2s_3 + \\
& c_7c_6s_5c_1c_3 - c_7s_6s_4s_1c_2c_3 - c_7s_6s_4c_1s_3 - c_7s_6s_1s_2c_4 - \\
& s_7s_5c_4s_1c_2c_3 - s_7s_5c_4c_1s_3 + s_7s_5s_1s_2s_4 - s_7c_5s_1c_2s_3 + s_7c_5c_1c_3 \\
m_{22} = {} & -s_7c_6c_5c_4s_1c_2c_3 - s_7c_6c_5c_4c_1s_3 + s_7c_6c_5s_1s_2s_4 + s_7c_6s_5s_1c_2s_3 - \\
& s_7c_6s_5c_1c_3 + s_7s_6s_4s_1c_2c_3 + s_7s_6s_4c_1s_3 + s_7s_6s_1s_2c_4 - \\
& c_7s_5c_4s_1c_2c_3 - c_7s_5c_4c_1s_3 + c_7s_5s_1s_2s_4 - c_7c_5s_1c_2s_3 + c_7c_5c_1c_3 \\
m_{23} = {} & s_6c_5c_4s_1c_2c_3 + s_6c_5c_4c_1s_3 - s_6c_5s_1s_2s_4 - s_6s_5s_1c_2s_3 + s_6s_5c_1c_3 + \\
& c_6s_4s_1c_2c_3 + c_6s_4c_1s_3 + c_6s_1s_2c_4 \\
m_{24} = {} & d_7s_6c_5c_4s_1c_2c_3 + d_7s_6c_5c_4c_1s_3 - d_7s_6c_5s_1s_2s_4 - d_7s_6s_5s_1c_2s_3 + \\
& d_7s_6s_5c_1c_3 + d_7c_6s_4s_1c_2c_3 + d_7c_6s_4c_1s_3 + d_7c_6s_1s_2c_4 + \\
& d_5s_4s_1c_2c_3 + d_5s_4c_1s_3 + d_5s_1s_2c_4 + s_1s_2d_3
\end{aligned}
$$

$$m_{31} = -c_7c_6c_5s_2c_3c_4 - c_7c_6c_5c_2s_4 + c_7c_6s_2s_3s_5 + c_7s_6s_2c_3s_4 - c_7s_6c_2c_4 + s_7s_5s_2c_3c_4 + s_7s_5c_2s_4 + s_7s_2s_3c_5$$

$$m_{32} = s_7c_6c_5s_2c_3c_4 + s_7c_6c_5c_2s_4 - s_7c_6s_2s_3s_5 - s_7s_6s_2c_3s_4 + s_7s_6c_2c_4 + c_7s_5s_2c_3c_4 + c_7s_5c_2s_4 + c_7s_2s_3c_5$$

$$m_{33} = -s_6c_5s_2c_3c_4 - s_6c_5c_2s_4 + s_6s_2s_3s_5 - c_6s_2c_3s_4 + c_6c_2c_4$$

$$m_{34} = -d_7s_6c_5s_2c_3c_4 - d_7s_6c_5c_2s_4 + d_7s_6s_2s_3s_5 - d_7c_6s_2c_3s_4 + d_7c_6c_2c_4 - d_5s_2c_3s_4 + d_5c_2c_4 + c_2d_3 + d_1$$

Geometric Jacobian

$$\mathbf{J} = \begin{bmatrix} \mathbf{J}_v \\ \mathbf{J}_\omega \end{bmatrix}$$

$$\mathbf{J} = \begin{bmatrix} m_{11} & m_{12} & \dots & m_{16} \\ m_{21} & m_{22} & \dots & m_{26} \\ \vdots & \vdots & \ddots & \vdots \\ m_{61} & m_{62} & \dots & m_{66} \end{bmatrix}$$

where

$$m_{11} = -d_7s_6c_5c_4s_1c_2c_3 - d_7s_6c_5c_4c_1s_3 + d_7s_6c_5s_1s_2s_4 + d_7s_6s_5s_1c_2s_3 - d_7s_6s_5c_1c_3 - d_7c_6s_4s_1c_2c_3 - d_7c_6s_4c_1s_3 - d_7c_6s_1s_2c_4 - d_5s_4s_1c_2c_3 - d_5s_4c_1s_3 - d_5s_1s_2c_4 - s_1s_2d_3$$

$$m_{12} = -c_1(d_7s_6c_5s_2c_3c_4 + d_7s_6c_5c_2s_4 - d_7s_6s_2s_3s_5 + d_7c_6s_2c_3s_4 - d_7c_6c_2c_4 + d_5s_2c_3s_4 - d_5c_2c_4 - c_2d_3)$$

$$m_{13} = -s_1d_7s_6c_5c_3c_4 + s_1d_7s_6s_3s_5 - s_1d_7c_6c_3s_4 - s_1d_5c_3s_4 - c_2d_7s_6c_5c_4c_1s_3 - c_2d_7s_6s_5c_1c_3 - c_2d_7c_6s_4c_1s_3 - c_2d_5s_4c_1s_3$$

$$m_{14} = -c_1c_3d_7s_6c_5c_2s_4 - c_1d_7s_6c_5s_2c_4 + s_1s_3d_7s_6c_5s_4 + c_1c_3d_7c_6c_2c_4 - c_1d_7c_6s_2s_4 - s_1s_3d_7c_6c_4 + c_1c_3d_5c_2c_4 - c_1d_5s_2s_4 - s_1s_3d_5c_4$$

$$m_{15} = -s_6(c_5c_1c_2s_3 - s_5c_1s_2s_4 - s_5c_4s_1s_3 + c_5s_1c_3 + s_5c_4c_1c_2c_3)d_7$$

$$m_{16} = -d_7(c_6s_5c_1c_2s_3 + c_6s_5s_1c_3 + s_6s_4c_1c_2c_3 - c_6c_5c_4c_1c_2c_3 + c_6c_5c_1s_2s_4 + c_6c_5c_4s_1s_3 + s_6c_1s_2c_4 - s_6s_4s_1s_3)$$

$$m_{17} = 0$$

$$
\begin{aligned}
m_{21} = {} & d_7 s_6 c_5 c_4 c_1 c_2 c_3 - d_7 s_6 c_5 c_4 s_1 s_3 - d_7 s_6 c_5 c_1 s_2 s_4 - d_7 s_6 s_5 c_1 c_2 s_3 - \\
& d_7 s_6 s_5 s_1 c_3 + d_7 c_6 s_4 c_1 c_2 c_3 - d_7 c_6 s_4 s_1 s_3 + d_7 c_6 c_1 s_2 c_4 + \\
& d_5 s_4 c_1 c_2 c_3 - d_5 s_4 s_1 s_3 + d_5 c_1 s_2 c_4 + c_1 s_2 d_3 \\
m_{22} = {} & -s_1 (d_7 s_6 c_5 s_2 c_3 c_4 + d_7 s_6 c_5 c_2 s_4 - d_7 s_6 s_2 s_3 s_5 + d_7 c_6 s_2 c_3 s_4 - \\
& d_7 c_6 c_2 c_4 + d_5 s_2 c_3 s_4 - d_5 c_2 c_4 - c_2 d_3) \\
m_{23} = {} & -c_2 d_7 s_6 c_5 c_4 s_1 s_3 - c_2 d_7 s_6 s_5 s_1 c_3 - c_2 d_7 c_6 s_4 s_1 s_3 - c_2 d_5 s_4 s_1 s_3 + \\
& d_7 s_6 c_5 c_4 c_1 c_3 - d_7 s_6 s_5 c_1 s_3 + d_7 c_6 s_4 c_1 c_3 + d_5 s_4 c_1 c_3 \\
m_{24} = {} & -s_2 d_7 c_6 s_4 s_1 + s_3 d_7 c_6 c_1 c_4 + s_1 c_3 d_7 c_6 c_2 c_4 - s_2 d_5 s_4 s_1 + s_3 d_5 c_1 c_4 + \\
& s_1 c_3 d_5 c_2 c_4 - s_2 d_7 s_6 c_5 c_4 s_1 - s_3 d_7 s_6 c_5 c_1 s_4 - s_1 c_3 d_7 s_6 c_5 c_2 s_4 \\
m_{25} = {} & -s_6 (-c_5 c_1 c_3 + s_5 c_4 s_1 c_2 c_3 + c_5 s_1 c_2 s_3 - s_5 s_1 s_2 s_4 + s_5 c_4 c_1 s_3) d_7 \\
m_{26} = {} & d_7 (c_6 c_5 c_4 s_1 c_2 c_3 + c_6 c_5 c_4 c_1 s_3 - c_6 c_5 s_1 s_2 s_4 - c_6 s_5 s_1 c_2 s_3 + \\
& c_6 s_5 c_1 c_3 - s_6 s_4 s_1 c_2 c_3 - s_6 s_4 c_1 s_3 - s_6 s_1 s_2 c_4) \\
m_{27} = {} & 0
\end{aligned}
$$

$$
\begin{aligned}
m_{31} = {} & 0 \\
m_{32} = {} & -d_7 s_6 c_5 c_2 c_3 c_4 + d_7 s_6 c_5 s_2 s_4 + d_7 s_6 c_2 s_3 s_5 - d_7 c_6 c_2 c_3 s_4 - \\
& d_7 c_6 s_2 c_4 - d_5 c_2 c_3 s_4 - d_5 s_2 c_4 - s_2 d_3 \\
m_{33} = {} & s_2 (d_7 s_6 c_5 c_4 s_3 + d_7 s_6 s_5 c_3 + d_7 c_6 s_4 s_3 + d_5 s_4 s_3) \\
m_{34} = {} & -c_2 d_5 s_4 - c_3 d_7 c_6 s_2 c_4 + c_3 d_7 s_6 c_5 s_2 s_4 - c_2 d_7 c_6 s_4 - \\
& c_2 d_7 s_6 c_5 c_4 - c_3 d_5 s_2 c_4 \\
m_{35} = {} & s_6 (s_5 s_2 c_3 c_4 + s_5 c_2 s_4 + s_2 s_3 c_5) d_7 \\
m_{36} = {} & -d_7 (-c_6 s_2 s_3 s_5 + c_6 c_5 c_2 s_4 - s_6 s_2 c_3 s_4 + c_6 c_5 s_2 c_3 c_4 + s_6 c_2 c_4) \\
m_{37} = {} & 0
\end{aligned}
$$

$$m_{41} = 0$$
$$m_{42} = -s_1$$
$$m_{43} = c_1 s_2$$
$$m_{44} = -c_1 c_2 s_3 - s_1 c_3$$
$$m_{45} = s_4 c_1 c_2 c_3 - s_4 s_1 s_3 + c_1 s_2 c_4$$
$$m_{46} = -s_5 c_4 c_1 c_2 c_3 + s_5 c_4 s_1 s_3 + s_5 c_1 s_2 s_4 - c_5 c_1 c_2 s_3 - c_5 s_1 c_3$$
$$m_{47} = s_6 c_5 c_4 c_1 c_2 c_3 - s_6 c_5 c_4 s_1 s_3 - s_6 c_5 c_1 s_2 s_4 - s_6 s_5 c_1 c_2 s_3 - s_6 s_5 s_1 c_3 + c_6 s_4 c_1 c_2 c_3 - c_6 s_4 s_1 s_3 + c_6 c_1 s_2 c_4$$

$$m_{51} = 0$$
$$m_{52} = c_1$$
$$m_{53} = s_1 s_2$$
$$m_{54} = -s_1 c_2 s_3 + c_1 c_3$$
$$m_{55} = s_4 s_1 c_2 c_3 + s_4 c_1 s_3 + s_1 s_2 c_4$$
$$m_{56} = -s_5 c_4 s_1 c_2 c_3 - s_5 c_4 c_1 s_3 + s_5 s_1 s_2 s_4 - c_5 s_1 c_2 s_3 + c_5 c_1 c_3$$
$$m_{57} = s_6 c_5 c_4 s_1 c_2 c_3 + s_6 c_5 c_4 c_1 s_3 - s_6 c_5 s_1 s_2 s_4 - s_6 s_5 s_1 c_2 s_3 + s_6 s_5 c_1 c_3 + c_6 s_4 s_1 c_2 c_3 + c_6 s_4 c_1 s_3 + c_6 s_1 s_2 c_4$$

$$m_{61} = 1$$
$$m_{62} = 0$$
$$m_{63} = c_2$$
$$m_{64} = s_2 s_3$$
$$m_{65} = -s_2 c_3 s_4 + c_2 c_4$$
$$m_{66} = s_5 s_2 c_3 c_4 + s_5 c_2 s_4 + s_2 s_3 c_5$$
$$m_{67} = -s_6 c_5 s_2 c_3 c_4 - s_6 c_5 c_2 s_4 + s_6 s_2 s_3 s_5 - c_6 s_2 c_3 s_4 + c_6 c_2 c_4$$

Appendix E
Notation

Vectors and Matrices

$\mathbf{a}$	Column vector
$\mathbf{a}^{\mathrm{T}}$	Transpose of the column vector $\mathbf{a}$
$\mathbf{a}^{\mathrm{T}}\mathbf{b}$	Scalar product of column vectors $\mathbf{a}, \mathbf{b}$
$\mathbf{ab}$	Shorthand notation for $\mathbf{a}^{\mathrm{T}}\mathbf{b}$
$l : \mathbf{nx} - d = 0$	Line l with normal vector $\mathbf{n}$
$P : \mathbf{nx} - d = 0$	Plane P with normal vector $\mathbf{n}$
$\mathbf{M}$	Matrix
$\mathbf{R}(x, \alpha)$, $\mathbf{R}(y, \beta)$, $\mathbf{R}(z, \gamma)$	Elementary 3×3 rotation matrices
$\mathbf{R}^{\mathrm{T}}$	Transpose of matrix $\mathbf{R}$
$\mathbf{R}^{-1}$	Matrix inverse
$\mathbf{q}$	Quaternion
$\|\| \cdot \|\|$	Vector norm

Kinematics

B, S_0	Base coordinate system
S_i	DH-coordinate system i
$\mathbf{p}_i$	Origin of S_i (given as vector in base coordinates)
x_0, y_0, z_0	Coordinate axes of system S_0
x_i, y_i, z_i	Coordinate axes of system S_i
$a_i, \alpha_i, \theta_i, d_i$	DH-parameters

A. Schweikard, F. Ernst, *Medical Robotics*,
DOI 10.1007/978-3-319-22891-4

${}^{0}\mathbf{M}_1$	DH-matrix transforming fom S_0 to S_1
${}^{i-1}\mathbf{M}_i$	DH-matrix transforming fom S_{i-1} to S_i
l_i	Length of a link in a kinematic chain

Forces, Torques and Velocity Kinematics

$\mathbf{t}$	Joint torque
$\mathbf{f}$	Force vector
$\mathbf{m}$	Moment vector
τ	Magnitude of a joint torque
$\mathbf{v}$	Linear velocity
ω	Angular velocity
$\mathbf{J}_\mathbf{v}$	Linear velocity part of a geometric Jacobian
$\mathbf{J}_\omega$	Angular velocity part of a geometric Jacobian

Machine Learning

s_i, s_i'	Slack variables in linear programming
ξ_i, ξ_i'	Slack variables in quadratic programming
α_i, α_i'	Dual variables in quadratic programming, Lagrange multipliers
ε, C	Parameters of a support vector machine
F	Kernel function
$\frac{\partial f}{\partial x}$	Partial derivative of f with respect to variable x
∇f	Gradient vector of f
Λ	Lagrange function

List of Figures

A. Schweikard, F. Ernst, *Medical Robotics*,
DOI 10.1007/978-3-319-22891-4

List of Tables

A. Schweikard, F. Ernst, *Medical Robotics*,
DOI 10.1007/978-3-319-22891-4

Index

A. Schweikard, F. Ernst, *Medical Robotics*,
DOI 10.1007/978-3-319-22891-4

Printed in the United States
By Bookmasters